Introduction to Psychosexual Medicine

Third Edition

Introduction to Psychosexual Medicine

Third Edition

Edited by

Philipa A Brough

Margaret Denman

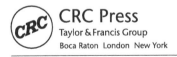

CRC Press
Taylor & Francis Group
Boca Raton London New York

CRC Press is an imprint of the
Taylor & Francis Group, an **informa** business

CRC Press
Taylor & Francis Group
6000 Broken Sound Parkway NW, Suite 300
Boca Raton, FL 33487-2742

International Standard Book Number-13: 978-1-138-09578-6 (Paperback)
                                       978-1-138-09579-3 (Hardback)

Library of Congress Cataloging-in-Publication Data

Names: Brough, Philipa A, editor. | Denman, Margaret, editor.
Title: Introduction to psychosexual medicine / edited by Philipa A Brough, Margaret Denman.
Other titles: Psychosexual medicine
Description: Third edition. | Boca Raton, FL : CRC Press, Taylor & Francis Group, [2019] | Preceded by Psychosexual medicine : an introduction / edited by Ruth Skrine, Heather Montford. 2nd ed. 2001. | Includes bibliographical references and index.
Identifiers: LCCN 2018043911| ISBN 9781138095786 (pbk. : alk. paper) | ISBN 9781138095793 (hardback : alk. paper) | ISBN 9781315105567 (ebook)
Subjects: | MESH: Sexual Dysfunctions, Psychological | Sexual Dysfunctions, Psychological--therapy
Classification: LCC RC557 | NLM WM 611 | DDC 616.85/83--dc23
LC record available at https://lccn.loc.gov/2018043911

Visit the Taylor & Francis Web site at
http://www.taylorandfrancis.com

and the CRC Press Web site at
http://www.crcpress.com

Contents

Part IV Applying the Skills to the Problem

Part V Effectiveness, Services and Training

Contributors

Susan V. Carr is a member of the Institute of Psychosexual Medicine (IPM), past council member and Scottish Training coordinator. As a consultant in Sexual and Reproductive Health in Glasgow, she led the Psychosexual and Gender Service and was a member of the multi-collegiate Advisory Group on the Treatment of Transsexuals in the UK. She then became lead consultant for the Psychosexual Service at the Royal Women's Hospital in Melbourne. She is currently immediate past president of the Australian Society for Psychosocial Obstetrics and Gynaecology. She has lectured extensively nationally and internationally, and authored various chapters on psychosexual topics.

Nicola Carter has been a member of the Institute of Psychosexual Medicine since 1997. She has been a general practitioner in Liverpool since 1990 and is a former fellow of the Faculty of Sexual and Reproductive Health. She is interested in the management of sexual problems in non-referral settings and has been working for 20 years within a specialist multidisciplinary team offering psychosexual therapy and erectile dysfunction prescribing services.

Nichola Chater is a member of IPM and also has a MSc in Multiple Sclerosis Service. She works as a consultant in rehabilitation medicine, part of Northumberland, Tyne and Wear NHS Foundation Trust. She is based at Walkergate Park Centre for Neurorehabilitation and Neuropsychiatry in Newcastle upon Tyne. Within her rehabilitation work, Dr Chater offers a clinic for addressing sexual problems related to neurological impairments.

Catherine Coulson qualified in Bristol in 1976. She has worked in infertility clinics and the IVF unit in Bristol for most of her career. Always fascinated with psychosomatic medicine, she undertook Institute of Psychosexual Medicine training and qualified in 1992. She has worked in specialist psychosexual clinics since 1990 and been a seminar leader on and off for 30 years. She is currently an examiner and chair of board of examiners for the IPM. She has coedited IPMJ in the past, contributed to undergraduate training, and written and presented on psychosexual medicine at medical and nursing conferences.

Fiona Cowan is a member of the IPM. She works in obstetrics and gynaecology and is an assistant Media and Communications Officer on the IPM Council and lead trainee representative for Health Education, Kent, Surrey and Sussex Deanery. Fiona has a keen interest in education, mentoring and psychosexual medicine. She has had several peer-reviewed publications and international presentations. Her articles on areas of psychosexual medicine feature in the *Institute of Psychosexual Medicine Journal* (IPMJ) and *The Obstetrician and Gynaecologist* (TOG). Fiona was awarded the prize for education at the RCOG World Congress for the presentation of her research on the importance of psychosexual medicine training for undergraduates and postgraduates in the UK.

Marian Davis has worked as a general practitioner for over 35 years. Training in psychosexual medicine and its focus on the doctor/patient relationship has informed her entire clinical practice. She has led IPM seminars since 1998 and really enjoys seeing colleagues develop their skills in this field. Her other passion is adolescent health and she currently chairs the Adolescent Health Group at Royal College of General Practitioners. Having left her practice, Marian is involved in a number of international projects including work to develop youth-friendly services.

Claudine Domoney is a consultant in obstetrics and gynaecology at Chelsea and Westminster Hospital, London, UK. She completed research in premenstrual syndrome and menopause, then became interested in sexual difficulties as they present in consultations. She holds membership of the IPM and was the Chair of the IPM. Subsequently she completed further training in pelvic floor dysfunction and surgery. Her interest in pelvic floor function covers physical, hormonal and sexual aspects, including postpartum problems. She provides holistic care for women suffering hormonal and pelvic floor issues.

Leila C.G. Frodsham graduated in 1995 and started training in 1998 in psychosexual medicine. She has worked in obstetrics and gynaecology for 23 years and as a consultant for 8 years. She leads the Psychosexual Service at Guys and St Thomas' and also works in medical education both there and at King's College London. She has done research in assisted conception and mother-to-embryo viral transmission risk. Her interests include improving childbirth experience, vulvodynia, ambulatory gynaecology and natural fertility. She has been on the IPM council for over 10 years as Programme Secretary, Chair and Media and Communications Rep. She is also a seminar leader.

Sandy Goldbeck-Wood is an IPM member and trainer. She is a clinician working in sexual and reproductive health, and editor-in-chief of *BMJ Sexual and Reproductive Health*. She publishes, researches and teaches on psychosocial aspects of physical health, medical humanities and methodological development within academic medicine.

Clare Gribbin has been a consultant obstetrician at Nottingham University Hospitals NHS Trust for 13 years. She specialises in maternal medicine and psychosexual medicine and runs a psychosexual clinic focusing on birth trauma service for women with post-traumatic stress disorders related to pregnancy. She completed membership of the IPM in 2002 and is a regular speaker on a variety of psychosexual and related topics both locally and nationally.

Annie Hawkins is a member of the Institute of Psychosexual Medicine has worked as an NHS consultant in obstetrics and gynaecology in London, Hampshire and Wiltshire. She has worked in obstetrics and gynaecology for 23 years and has a special interest in female reproductive hormones, including the treatment of premenstrual syndrome, premature ovarian failure and peri-menopause. She is also trained in the management of sub-fertility. She has an interest in psychological issues in gynaecology and obstetrics, is passionate about improving care for women, and combines a caring, listening, supportive approach with her medical knowledge to provide holistic care for her patients.

Catherine Hood has worked in the field of sexual health for over 20 years. She is an expert in psychosexual medicine and is a senior doctor at the St Pancras Sexual Problems Clinic, London, part of Camden and Islington NHS Foundation Trust. Dr Hood is a member of the IPM and a fellow of the European Society of Sexual Medicine. Dr Hood qualified in medicine from the University of Oxford. She subsequently lectured at the Oxford Medical School in Communication Skills, based in Ethox, the Oxford Centre for Ethics and Communication in Healthcare. In addition to her medical work, Catherine is an experienced broadcaster and writer and an international moderator and facilitator. She gives frequent lectures on sexual health, ethics and doctor–patient communication in the UK and abroad.

Gareth Hughes is a member of the Institute of Psychosexual Medicine. He recently retired from general practice in Jersey, where he has worked for the last 30 years; prior to that he was a general practitioner in Norfolk. He has been a member of the IPM Council and previous programme secretary.

Caroline Hunter has been a member of the Institute of Psychosexual Medicine since 1989. Before moving to Northern Ireland in that year, she was a member of Dr Tom Main's last seminar group in Hammersmith, London. She works in sexual health, taking sessions in genito-urinary medicine and is a senior doctor in a young people's clinic in Belfast. She is also a psychoanalytic psychotherapist and has her private practice, specialising in those with psychosexual problems. She is an IPM seminar leader, examiner and member of the IPM training committee.

Jasmin Khan-Singh graduated from Southampton University and is a member of the Institute of Psychosexual Medicine. She works in psychosexual medicine and sexual and reproductive healthcare in South Wales and has also worked as a community paediatrician. She has a special interest in medical education and is a fellow of the Academy of Medical Educators, attributed mainly to her work as the Director of Training for the IPM (2008–2013). Currently, she holds local, regional and national roles as a seminar leader, trainer, regional assessor, general training and programme director and examiner for both the IPM and the Faculty of Sexual and Reproductive Healthcare. In 2018, she started providing psychosexual support for a brand-new Female Genital Mutilation Support Service, in Cardiff, Wales.

Nikki M.W. Lee is a specialist trainee in obstetrics and gynaecology in London. She was born and raised in Hong Kong and did a Bachelor of Arts at the University of Pennsylvania, majoring in Health Communication. She did her undergraduate medicine degree at Barts Hospital and The London School of Medicine and Dentistry. She is undertaking training in psychosexual medicine and has recently written an article on dyspareunia.

Sally Soodeen is a former general practitioner who now works in sexual health and psychosexual medicine in Bristol. She is a member of the Institute of Psychosexual Medicine. She enjoys teaching and writing and is interested in the effects of pornography on sexual health.

Andrew Stainer-Smith is a general practitioner in Devon. He has led a specialist service for organic and psychosexual problems for many years in Exeter. He has been Chair of the IPM and a training group leader. His special interests are in the psychodynamics of the consultative process, changes in the practitioner during training and the history of the development of psychosexual medicine.

Gillian Vanhegan has worked in sexual and reproductive health for more than 30 years. She has a special interest in psychosexual medicine, especially vaginismus. Currently she works as an associate specialist in the NHS in London and also has a private practice. She is a member of the Institute of Psychosexual Medicine and has presented papers on psychosexual medicine, both nationally and internationally. Her current roles at the IPM are as a member of the Training Committee, council member and as an examiner. She is a past Chair of Council.

Ian K. Walsh is a clinical academic urologist at Belfast Trust, Kingsbridge Private Hospital/3fivetwo Healthcare and Queen's University, Belfast, and was previously a visiting professor in neuro-urology/reconstruction at the University of California, Davis. He has produced two theses and over 100 publications and is a higher education authority senior fellow. Mr Walsh is the Chairman of the Scientific Committee of the Irish Association of Sexual Medicine and a founding member of the British Association of Urological Surgeons Society for Female, Neurological and Urodynamic Urology, as well as co-editor of The *Journal of Psychosexual Medicine.*

Catherine White is a member of the Institute of Psychosexual Medicine (IPM). She works in integrated sexual health and psychosexual medicine. She is a clinical lead for psychosexual medicine within Manchester Sexual Health and Deputy Regional Coordinator for the IPM for the North West. Catherine was a general practitioner for 20 years alongside her other role but retired from this in 2016 in order to focus on her passion.

1

The Institute of Psychosexual Medicine Approach to Psychosexual Medicine as Practised by Health Professionals

Margaret Denman

The Buddha (480–400 BCE), founder of Buddhism, is said to have described the mind and the body as depending on each other in a way that two sheaves of reeds were to stand leaning against one another

The Institute of Psychosexual Medicine (IPM) was founded in 1974 by the psychoanalyst Tom Main, and he became Life President until his death in 1990. He was a colleague of Michael Balint, who wrote the seminal book *The Doctor, His Patient and the Illness* (1). This was based on transcripts from a series of seminars held with a group of London general practitioners (GPs). The format was case presentation and discussion. The seminar group became aware that they had patients in whom no physical cause could be found for their disease, and they came to accept the existence of psychosomatic illness. The GPs realised that to help these patients they had to deviate from the standard hospital-based tradition of investigation and treatment. Balint developed the concept of the 'doctor as the drug', also using this model of case presentation to a group, and Main held seminars with GPs and family planning doctors. Patients in family planning clinics were increasingly presenting with sexual difficulties, and the doctors felt ill-equipped to help them. Main's groups began to specialise in this field, and from these seminars the IPM evolved as discussed in his book *The Ailment and Other Psychoanalytic Essays* (2).

The IPM is still primarily a teaching organisation where doctors, and increasingly other allied health professionals, can learn by case presentation to a seminar group with a trained leader. This leader does not supervise or teach but allows a safe space in which the material can be discussed with an emphasis on looking at what happened in the room between that healthcare professional and that patient on that day. The leader and the group members all start from a place of ignorance with each new piece of case material presented. Feelings are looked at, but personal experiences and revelations are discouraged. The leader studies and manages the atmosphere in the group and, at times, will relate this back to the case material presented.

Building on their medical training and knowledge, this experiential learning allows doctors, nurses and physiotherapists to gain skills that enable them to treat patients with all types of sexual difficulties. These are mainly patients that they come across during the course of their day-to-day clinical work, while those with further training may treat patients in specialised psychosexual or sexual problem clinics. Clinicians are encouraged not to imitate their leader or other members of the seminar group but to learn to work in their own individual ways.

What does *psychosexual* mean? There are various definitions, but I like to think of it as:

The psychological and emotional attitudes concerning sexual thought and activity.

Increasingly we are understanding the scientific connections between the mind and the body. Since time immemorial people have been aware of the connections. Our language is littered with expressions such as 'butterflies in the stomach', 'gut reaction', 'pain in the neck' and many more. A blush of embarrassment is an instantaneous physical response to a psychological stimulus. We can see that many diseases, for example migraine and eczema, can be exacerbated by stress. On a more scientific level studies are showing that stress and depression can affect white cell function. Neuroimmunologists are increasingly studying the effects of stress on health at the hormonal and molecular levels. For sexual activity to be successful and fulfilling, the body has to be functioning and there needs to be no psychological or emotional barrier affecting libido or limiting sexual enjoyment. Patients do not like being told that their disease is 'in their head', but can often accept the explanation that the mind can affect the body, or that they are feeling their mental anguish as a pain or dysfunction in their body. This approach helps patients understand the concept of a psychosomatic or a psychosexual problem, i.e. their psychological and emotional attitudes are affecting their sexual thought and activity. Elsewhere in this text authors will discuss the physical aspects of the sexual response, the psychological components and their interaction.

As medical professionals, we have a duty to first exclude any physical disease. We are licensed to examine our patients and need to do this. Unlike psychotherapists and counsellors, IPM-trained clinicians also have to manage the physical aspects of the sexual problems that their patients present. It is not possible to look at the psychological issues until physical problems have been considered. Physical sexual difficulties may cause primary sexual difficulties sometimes leading to secondary psychosexual problems in the patient and sometimes their partner. The power of the IPM training is that one health professional can learn to manage both the mind and the body and thus help the patient to see the link between them.

You will discover as you delve into this text that the IPM training puts an emphasis on observation of the patient's behaviour during the genital examination. This information can help the health professional unravel the patient's problem. Because this is an important part of the jigsaw, the IPM does not train therapists who cannot examine their patients. The doctor or allied health professional who is treating and examining the body is also exploring the mind. This consolidates the link between the two.

As soon as health professionals start doing clinical work they are trained to ask questions. Of course, this is often necessary to exclude disease and make a diagnosis, but may allow the patient's agenda to escape. The following chapters show how the IPM training empowers patients to have a voice. The patient, not the health professional, is the expert in his or her problem and the feelings about it. The text also demonstrates how the health professional studies what is happening between them and the patient in the consulting room and, using this information, learns to reflect and interpret what is going on. At times this can also be related back to the patient's sexual life. To help illustrate this psychodynamic method of 'brief interpretive therapy' subsequent chapters contain case histories. These case histories are almost entirely fictional but based on situations that the authors have come across during their working lives. Anyone who thinks that they can recognise themselves can be reassured that no one else will be able to do so. It is more probable that they are identifying with similarities in the story of some other person. Although some patterns arise, it is shown that is impossible to have a preconceived theory of causation or generalise about an individual's sexual problem based on their gender, age, sexual orientation, culture, social status or religion. Every human being has a different experience of life and reacts to it in his or her own unique way. This will become apparent as you experience the diversity of case histories described in this book and the unique experience of each health professional/patient interaction.

As a multi-author book there is inevitable overlap between chapters, but it will be appreciated that each contributor has interpreted the material in his or her own way. Each chapter stands alone.

REFERENCES

1. Balint M. *The Doctor, His Patient and the Illness*. London: Pitman, 1957.
2. Main T, ed. by Johns J. *The Ailment and Other Psychological Essays*. London: Free Association Books, 1989, Chap. 15.

2

Identifying and Managing Problems in Different Settings

Margaret Denman

Different Types of Sex Therapy

This book mainly demonstrates how the Institute of Psychosexual Medicine (IPM) method of brief interpretive therapy is used to help patients with sexual and psychosexual problems. There are, of course, many other types of therapy for people with sexual difficulties. Counsellors, psychologists and psychotherapists treat people with psychosexual problems using a whole variety of skills. These include cognitive behavioural therapy (CBT), psychoanalysis, hypnotherapy, eye movement desensitisation and reprocessing (EMDR) and many others. The College of Sexual and Relationship Therapists (COSRT) (1) trains both medical professionals and counsellors. Most Relate (2) sex therapists are COSRT trained. Their emphasis is on couple and relationship therapy, whereas the IPM training is usually one-to-one, the patient not necessarily having a current partner. Clients need to self-refer to Relate. COSRT counsellors have many skills, but mainly use behavioural therapy based on *sensate focus*, a term usually associated with a set of specific sexual exercises for couples but sometimes for individuals. The term was introduced by Masters and Johnson (3), and was aimed at increasing personal and interpersonal awareness of self and the other's needs. This method is most helpful with motivated couples but can also be used with an individual in order to put them in touch with their sexual feelings.

Sensate focus and the other methods mentioned are useful but tend to be structured around longer programmes of intervention and are therefore more time consuming for the therapist and client. They do not fit in with the day-to-day work of busy National Health Service (NHS) medical professionals, where the psychosexual counselling is often taking place alongside the management of other medical problems and is often brief. The IPM training and method provide skills that clinicians can use during any short or long consultation in a multitude of settings.

Different Settings

Specialist psychosexual services are discussed elsewhere in the book. Patients will have self-referred or been referred into these clinics. In most other settings where doctors, nurses, physiotherapists and other healthcare professionals (HCPs) work, some of the patients they encounter will have sexual problems. This chapter cannot cover all of these but will highlight the areas in which sexual problems are most prevalent. Patients in a variety of settings are discussed throughout the book. Problems can be physical, psychosexual or mixed. While in a diabetic, neurology or cardiology setting they are more likely to be physical, it may be more common to find psychosexual problems in sexual health or fertility clinics. It is imperative in any setting that physical causes are excluded. All practitioners entering IPM training must have the necessary medical knowledge and be able to examine their patients.

Most types of problems will be encountered in most settings, although gynaecologists will rarely talk to their patients about erectile dysfunction (ED) and urologists are less likely to hear about tocophobia. But in all settings patients may discuss their partner's problem. For example, a man in an andrology clinic may admit his wife has vaginismus or a woman being investigated for painful sex in a menopause clinic might discuss her husband's ED. In any setting, a relationship problem might be revealed and signposting to Relate or another organisation often useful. Loss of libido is often related to relationship or situational difficulties. It is also of paramount importance that the HCP assesses the patient's mental health. A patient with severe mental illness, personality disorder or learning difficulties may not find the IPM approach useful.

Couples

Although the IPM training concentrates on the relationship between the HCP and the patient on a one-to-one basis, couples are sometimes seen if they present together. Observing how they behave with each other may be useful. It does, however, make the work more difficult as there will then be a myriad of relationships going on in the room, and it may be necessary for the professional to separate them upon identifying who has the problem. Once separated, the patient may be liberated to divulge the root cause of their problem. On occasions, both members of the couple have difficulties and may need to be seen apart, possibly presenting the HCP with confidentiality issues. Relate sex therapists work with couples, as do a lot of others with COSRT training. If the main problem is the relationship itself, signposting to Relate or another type of relationship counselling is often useful.

Non-Medical Settings

Aphrodisiacs and Sex Toys

It is important to recognise that HCPs and counsellors do not have the monopoly on the treatment of sexual problems. For centuries, populations have believed that certain substances have aphrodisiac properties, enhancing both sexual desire and performance. Some ginseng reaches astronomical prices in the East, and sadly rhinoceros horn is still illegally sought after, demonstrating the power of placebo. Many types of products, including hormones, are bought on the Internet – often less embarrassing than speaking to a pharmacist or HCP. Lubricants and exotic pleasure-enhancing condoms are usually obtained in this way.

Sildenafil in the form of Viagra Connect 50 mg has just become available over the counter in UK pharmacies. Training has been provided for pharmacists and a standard questionnaire provided.

Vacuum pumps for ED and 'cock rings' to enhance erection are among many products available online and in sex shops. Some shops have special discreet areas where people can go and discuss their problems. Vibrators are also bought in this way. It is worth remembering that our patients may have been down some of these routes before we see them.

Patients may also be using recreational drugs. Some of these may enhance sexual pleasure while others depress sexual activity and libido. Alcohol will also have an effect. All of this needs to be discussed in a non-judgemental way.

Sex Workers and the Internet

Sex workers also have a role helping their clients, mainly men, with sexual difficulties, and they can adapt to the need for fetishes and other ritual behaviours often not tolerated within other relationships. It is possible that some women with sex addiction become sex workers. The Internet now provides an enormous wealth of information which is, on the whole, helpful. But the ease of exposure to sexual activity in the form of pornography can sometimes be damaging – as is seen in the chapter on Internet porn. This can be harmful when seen by adolescents, as the material seen raises expectations about unrealistic, perfect genitals. They may witness a variety of vigorous and even violent activities that may not be acceptable once they try to form a relationship. Once again, we need to explore our patients' experiences, sources of information and expectations.

General Practice

The original IPM seminars were made up of general practitioners (GPs) and family planning doctors. GPs and practice nurses are often the first port of call for someone with a sexual problem, whether it is physical or psychosexual. Appointments are available without referral and the patient often knows the doctor or practice nurse. It is sometimes more difficult to discuss a sexual difficulty with a familiar doctor or nurse who may also treat the rest of the family. Patients will sometimes pick an unknown doctor, an anonymous locum or even the new GP registrar. It may seem easier to talk to the nurse, who seems less hurried when doing a cervical smear, talking about contraception or doing a diabetic check-up. Sadly, asking about ED in diabetic men is now no longer part of the GP's quality and outcomes framework (QOF). Disclosing a sexual difficulty for the first time can be frightening, and patients will often come with a series of trivial complaints, known as calling cards, that they can use until they feel comfortable enough to disclose their real anxieties. During this process they assess the health professional's receptivity and possibly hope that the HCP will take the lead and open up the discussion. This is a well-known phenomenon in general practice and is known as 'the hand on the door' syndrome as the real problem may not be revealed until the patient is on their way out of the consulting room. An astute practitioner will sense that there is another agenda and facilitate disclosure through the use of statements or open questions. The patient will be weighing up how sympathetic or open the HCP seems and will also be aware of the apparent pressure of time.

Once a sexual problem has been disclosed in general practice then it is up to the doctor or nurse to decide how to manage it. They can allow themselves to 'run late' and talk to the patient there and then or make another appointment, risking the patient not coming back. Some GPs can offer extended appointments to discuss emotional problems. It may be that they see their patients for lots of short appointments and help in this way. Once the problem has 'improved' they will find that mentioning it will seem prurient and the patient will not want to discuss it again. GPs often refer within the practice to colleagues who have more skills or may need to refer outside the practice. However, it is most important to try and stick with the patient for as long as possible as they might feel rejected if immediately referred on. They have plucked up their courage and picked this doctor or nurse. Getting problems at an early stage can be helpful, and the professional must always ask why now, why has this patient presented now and has the patient been sent? What happened in the patient's life when the problem started? Referral to a psychosexual clinic signposting to Relate may be necessary if the primary care professional feels that they cannot manage the patient. While most GPs prescribe phosphodiesterase type 5 (PDE5) inhibitors, many do not have the skills or knowledge to manage male physical sexual difficulties that do not respond to this class of drugs.

Unbeknownst to them, a lot of GPs will be making referrals for undisclosed psychosexual problems presenting, for example, as infertility, pelvic pain or recurrent vaginal discharge. It then depends on the patient's experience in secondary care as to whether or not the real problem is exposed.

Sexual Health Clinics

Once again, these clinics are available without referral. Appointments can be made and there are also drop-in sessions. Dealing with contraception and sexually transmitted disease, these clinics may appear to be a setting in which sexual problems can be discussed more freely in a non-judgemental and anonymous way. Even so, calling cards may have to be used by the patient, such as recurrent vaginal discharge or an insignificant rash. The practitioner should be alerted to women with recurrent pelvic pain for which no cause is found. They should also consider a sexual problem in men with recurrent prostatitis not responding to antibiotics or unexplained testicular pain. These symptoms may, in some patients, be somatisations of their sexual and emotional distress. Sensitively enquiring about their current sex lives or commenting on how they seem in the room or during the examination may open up a discussion about their underlying problem.

When swabs are being taken for sexually transmitted infections, it is common to have another practitioner in the room. This third person may inhibit disclosure, and it may be necessary to ask them to leave once specimens are retrieved. If a chaperone is necessary they must be asked to remain as quiet as possible during the examination and may be asked to leave the room afterwards.

The hopes or fears of people with HIV or recurrent herpes must be discussed in terms of sexual activity, and these conditions in particular can provoke sexual problems post-diagnosis. Anxiety about how someone contracted a sexually transmitted infection may lead to relationship difficulties, loss of libido or sexual problems. Even the knowledge that an abnormal smear is caused by papilloma virus can create shame and/or subsequent anxiety. Disclosures of sexual difficulty may seem to make consultations longer, but in the long run may prevent patients from going from one health professional to another in search of someone who might actually listen to their real problem.

Gynaecology

Most patients going to a gynaecology clinic have been referred there by their GP or another doctor. The overt symptom may mask an underlying sexual problem. Conversely, a physical problem may be causing a sexual difficulty or fear that had not been disclosed to the referring doctor. It is also important to remember that gynaecological procedures can lead to sexual difficulties. For example, a woman may worry that sex may be impossible after a prolapse repair or that she will not have any pleasure after a hysterectomy. Women treated for cancer may have fears and may also have physical difficulties following surgery, chemotherapy and radiotherapy. Exploring the patients' sexual fears can both prevent problems and limit the number of women returning to clinics for needless investigations for unknown causes of pelvic pain or vaginal discharge.

Davies and Frodsham (4) found that a high rate of negative laparoscopies (47%) for pelvic pain disorders suggests other less invasive interventions are preferable in the first instance. By exploring the patient's sexual pain disorder more holistically, with active listening and engaging the patient in a psychotherapeutic consultation with a range of management methods including medical management and CBT strategies, then this could improve patient care and decrease the potential morbidity of surgery in patients presenting with sexual pain disorders.

Physiotherapists in gynaecology departments are well placed to discuss sexual difficulties when they are referred women with urinary and other problems. They have the skills needed to help women with vaginismus, and this is often best not done in a purely behavioural way. Their techniques can be combined with IPM methods and many physiotherapists find seminar training useful.

Doctors and nurses working in fertility clinics will also find that patients may not have actually consummated their relationships, having misled their referrer. This is not always intentional, for there are still patients whose lack of knowledge is extreme. Sometimes, it is not until the woman is examined that vaginismus is discovered. Erectile difficulties may also be disclosed at a late stage. Couples/patients do not always want help with the psychosexual issues; it may be only that a child is desired.

Women may be referred to the colposcopy or gynaecology clinic for a smear when the practice nurse and/or the GP have found the smear impossible. Occasionally this is a vagary of anatomy, but more often than not, it is due to vaginismus. Discussing the underlying reason for the vaginal tightness is more productive than pressing ahead regardless. Forceful or insensitive attempts to do smears or vaginal examinations can also be a cause of sexual problems in the future. Colposcopy and the treatment of abnormal smears can leave women with fantasies about their remaining anatomy and their infectivity.

Termination of pregnancy and natural miscarriage are deeply emotional events for some women. There may be fears and fantasies about the surgical interventions and subsequent fertility. Sexual difficulties may follow these events.

Women will expect their gynaecologist to be able to talk about sexual problems. Ideally, they should be thought about and discussed in relation to most gynaecological disorders and procedures, regardless of the patient's age, appearance, sexual orientation or partner status.

Obstetrics

Sexual problems are not so prevalent in antenatal clinics but may become an issue when it is realised that a woman has fears about vaginal examination during labour. This may occur in women who have become pregnant without full vaginal penetration or with *in vitro* fertilisation (IVF) and may be a cause of tocophobia. Sometimes this is discovered early in the pregnancy and help can be put in place.

Post-natal clinics provide an ideal scenario for 'preventative care' before sexual problems become too entrenched. Women may suffer from post-traumatic stress disorder (PTSD) following a difficult labour leading to anxiety, depression, sexual problems and fears relating to another pregnancy or delivery. This will be expanded on in the chapter on tocophobia.

It is important not to generalise – a woman who has had an enormous tear and perineal infection may have no problem, while a woman who has had a medically insignificant event may be unable to resume intercourse after the birth of her child.

Surgery and Urology

Urologists are hopefully aware of sexual problems when treating men with prostatic problems and other issues that may affect erectile function. Although difficult, the subject should be raised and, if possible, an open and empathic conversation exploring fears and concerns pre- or post-surgery may dispel anxieties. Ideally the patient is given advice in the clinic or signposted to somewhere they can get help. Women with urinary incontinence may be concerned about leakage during intercourse. Both men and women with catheters will need advice. Major abdominal surgery and bowel conditions can often affect sexual function both physically and psychologically. If it is hard for doctors and nurses to discuss these problems, imagine how much harder it must be for a patient to raise the subject.

General Medicine

Many medical illnesses affect sexual function – most notably diabetes and cardiovascular disease in men. Little research has been done on the effect of these illnesses on women. Many neurological conditions and chronic illnesses affect sexual function and pleasure, and it is up to the physician to bear this in mind. As discussed later in the book, many prescribed drugs can affect sexual function in men and women, and it is the duty of the prescribing doctor or nurse to discuss this. Rehabilitation services are well placed to discuss sexual matters as health professionals often have more time with the patient. It may be the last thing on the HCP's mind when the patient has faced life-threatening illness or is coping with severe disability – it may be the uppermost thing on the patient's mind who may be waiting to pluck up courage to discuss the problem.

Mental Health

Mental health disorders and the drugs commonly used to treat them have significant effects on libido and sexual function in men and women. It is important that this is borne in mind and discussed with the patient. If using IPM methods, as demonstrated throughout this book, it is important to assess whether the patient is suitable for brief interpretive therapy. This may not be possible if the patient is significantly depressed or suffering from a psychotic illness. Helping people with personality disorders may also prove difficult. Similarly, these methods are not suitable for treating people with fetishes and sexual obsessions.

Cultural and Religious Differences

Some cultures and religions have fixed rules surrounding sexual intercourse. In most religions this is banned until after marriage. Some religions, such as Roman Catholicism, restrict the use of contraception and abortion. Orthodox Jews are supposed to avoid intercourse during menstruation or any other type of vaginal bleeding and for seven days following this. A cleansing ceremony or *mikva* is then performed.

Many Muslim groups also ban sexual intercourse when there is bleeding. (This must be borne in mind when suggesting contraceptive measures that may cause irregular bleeding.) HCPs working with Southeast Asian men may come across the Dhat syndrome where loss of energy, weakness and anxiety may be attributed to loss of semen by nocturnal emission or masturbation. In fact, many religions ban masturbation. Homosexuality is also taboo in many cultures and is still illegal in many parts of the world.

Doctors, midwives and nurses working with some communities must be on the lookout for the possibility of female genital mutilation (FGM) and the effects that this has on sexual function, as well as the other more obvious problems such as urinary leakage and difficulty with labour. Women from these cultural groups may find it particularly difficult to talk about sexual difficulty.

While it is useful to hold these differences in mind and to be sensitive and informed about these issues, it is important to see the person in front of you and make no assumptions. All individuals are different, and they may not adhere to the expectations of their religion or culture. We must not generalise about someone or imagine anything about their sexual life or desires because they are dressed in a certain way or come from a specific part of the world. Similarly, it is not useful to jump to conclusions about a woman who may be dressed in an overtly 'sexy' manner – she may have no libido or have vaginismus. Generalisations or pre-conceived ideas about human sexual behaviour do not help, and these prejudices must be set aside if the HCP is going to enter the patient's world.

Conclusion

Patients in many medical environments may be experiencing sexual and psychosexual problems. All the possible scenarios cannot be covered in this book, but many examples and case histories are described in a variety of settings. Patients may have fears about resuming sexual activity after surgery, cancer treatment, infection, cardiovascular events or in many other situations. A man may fear that resuming intercourse might be damaging or painful after his partner's hysterectomy. There may be a terrified woman who avoids sex in case it may precipitate another stroke or heart attack in her partner. We tell our patients when they can drive again and when they should go back to work, but we are not very good at telling them when they can resume sexual activity and what they might expect. No assumption must be made that someone is too old, too disabled or too ill to have sexual needs. Likewise, not having a partner should not preclude any discussion of sexual function. While all HCPs do not wish to train in this area, we owe it to our patients to have a basic understanding of human sexuality and to have the courage to enter into a dialogue with them about their problems. If the problem cannot be managed by the HCP then they can then refer or signpost to another agency – many of which are included in the glossary. Referring too quickly may be detrimental as the patient has chosen this particular HCP, in this particular setting, having possibly taken a long time to pluck up the courage to disclose their problem. If possible, it is often beneficial for the patient if this HCP can work with them initially before passing them on to another professional where they will have to start all over again. Nurses, doctors, midwives and physiotherapists, unlike many other sex therapists and psychologists, are in the privileged position of being able to examine their patients. They are therefore well placed to explore the psychosomatic, psychosexual problem, thus demonstrating to the patient the link between the mind and the body.

REFERENCES

1. COSRT. The College of Sexual and Relationship Therapists, London, UK. Available from: www.cosrt. org.uk
2. Relate – Relationship Counselling. Available from: www.Relate.org.uk
3. Masters W, Johnson VE. *Human Sexual Inadequacy*. New York, NY: Little, Brown and Company, 1970.
4. Davies JC, Frodsham LCG. Sex: What a pain! The investigation and management of sexual pain disorders in a district gynaecology department [Abstract]. In: *Abstracts of the RCOG World Congress 2013*, 24–26 June; Liverpool, UK. *BJOG*. 21 June 2013. Pages 490–491. Abstract number–EP10.14.

3

When Bodies Speak: Psychosomatic Illness as Hidden Communication

Sandy Goldbeck-Wood

Introduction

In this chapter, I present psychosomatic symptoms as a form of partial or blocked communication – a muffled cry for help that needs creative and open-minded attention in order to be understood. I show how with the right stance and skills, psychosomatic symptoms, exemplified here by psychosexual symptoms, can be read as a hidden story in need of a listener.

First, we should acknowledge that this is an area where terminology has been difficult. *Psychosomatic* means different things to different people. Although innocent enough in its etymological origins, where it simply points to the indissoluble connection between mind and body, the word *psychosomatic* has frequently been used in confusing, stigmatising and uninformative ways. Some commentators have used it to refer to purely symbolic, historically called *hysterical* illness, while others use it more broadly to refer to all illness where there is a significant interplay between emotional and physical distress. Worse, clinicians uninterested in mind-body connections but reluctant to admit lack of understanding have used it to imply 'illness which is not real' or 'illness in which I am not interested'. This makes it, in turn, difficult to raise as a possibility with patients, who understandably resist a diagnosis which they fear may condemn them to therapeutic disinterest and nihilism.

This 'terminology-creep' is particularly unfortunate given that all illness is to some extent psychosomatic. We blush with shame, and tremble with anxiety. Myocardial infarction is associated with *angor animi*. And while it is of course possible to deliver a distressed baby or remove a tumour without recourse to a psychosomatic model, no competent or humane clinician would delude themselves that obstructed labour and cancer are purely biomedical phenomena, free of psychological and social dimensions. The fact remains that while many illnesses can be treated successfully by a combination of biomedicine and ordinary human kindness, many others simply cannot helpfully be thought about at all without a psychosomatic model. This includes most of those we call 'medically unexplained' symptoms, almost all sexual problems and much multi-morbidity. Rather than invent new words, I propose for the purposes of this discussion to reclaim the term *psychosomatic* at its face value, to mean illness where mind and body are interacting to produce symptoms – illness where we cannot helpfully split the two.

Sandor Ferenczi, the Hungarian psychoanalyst often regarded as the father of psychosomatic theory, argued that 'When the psychic system fails, the organism begins to think' (1). In his account, unprocessed psychic distress manifests as real, often incapacitating physical illness, as the body is left to 'articulate' what cannot be expressed any other way. This focus on *symbolic* forms of bodily communication has formed a core element of psychoanalytic and psychodynamic approaches, and the cases which follow illustrate its diagnostic and therapeutic potential. But we should remember that chronic distress, as well as causing emotional and psychosomatic distress, also impacts the body in literal, biological ways. Dysfunctional or abusive relationships, chronic overwork, lack of control over one's own destiny, loss of meaning in life, and other forms of chronic stress eventually overcome the body's ability to cope, driving risk, disease and death. The psycho-neuro-endocrinological and epigenetic mechanisms by which this occurs are increasingly well understood (2,3). The ways in which life experience affects health, biography affects biology, is not only relevant to those of us interested in psychosomatic illness in a narrow sense but affects all of health practice and policy (4).

We could think of psychosomatic communication as a theatrical gesture – a piece of improvised, incomplete poetry or theatre – an instance of what the philosopher Julia Kristeva called *semiotic* communication where ordinary *semantic* reporting has proved impossible (5) – a sort of non-verbal cry for help like that of Stevie Smith's struggling, misunderstood man who was *Not Waving but Drowning*. Understanding psychosomatic symptoms as incomplete creative communication is useful because it explains why empathic imagination is essential to treatment, and why non-creative, purely scientific or reductive approaches simply do not work.

A theatrical performance or poem gains its power by embodying something emotionally resonant in physical terms and addressing an audience or reader in emotional and physical terms at the same time. These holistic forms of expression invite, or perhaps force, the observer or reader to feel and think in parallel. But unlike a successful poem or piece of theatre, which we can enjoy as a complete communication on several channels at once, a psychosomatic symptom is neither complete, nor heard. Precisely the reverse – the story has become somehow blocked and is not making sense either to the patient or other practitioners. External help is needed because the block is causing distress, and that help involves creativity. The task of psychosexual medical treatment is to help a person first complete the job of expressing, and then hearing, their own story.

In psychosexual medicine, this is done using the combined skills of medicine and psychodynamic therapy, in a process which requires the practitioner to think and feel at the same time. The practitioner reflects on and integrates both subjective and objective data, using two different ways of 'listening' based on two different theories of knowledge or epistemologies. The empirical approach of biomedicine which captures and analyses objective, external data is complemented by the hermeneutic approach of psychotherapy which captures and analyses internal and subjective data. Each approach is relevant to understanding illness and health (6), but the two have been split during the history of philosophy (7). But many areas of health, including medically unexplained symptoms, multi-morbidity and psychosexual medicine demand an integrative approach. Let us look at some examples.

CASE 1: WOMAN WITH DARK GLASSES

'Can I help you?' I heard the receptionist say, as I walked towards the clinic waiting room to meet Emily and Dave, and I heard Dave reply, 'Well, I certainly hope so – no one else has been able to'. I feared a challenge.

Emily was not, in fact, wearing dark glasses – that bit is an elaboration, in memory, of her extreme fragility and defencelessness – though she may have been walking with a stick. But she rose to her feet slowly and with some difficulty, as though arthritic or elderly; and Dave, at 50-something 10 years her senior, sprang to her aid.

The referral had been for Emily, whose long-standing difficulties in having sex were now interfering with the couple's desire to have a family. But they had made it clear on the phone that they would both like to attend. I invited them both to tell me about what had brought them. 'It's me', said Emily, confessional: 'I find sex painful. Impossible. The thing is, I go to the chronic pain clinic…'.

A story unfolded which seemed much wider and more intractable than a specific sexual difficulty – a story featuring several kinds of musculoskeletal pain which made sex uncomfortable in her whole body as well as vaginal pain, pretty much everywhere, on penetration. My heart began to sink. There were several doctors and even a counsellor in the story, all of whom had failed to help – some were characterised as well-meaning but impotent, others as unkind or uninterested. I saw pitfalls everywhere, and feared walking across land mined territory only to join the company of inadequate colleagues.

Conscious that I was working with a couple, I made repeated efforts to turn the conversation to Dave, but he simply referred me back to Emily's distresses. Sadly, tenderly, he described how Emily had to give up her work as a textile designer, and her piano playing, at which she was very talented, he said. The three of us agreed that somehow or other Emily's passions had become stymied, right across the board.

On enquiry, Dave said he loved Emily, would love to be able to make love with her, but was reluctant to push, when it clearly caused her so much pain. Endorsing Emily's account of the many unhelpful doctors, he nevertheless praised 'Steve the physio'. I leaped to enquire more about Steve – keen for a hint about how to work with Emily.

Steve the physio had, according to Emily, been gentle but also persistent, according to Dave. As the two of them described his work with her, I imagined someone focussed, attentive, compassionate, and hard to live up to. I reflected back to Emily my impression that gentleness was extremely important to her and earned a glance of what may have been gratitude, certainly it felt like momentary contact. I felt I had scored a first point in what promised to be a tricky chess game.

What was it about gentleness? Had gentleness been lacking somewhere in Emily's life, I wondered? She began to describe her mother – a critical tyrant: measuring the milk in the bottle in the fridge lest her daughter take too much; criticising her for holding a pen the wrong way or for inadvertently dirtying the waste bin while throwing something away. 'Hypersensitive', said Emily – ever since an episode of severe postnatal depression following Emily's younger sister's birth. Intolerant of vulnerability in her daughter, even when ill or in pain, she accused her, wherever it showed of 'hypersensitivity'. Did Emily feel angry? 'Seething!' she said.

I felt relief. I wondered, aloud, whether perhaps Emily's whole body was now seething; whether her body was saying, 'I'll give you hypersensitivity!' Emily's assent encouraged me, but we still seemed a long way from our agreed subject matter – sex. My role here was to offer a brief, four-session, psychodynamic, psychosexual intervention, not long-term psychotherapy. My anxiety about the scope of the work and the timescale grew.

I became a bit more explicit and pushy – wondered aloud whether anyone had ever hurt her sexually. 'No, nothing like that', she assured me. Physical examination – given painful sex, this was medically indicated and expected of me as an IPM trained doctor – was smoothly declined, 'perhaps another time'. I was getting nowhere and starting to feel disempowered: unsure what Emily's many present physical problems and past psychological distress might have to do with the sexual difficulty; aware that while she might benefit from long-term psychotherapy, we had just four sessions to focus on sex; and that, while they had come as a couple, we had despite my best efforts spoken only of Emily. I reflected this imbalance back, suggesting Emily might come on her own next time. Dave leaped at this idea, but Emily resisted it, wanting him at her side – her protector: perhaps also her defence against working, I feared.

So, I was surprised when at our next meeting only Emily stood up in the waiting room, after all. She explained she had come alone to answer my question about whether anyone had hurt her sexually. To tell me something that Dave did not and must not know. She said that since we only had four meetings, she had, 'better get on with it'. But she then stopped. Prevaricated. Didn't know whether she would be able to tell me; insisted it felt too difficult. I sensed both a kind of game-playing, in the prevarication, and also a genuine difficulty in approaching something distressing. Feeling tantalised, I registered an impulse to try and 'wrest' her story from her, by brute force, as it were. Instead, I acknowledged the difficulty in speaking, and waited.

Between sobs, a halting, sketchy story emerged of a relationship with a lecturer by whom Emily had been bullied, undermined and 'forced to do things she did not want to' – yes, sexually, she admitted, on direct questioning. Already in her early 30s at the time, though a virgin, she excoriated herself for having been 'stupid' enough to allow these shadowy, unspoken, unspeakable things to happen. She became withdrawn and distant, hunched, fearful and inarticulate; she shook and sobbed, and would or could not make eye contact. For the remainder of the meeting she seemed to regret bitterly having told me her still-sketchy story.

Just as Emily felt 'stupid' for not stopping the abuses she had suffered, I was left after this second consultation feeling vehemently self-critical: why had I failed to make clear, crisp connections between Emily's distress and her sex life? And to make her tell me more of what actually happened with the bullying lecturer? Why had I got mired with her in this 'distress of uncertain analytic significance', and why, for goodness' sake, had I, a psychosexual doctor and gynaecologist, again failed to examine her (though to do so, given her 'abused child' state, had seemed inconceivable)?

To my surprise, Emily seemed somehow different at our third meeting. Neither the defensive, brittle woman-child hiding behind Dave, nor the broken, lonely, abused child of our last meeting, she seemed more adult and composed; said she felt better, and thought she would 'come through this'. She seemed in touch with her creative, reflective self, had come with dreams suggesting healing, and about challenging her abuser. She took more charge of the consultation, and seemed in touch with space, strength and self-compassion.

From this situation, we were able to wonder how Emily could still have been so defenceless in her 30s? The tyrannical mother re-entered the conversation: Emily, smacked for holding the mop the wrong way while cleaning the floor. Emily, buying her own food and keeping it on her window ledge, to avoid criticism; Emily, terrified to remove a sweltering wool coat on a long, hot bus ride on a summer school trip, lest her mother, who had expressly forbidden its removal, find out and punish her. Criticising her father's impotent attempts to mediate, she wept: 'I was only little – I just didn't know how to stop it'. Still 'only little', therefore, when it came to resisting further, sexual bullying from a man in authority whom she should have been able to trust. Emily – twice bullied where most she would have needed gentleness. And now Emily, locked inside a woman's body 'seething' with a little girl's anger and pain.

Our final meeting yielded the long-postponed examination, which felt like something of an anticlimax – little more than an epilogue. I had expected clamped legs and shrinking up the examination couch – but Emily tolerated examination with no more than a slight wince. We agreed that it wasn't as bad as either of us had expected. 'Tolerable discomfort', was the phrase we agreed upon, and it seemed also to describe where Emily was left with her abusive history.

Summing up the work done, Emily said she had known from the beginning that she needed to face this story. She had revisited it, privately, numerous times since our first meeting, and found each facing slightly less painful than the last. She was singing and playing her piano again, interested in a more equal relationship with Dave, less child-like, more challenging. What about sex, I wondered? She pulled a face, as though this was a question, and intrusion, too many, 'we're having much more closeness and non-genital sexual contact'. And penetration? I probed, gently, because this was the problem she had brought at the beginning …. well … she could imagine it. A shy smile. 'Does Dave know that?' 'I guess I'll need to tell him. In my own space, in my own time', was the message I was hearing, loud and clear, from this now more assertive, more adult woman.

I would not, at my heart-sinking first encounter, have expected Emily to make the progress she did, in the four meetings available. Had I known in advance the extent of her problems, I might well have wondered whether such brief work was suitable at all. Yet, modest as they were, set against a lifetime's suffering, these four sessions felt like a significant opening up of space and reclaiming of adulthood, relative to our first meeting.

What did she think had helped? A balance of gentleness and persistence in our conversation, she thought. In the tradition of Steve the physio, then. Maybe also the knowledge of the strict time limitation, we both agreed – certainly she had referred to it so clearly as the work evolved that I had at one point decided against my impulse to offer her extra sessions, for fear of disrupting her obvious use of the time frame's rigor. Indeed, although Emily and I each worked hard with the 'content' of the material she brought – she to face pain formerly locked in her body, I to tolerate the anxiety of work which threatened to disempower and overwhelm me – I think 'the frame' was the mysterious third element in this work. As therapeutic as any specific intervention I offered or might have offered was the firm boundary: a firmly contained space in which openness to Emily's broad, intractable, more-than-sexual problems, coupled with a commitment to returning to the question of sex, drove the work forward. Also, as an obstetrician, I imagined this frame as a kind of contracting uterus: a benignly rigorous maternal space, such as Emily had lacked. Not just cosy, uncomfortable for both parties, but containing, safe and essential to progress.

How was Emily's hidden story expressed? What kinds of clues did she present, how did she engage her doctor, and what kinds of responses did she elicit?

Radical Openness

Long before Emily entered the consulting room, her difficult lived experience was communicating itself through her general practitioner's referral letter, her husband's despair-laden opening comment, and her own pained body language. She was offering unconscious clues about her extreme vulnerability, and about her husband's assigned role as her asexual protector. These clues were far from a full story, without her own verbal account, but could, with the use of a kind of radical, imaginative openness, be gathered as up-front, contextual evidence – factual material with emotional resonance, presenting themselves to the practitioner's awareness in the form of vague feelings which could be noticed and stored for future reference. I read her clues as an early warning against approaching too close.

Using Intersubjectivity

This broad welcoming of subtle clues, accompanied by emotional self-scrutiny, forms a way of 'reading' the other person in the light of one's own responses. In psychoanalysis this is called *countertransference* – a form of emotional imaging which, like radiological imaging, does not identify a problematic structure with 100% certainty, but is a useful guide to the right kind of further investigation. Right from the beginning of the encounter, the practitioner is capturing objective clues together with the subjective responses they produce, in a process which is neither objective nor subjective but intersubjective. She is observing and interacting, thinking and feeling at the same time. Subjective responses are not treated as contaminants to be ignored, denied or 'risen above' but as sources of potential information, in a carefully qualified, provisional, hypothesis-generating sense. Maintaining a clear sense of what originated as fact and what as feeling, the practitioner holds the two side by side in awareness, allowing potential connections to emerge which can be offered to the patient as hypotheses. The practitioner allows feeling to illuminate fact, fact to illuminate feeling, and an inner dialogue between objective and subjective truth to emerge.

Applied Sensitivity

This process may be subtle, but it is not magic: it is sensory, not extra-sensory. It is based firmly on observation, but includes observations normally ignored in everyday life or ordinary medical practice. It is sensitive, in that like an ultrasound scan it involves tuning up reception of a particular set of real but subtle signals of a kind easily swamped by other data, if not actively sought. Emily's subtle injunction to 'stay away', alongside the invitation to come close which is implied by seeking an appointment, was a useful beginning.

Spaciousness

The practitioner's stance could be understood as one of 'hosting' some unresolved subject matter and difficult feelings, to give the patient space to complete the creative work of integrating them. From early in the conversation, the practitioner was preparing inside herself a space for something whose identity she could not possibly yet know but had allowed herself to sense 'between the lines' of the patient's clues. She was agreeing to encounter this unknown element with warm, open-minded curiosity – tolerating the discomfort of sensing something she could not yet name. It was impossible to understand in advance the connection between this 'space' and the lack of accommodation which Emily's childhood needs had been given. Winnicott uses the word 'holding', Bion 'containing', for these 'hosting' roles, which characterise all psychologically developmental relationships, whether between practitioner and patient, parent and infant or teacher and pupil (8,9).

Insightful Interpretation and Therapeutic Endurance

Insightful interpretation is often how we think of therapeutic work, and this can be the most satisfying and flattering part for the therapist. The conversation with Emily certainly offered occasional, pleasurable moments of interpretive success, such as articulating *gentleness* as a key, missing dimension in Emily's life – moments which restored a sense of therapeutic competence and agency and mitigated the struggle and mess which characterised other moments.

But the work also brought several prolonged phases of confusion, 'not knowing what was happening', 'not knowing how to move forward', and 'not being able to imagine a satisfactory outcome in the time available'. This therapeutic persistence in the face of difficulty or 'hanging in' can be one of the most challenging, important effective and underreported interventions in therapy. We may overlook it for various reasons. These might include perceptual bias – just as a figure in a painting strikes us more readily than the background, elegant interpretations, obvious defences and neat breakthroughs may stand out more than the texture or 'background' of 'mute process'. There may also be narcissistic bias in what we choose to report – a natural if unconscious desire to look good, sound insightful and present work as though we know what we are doing. But in overlooking this I suggest we overlook one of the greatest therapeutic gifts in a therapeutic encounter – moral solidarity and emotional role modelling.

What are we offering, when we persevere in the chaotic-seeming passages of an encounter, allowing the patient to make us feel uncomfortable without turning away, tolerating our own uncertainty? One thing we offer is our own vulnerability, as a form of therapeutic role modelling. By not attempting to remain (or pretending to be) strong and all-knowing, the practitioner who is secure enough to struggle visibly and authentically alongside the patient, offers moral solidarity. The patient is not alone in floundering. She can sense that it is not she who is stupid (the practitioner is after all also puzzled) but the material which is difficult. But as the work proceeds, she can also experience that 'it is OK to flounder', that floundering can be tolerated, survived, met with creative exploration and curiosity, and lead to greater self-awareness. Consider the place of therapeutic vulnerability encountered in Case 2.

CASE 2: ON WOMEN AND GEARBOXES

'Hello Sandy, I'm Bob'. He was nice-as-pie, well-presented with a warm smile and a firm handshake. I had no idea why the receptionist had thought him angry. 'How can I help? Your doctor has written that there have been some problems with sex'. 'No – not problems really – I'm just not interested. I've come because I'll get earache otherwise!' he quipped. 'Well – she cares; wants some attention: all I really want, to be honest, is a good armchair'. They were married with two grown-up kids, and a granddaughter they adore, he related; he plays bass guitar in a band and has motorbikes. Life was pretty good. So why was he here, then? The conversation felt like jousting – a bit like a lad's game. 'Search me!' he shrugged, then added, breezily, 'I'm probably wasting your time... feel a bit of a fraud!'

'But something brought you!?' I challenged. 'Yes, I've no idea really'. I was having to work harder than usual to get this conversation going and felt 'at sea'. Retreating into the familiarity of a more medicalised sexual history, I elicited a flat, factual account of vasectomy, and also diabetes, meaning that now 'the mechanics didn't work very well', and it was hard to 'get a result'. He didn't say what counted as a 'result' and for now, I didn't ask. Yes, he had tried Viagra, but it gave him a headache and was not worth the bother. The alternative phosphodiesterase inhibitors I mentioned – retreating into biomedicine – those with fewer side effects, raised no interest either. He had no idea what the problem might be and did not seem interested in finding out.

It sounds like you're 'out to pasture', I needled, searching for a response, wondering where his feelings were. 'Yes, that's about right', he smiled, completely unruffled. I tried another tack: if someone could wave a magic wand and fix the erection problems or headache, did he think this would make a difference to his desire for sex? Was it, I wondered privately, all too painful because of the erection problems – was that why he had given up? I felt I was practically 'swinging from the chandeliers' in an attempt to get a response, but all he said was: 'In all honesty? No'.

Bob was firmly in control of the conversation, and I was frustrated and anxious, disempowered in the face of a pleasant man seeking treatment but denying any real problem or feelings. Observing my own discomfort, I commented that she cares, and I seem to care, but not him. 'Oh, right! Was that the wrong answer?' he said, blasé. Feeling patronised and a little irritated, I nonetheless battled on, 'What constitutes, "a result"?'

There was a long pause. Then hesitantly, Bob said: 'The thing is, I've never been able to orgasm Linda'. His words were powerful, and vulnerable, and shifted the atmosphere in the room: suddenly he seemed uncomfortable, while I registered relief and a sense of connection – with his feelings, and with a story, which might begin to explain his presenting complaint: a story not, after all, only about erections, but about something less technical and more emotional, to do with his relationship with his wife's pleasure. 'I've been married to Linda 26 years', he said, 'I love her. We used to have a lot of sex – used to be at it like rabbits. But I can't orgasm her. Not really. I could count the times on the fingers of one hand. She can do it herself; we got into a habit early on – I just felt in the way and let her get on with it'. It was clear, he said, that she would like him involved in her orgasm, but he was not interested.

'What did that feel like?' I asked, more gently, feeling for a moment that we might now be on track. 'I think it's just how it is', he said, calmly closing things down. 'Yes, but what does it feel like to be in that place?' I pointed to a place on my own chair, as if to indicate physically what I meant by being in a situation. 'Well I just can't be bothered'. Dissatisfied with his slippery response, I tried a third time: 'Yes, but how does it feel…' this time he completed my sentence for me, 'to be superfluous to requirements?' he said, his words hanging painfully in the space between us, as though I had wrested them out of him by force. 'Nauseous', he said.

'Well sometimes it had happened', he said, taking a step back. 'What did that feel like?' I wondered. 'Good', he said flatly. I said I imagined it might be touching, or quite special – something good, that didn't happened much. Oh, I'm not very emotional, he said, unmoved. Then as if catching some dissatisfaction in me, he said: 'Am I saying the wrong thing again?' There seemed to be both pain and pleasure in the room, now, but it was I who seemed to be feeling them, while he remained flat. I reflected that it seemed a struggle to get 'hold' of him in the conversation and felt a bit anxious. I wondered whether he felt anxious in relation to Linda.

Partly as a matter of clinical routine, partly in escape from this difficult conversation, I proposed physical examination – 'no problem' for Bob, who stretched out on the couch, arms above his head, teasing me that he hoped my hands were warm, maintaining control even while undressed. I was more than usually businesslike and brief, perhaps in response to some embarrassment of my own at the intimacy of genital examination; perhaps also reflecting this mechanically minded man's discomfort about sexual relating. Abdominal and genital examinations were unremarkable. Except that at the end, Bob sat up abruptly and said: 'I've really got to sort this out, haven't I?'

I asked him where he felt his passion went, if not into sex. 'I'm not passionate', he said. I wondered, privately, if 'not caring' is a way of expressing anger at feeling superfluous. 'It's funny that I can't be bothered', he volunteered suddenly, 'because I'm not like that about mechanical things … gearboxes, for example. I do prefer mechanical to biological systems. I'd be perfectly happy to stay with a gearbox problem 'til it is fixed – with Linda's orgasm, I can't be bothered'. He said it almost smugly, and I, maybe irritated on Linda's behalf, or maybe on my own, played devil's advocate: 'Why? Was it that gearboxes were more interesting or important?' 'Of course not!' he threw back, needled.

We explored the higher stakes, lower confidence and more uncertain outcome associated with the orgasm, compared with the gearbox. The way uncertainty combined with a sense of responsibility and wanting to get it right made the sexual exploration harder to stay with than the mechanical one – 'harder to know where you were'. I knew the feeling, from the here and now of the doctor-patient relationship. I wondered aloud whether the key task might precisely be to stay with not knowing how to do things. Bob shifted the conversation to manuals. Slightly boastfully, he told me he never used manuals because he doesn't need them. And that if a thing is user-friendly, you shouldn't need one. He was back in his element, and away from the sore spot of Linda's orgasm, and from contact with me.

I commented on his language: 'user-friendly' … 'getting a result' – clinical, distancing terms, I suggested. 'Oh, have I said the wrong thing again?' We seemed to be handing the discomfort back and forth between us – the more I found my feet in the conversation, the more uncomfortable he became, and vice versa, until tapping on the table nervously, he said 'I'm tapping on the table'. 'Are you anxious?' I asked. 'Yes'. 'Do you know why?' 'Well, some of the things you've said…' 'What have I said that's made you anxious?' 'Well, we've talked about why I'm here. I suppose. That, and the gearbox conversation'. 'Well, I suppose maybe that's some sort of a result', I quipped, laddishly, nervously.

Almost to my surprise, he accepted my offer of a series of further appointments. In the waiting room, in front of the receptionist, in a gesture that seemed suddenly, uncharacteristically intimate, he said 'thanks for listening'.

This initial session had felt like a long football match, and Bob had been a slick opponent, skilled at maintaining the upper hand without obvious aggression. Humour had proved a powerful defence against intimacy, at times charming, at times irritating, heading off my initiatives and hypotheses. As my best efforts failed and I feared letting this likeable man down – as he, perhaps, feared letting his wife down – my anxiety had mounted. But all of this anxiety and resistance – Bob's anxiety, resonating in me, as we struggled together – was the clue to the problem.

Achieving Therapeutic Intimacy

Each of these two individuals presented a hidden story in a kind of camouflage. Each presented a physical block to something they consciously desired – having a family in the one case, marital harmony in the other. In neither case was *the relational intimacy of sex* presented directly as a lost pleasure in its own right, rather its absence figured as a mere obstacle to something else – a 'thing' brought to the doctor for removal or treatment, almost like an inconvenient foreign body. But in both, a more or less dissatisfied partner waited in the wings, unable to get close; in each case, it was the relational context in the treatment room, the rapid establishment of a kind of therapeutic intimacy against the odds and within a time constraint, that melted the frozen 'thing', the physical block or symptom, back into palpable distress, and an audible call for help. Part of the doctor's job was to re-experience in the doctor-patient relationship, and tolerate, what *being kept at a distance* felt like, but not to give in, using the therapeutic role to sustain the pressure of warm curiosity and keep pushing for intimacy of real contact.

Both encounters involved the re-establishment of a free flow of feeling and thinking, around a block, where things had become two dimensional and fixed. The process in both cases required the practitioner to use her creative, spontaneous self to establish a climate of 'playing with' the material. The feelings initially 'in play' in the room are those of the practitioner, accompanied by her imaginative hypotheses as to what the patient might be feeling. These hypotheses are sometimes right and sometimes wrong, but collectively begin to set a tone, and the terms of engagement. The practitioner's sustained, warm, at times insistent search for meaning in the patient's story begins to create pressure towards intimacy.

Space and Containers

Here, Bion's word *containment* helps us, with all its connotations of firm but flexible boundaries, and three dimensionality. Like the psychic growth or learning of an infant, the therapeutic process requires a chamber or space into which material which cannot yet be borne or integrated can be safely placed, or projected (10). Beginning literally in the form of a physical room and an agreed time frame, that space establishes itself as a relational space between carer and patient, and then if all goes well, a psychological space within the patient. In the process known as *projective identification*, the patient uses or borrows the therapist's own mental space as a temporary repository for their own frozen feelings, managing to make their therapist 'feel their discomfort'. This requires a capacity and willingness on the therapist's part to take in or 'introject', feelings generated by the patient, and to tolerate them without retaliating or collapsing for long enough to allow new thoughts to emerge. This 'firm elasticity' of the therapists's mental space which expands to receive the patient's story allows tough material to be reviewed, rearranged and broken down into something more digestible and useful.

The Boundary

A space has a boundary, and in brief psychodynamic work, this can feel quite tight. Time pressure can sometimes feel extreme relative to the burden of distress, especially in a publically funded health setting where patients may have waited many months for treatment. Establishing the therapeutic alliance rapidly and efficiently is of the essence. Without the luxury of the extended development and analysis of a transference relationship, such as is possible in long-term psychotherapy, a reflective space with future potential for the patient must be opened and used within a few sessions. Rather than aiming to deliver a set of doctor-centred interpretations relating to a single set of circumstances, issued like a medical prescription, the patient ideally needs to leave treatment with a strengthened sense of their own capacity to interpret their own experience. Emily appeared well aware of this urgency, and her awareness seemed actually to drive the work forward.

At times, the intensity of this can feel almost surgical, as the need to move swiftly but atraumatically through layers of resistance and confusion – 'to cut to the chase' – can feel urgent. But if surgical and obstetric analogies make the work sound tense and pressured, the work also contains playful elements – a kind of serious play. The ability to play has been identified as an absolute precondition for psychic growth and development in adults as well as children. So, this is work which connects therapeutic and creative activities.

We might think of this kind of intense, serious-playful work as a kind of poetry. Psychosomatic symptoms present a kind of disturbing but promising poetic raw material which through careful listening and reconstruction by two people in intimate dialogue can be made clear and coherent. Practitioner and patient embark on a swift but careful journey towards the place where important knowledge lies hidden – the point of maximum sensation. Time limitation can be a tough ally, helping the hidden story to emerge.

REFERENCES

1. Ferenczi S, ed. by Dupont J. *The Clinical Diary*. London: Harvard University Press, 1988.
2. McEwen B. Brain on stress: How the social environment gets under the skin. *PNAS* 2012;109(Suppl. 2): 17180–17185.
3. Murphy T, Mill J. Epigenetics in health and disease: Heralding the EWAS era. *The Lancet* 2014;383(9933):1952–1954.
4. Kirkengen A. *The Lived Experience of Violation: How Abused Children Become Unhealthy Adults*. Bucharest: Zeta Books, 2010.
5. Kristeva J. *Revolution in Poetic Language*. New York: Columbia University Press, 1984, 19.

6. Antonovsky A. The salutogenic model as a theory to guide health promotion. *Health Promot Int* 1996;11:11–18.
7. Descartes R, ed. by Cottingham J. *Meditations on First Philosophy.* Cambridge: Cambridge University Press, 1996.
8. Winnicott D. *The Maturational Processes and the Facilitating Environment.* London: Hogarth, 1965.
9. Bion W. A theory of thinking. *Int J Psychoanal* 1962;43.
10. Winnicott D. *Playing and Reality.* New York: Routledge, 1971.

4

Talking about Sex

Catherine Hood

Introduction

How good is your sex life? Think about that question for a while. While contemplating, you can start to understand some of the difficulties involved in talking about sex.

How are you going to measure and communicate your satisfaction? Marks out of 10? Thumbs up, thumbs down? Smiling or frowning emojis? What most people value in their intimate lives are qualitative attributes, not quantitative. These are harder to express, very individual and more difficult to objectively measure.

The next question you may contemplate is: How good *should* my sex life be? We all have expectations of what a healthy sex life looks like. These expectations are formed by our personal beliefs, early learnings, what our community thinks and what the wider world tells us through all elements of media from the printed word, television, film and more recently, social media, the Internet and pornography.

The reality is that no two sex lives look the same, and there is no standard. Despite this, when discussing your sex life with another person, it is difficult to escape a sense of internal and external judgment. As a healthcare professional listening to an individual or couple you have to beware of making too many assumptions of what 'normal' should be and respectfully hear each person's most intimate desires, even if they do not match your own.

Going back to the original question, the third aspect that will almost certainly be going through your mind is that your intimate life is deeply personal. Opening up and discussing your sex life can make you feel very vulnerable. To some degree you are revealing the true essence of who you are. This vulnerability must be respected in the consultation room.

However, our intimate lives are a vital part of our well-being. The way we choose to share and express ourselves with loved ones is linked to happiness and self-esteem. Intimacy brings enjoyment, affirmation and a deep sense of connection. It is important and when things go wrong, it is essential to know who to turn to for help.

Discussing Sexual Issues

If you look at the Internet, magazines and television, the level of sexual content would make you assume that twenty-first century patients find discussing sex as easy as talking about other areas of their lives. This is not the case. The reality is that patients will not always talk about sexual issues even when problems are significantly affecting their quality of life.

The large 2013 National Survey of Sexual Attitudes and Lifestyles (Natsal) in Britain interviewed 15,000 men and women (1). Almost one in six reported a health problem affecting their sex life in the preceding year, yet of these people, less than one in four men and one in five women had sought any help from a healthcare professional.

This reluctance to seek help could be because some individuals are not particularly distressed by their sexual issue and thus not motivated to get advice. Indeed, the Natsal survey revealed that despite high numbers of sexual problems being reported (around 40%), only roughly 10% of individuals are distressed or worried about them.

However, many studies have shown that patients with sexual issues would like to talk to their doctors about their troubles but there are barriers to communication (2–5).

Research also reveals that healthcare professionals could do much more to pick up on sexual issues in their patients.

A large global survey of older people aged 40 to 80 revealed that less than one in ten had been asked about their sex lives in the previous three years despite more than half of them reporting a sexual concern (3). Perhaps healthcare professionals are sometimes guilty of making assumptions about the sexual activity of this population group, thinking this is not an important area to explore (4).

Even with population groups that you might expect to discuss sex with, these conversations are often not being done routinely (5–8).

In a survey of physicians who routinely review adolescents, a patient group you might expect to have high sexual activity, one-third of consultations had no mention of sexual behaviour. In the consultations where sex was discussed, the average conversation lasted for 36 seconds and only 4% had a long discussion with their doctor on this subject. Of note, none of the adolescents initiated the discussion (6).

Obstetrics and gynaecology is a specialty where you might expect regular discussions about sexuality as part of the medical history. However, a large US survey (7) revealed that more than one-third of obstetrics and gynaecology physicians did not routinely ask about the sexual activities of their patients and fewer still asked about sexual experience. Only 40% of doctors in the survey asked routinely about sexual problems and 28.5% about sexual satisfaction.

So, we have a situation where people are reluctant to raise their problems when they have them and healthcare professionals are reluctant to routinely ask questions about sex and even less willing to allow discussions around the qualitative and emotional aspects of sexuality. The inevitable conclusion is a perfect collusion of silence.

Presentation of Sexual Problems

One of the features of a psychosexual consultation is that you can never completely predict when a sexual problem will present itself.

On entering the United States, one psychosexual doctor was asked about her speciality by the homeland security guard at the passport desk. When she revealed her specialism, the guard started to tell her all about the sexual problem he was having with his wife.

However, not all people are as forthcoming about their sexual difficulty. A patient may hint at a sexual problem in an otherwise seemingly unconnected consultation. In such situations the doctor has to be aware of the possibility of a hidden sexual issue that may require discussion.

For example, a patient may make a sideways reference to their partner not showing interest anymore. A new father may allude to lack of time with his partner since the arrival of their child. A woman may make excuses for repeatedly cancelling a smear test.

Sexual problems can cause a lot of anxiety and distress. Low mood and anxiety may be the presenting feature, and physicians need to be aware of this potential underlying cause or association.

Sometimes sexual problems present as more general physical concerns. A man may talk of a lack of energy or power, or a woman may complain of abdominal pains or vaginal discharge when in fact the problem is less physical but more psychosexual in nature.

The pressure to conceive can also trigger or reveal underlying sexual difficulties. It is not unusual for couples to be referred for specialist fertility support when the lack of conception success is due to the fact that they are simply not having sex.

Door Handle Questions

There are some issues that are too embarrassing or difficult to broach during the consultation but too important to leave unsaid; sexual problems may fall into this category. The patient will wait until the very end of the consultation, often just as they are leaving the room, before asking 'one further question, doctor'.

This can trip up the unsuspecting physician as the time for discussion is now very limited and you have an awkward situation with a very important concern only being revealed when there is no time to adequately deal with it. In this case it is important to acknowledge the problem and arrange a separate appointment to allow the time to explore the issue in greater depth.

Proactively Asking about Sexual Experience

Ideally healthcare practitioners will feel comfortable routinely asking questions about sexual matters.

There are some settings where the patient may expect to be asked about their intimate life: In a specialist sexual and family health clinic or psychosexual service, for example, or in general practice or other specialities like urology, andrology, obstetrics and gynaecology where the presenting complaint has a sexual element.

In other settings the patient may not be expecting a discussion, and it is important that the healthcare practitioner can broach the subject and be prepared to explain why potentially intimate questions are important in this context.

If a doctor is to prescribe a drug or recommend a procedure that may affect sexual function, then the doctor must feel confident to raise the issue with the patient (4,5). Not doing so can engender a lot of anger if the patient subsequently suffers sexual dysfunction as a result of the treatment.

For example, a woman undergoing pelvic radiotherapy for bowel cancer needs to be warned about the impact on the vagina and the need to use dilators. A man undergoing prostatectomy should be offered a discussion about the risks of erectile dysfunction and the effect this may have on his relationships. A young person considering treatment for acne should be able to discuss the dangers of getting pregnant while on some of the medications.

Sexual problems are common in the context of chronic disease, but again, often not discussed in the healthcare setting (8,9). The association between cardiovascular disease or diabetes and erectile dysfunction is well known. Less obvious are the sexual problems associated with joint pain and chronic arthritis, chronic skin conditions, numbness and neurological conditions, or from the diagnosis and treatment of cancer.

Other common conditions that have been linked to an increase risk of sexual dysfunction include repeated urinary tract infections, sexually transmitted infections, irritable bowel syndrome and thyroid disease to name but a few.

Barriers to Communication

To facilitate discussion around sexual function you need to be mindful of the barriers.

Table 4.1 lists some of the potential barriers that inhibit both patients and healthcare professionals (HCPs) from discussing sexual problems. These have been cited many times in the literature. You will notice that there are several similarities between the lists.

TABLE 4.1

Barriers to Talking about Sexual Problems

Issues that May Prevent Patients from Talking about Sexual Problems	Issues that May Prevent HCPs from Talking about Sexual Problems
• Confidentiality	• Confidentiality (interruptions)
• A fear of judgement	• Perceived lack of time
• Shame at being sexual	• Not wanting to cause offence or embarrass the patient
• Feeling rushed	• Discomfort with the subject matter
• Difficulty bringing up the subject	• Lack of training in this area and uncertainty of what to ask
• Not wanting to embarrass the HCP	• Language barriers
• Discomfort with the subject matter	• Cultural differences
• Not believing there is a solution to their problems	• Presence of a partner or relatives in the room
• Language barriers	• Perceived relevance of the questions
• Cultural differences	• Not knowing what to do if a sexual problem is disclosed

Arguably the most powerful inhibitor to a discussion about sex is a perceived lack of confidentiality. To facilitate these discussions healthcare professionals should look at the environments in which they work and make them more conducive to discussions about intimate life.

Posters in the waiting room about contraception or sexual issues can help give a message to patients who are waiting that these conversations are encouraged and welcomed. It is important that these focus not only on young people but on older patients too.

In the consultation room, interruptions from telephone calls or other healthcare staff entering the room should be kept to a minimum, and having these conversations on open wards when the discussion may be overheard by other patients should be avoided.

Another powerful inhibitor is the fear of causing offence. In a Swiss study of over 1,400 male patients attending their family practitioners, 90% wanted their doctor to ask them questions about their sex life (10), and 85% said they would not feel embarrassed to be asked sexual questions but 15% would feel uncomfortable. Of this 15%, despite their feelings of embarrassment, three-quarters said they would still like their physician to ask about their sexuality.

Patient willingness to be asked these questions has been observed in other studies too (2,4,5,7,8). In other words, sometimes we have to risk a little embarrassment on both sides. A little discomfort does not mean an individual does not want to talk about this issue; on the contrary, he or she may feel relieved that the subject has been raised.

The other consistent concern among physicians is that permitting a discussion about sexual issues is going to result in a tide of emotional worries that will overwhelm the consultation, resulting in an emotional patient who is difficult to contain and an overrunning clinic, opening the 'can of worms'. Asking about a person's sexual activity, sexuality or sexual experience does not have to take a long time.

Patients come into the consultation with a well-formed experience of their illness, how their problems are affecting them. Research shows that eliciting all of a patient's concerns early in the consultation can actually save you time in the long run and reduce follow-up appointments (11,12). In addition, not allowing a sexual concern to the expressed will not make that problem disappear; it will keep it hidden and potentially increase the distress felt by the patient. It will also deny the patient the support and help that is available, as most sexual problems can be improved with a supportive approach or referral to the relevant specialist.

Starting the Discussion

Having a discussion about sex and sexuality with a patient can be difficult but it is probably not as difficult as you think, you just need to know where to start.

The principles of patient-centred medicine encourage a doctor to allow a patient to lead the way in opening up about issues they want to discuss in a consultation (11,12). However, healthcare professionals have to be mindful that patients, as we have already discussed, will not always volunteer information about their private sexual lives, even if they are experiencing problems. This is one area where you have to take the lead.

Every healthcare professional should have a few opening phrases they can draw on to begin the discussion about intimacy. View it as opening a door to a conversation; the patient can then decide whether they want to explore this subject further or shut the door on it for now. Even if on the first occasion they do not want to discuss these issues, once you have shown them that you are willing to have a non-judgemental discussion about sex and sexuality, they may feel empowered to open the door to the discussion themselves at any subsequent meeting.

Table 4.2 shows some phrases that have been shown to work. It is important to practise these phrases and make them your own so you feel comfortable using them. A good tip is to consider asking about sex as another routine part of the healthcare checklist. The more comfortable you are with initiating the discussion about sex, the more comfortable the patient will be with responding.

TABLE 4.2

How to Initiate a Discussion about Sex

Helpful Phrases to Initiate a Discussion around Sex and Intimacy
• I'd like to ask a few questions about your sex life, would that be okay? • Are you sexually active at the moment? • Do you have any questions or concerns relating to your intimate or sexual life? • If you're sexually active, has the operation/illness affected your ability to be intimate? • Sometimes individuals with symptoms like yours experience difficulty in their sex lives, is this something that has been an issue for you? • These tablets are known to cause problems with sexual function for some people, has this been a problem? • Sex may not be an issue for you at the moment, but I'm happy to discuss any questions you have about this.

Making Assumptions

One of the main reasons why many sexual problems remain undetected in patients is that healthcare practitioners make assumptions about a person's sexual activity and so do not ask the questions.

Common assumptions made are assuming sexual preferences, that a person is heterosexual or homosexual without checking, that sex stops when individuals reach a certain age, that people in long-term relationships do not have multiple partners and that disabled people are not interested in sex.

A sexual drive is a natural part of every person's life. Always ask and never assume; if you do not ask the question and if you have not heard the answer, then you do not know what is happening in a person's private life. Opening a discussion about sex should become part of the routine consultation for everybody.

The Psychosexual History

Once the discussion about sex has been facilitated, what is it that the psychosexual practitioner needs to explore? Traditionally, sexual problems were seen as being either psychogenic, organic or of mixed aetiology. This model has evolved and there is increasing recognition that sexual problems may have multiple contributing factors: biological, cognitive, emotional and behavioural, contextual and interpersonal (13,14).

It may seem like a lot to achieve, but exploring all of these areas with an individual or couple will give you and the patient(s) a greater understanding of the many factors contributing to the sexual issue and in turn help identify possible areas that can be changed to improve the situation.

Table 4.3 shows specific issues you might want to explore during a consultation. These should be viewed as areas for discussion rather than as a list of questions. The psychosexual consultation should steer away from too many questions. Asking multiple questions can turn the consultation into an interview and inhibit the most important skill of the psychosexual practitioner, which is the ability to listen.

The number of areas you delve into in the consultation and the degree to which you explore these issues with an individual will depend upon the context of the consultation. To explore everything can take time, but an in-depth discussion is not always required. If you are time limited, then explore only as much as will allow you to come to a decision about the next step, whether that is to arrange a longer follow-up appointment or to do an onward referral where the issues can be explored in greater depth.

Sexual Function and Screening Checklists

There are multiple screening checklists and questionnaires published to help assess sexual function. Some may be useful to incorporate into clinical practice to ensure that sexual problems are not missed. They can also be used as assessment tools to allow greater understanding of a person's sexual difficulty.

TABLE 4.3

The Psychosexual History

Parameter	Possible Areas to Explore
Sexual	• Nature of the sexual problem – what happens, how often, in what circumstance and with whom • Duration and onset • Individual sexual practices, e.g. penetration, oral sex, foreplay techniques • Previous sexual problems/traumas/events • Initiation in sexual activity • Libido • Arousal • Lubrication • Ejaculation • Orgasm • Sexual pleasure and satisfaction • Sexual pain or discomfort • Impact of different sexual positions • Masturbation • Exploration and understanding of genital anatomy • Fantasy • Use of pornography • Sexuality • Gender
Biological	• Morning erections/night-time emissions • Fertility and obstetric history • Menstrual history • Contraception history • Additional and/or associated medical history, e.g. sexually transmitted infections, frequent urinary tract infections, diabetes, cardiovascular disease, thyroid disease, surgery/radiotherapy for cancer treatment, etc. • Drug history
Psychological	• Emotions associated with the sexual problem, e.g. anxiety, guilt • Previous sexual or relationship trauma • Sexual confidence • Difficulty with intimacy • Poor self-image • Desire for conception • Other contributing psychological issues, e.g. anxiety, obsessive-compulsive disorder, personality disorders
Cultural/ Social	• Upbringing and attitudes to relationships and sex • Current and past relationship to parents and siblings • Religious beliefs • Cultural traditions
Relationship	• Current partnership – duration • Attitudes towards partner • Quality of communication in the relationship • Commitment to the relationship • Sexual problems in the partner • Other partners • Problems in previous relationships • Response of the partner to the sexual problem

While these screening tools may be of help, they should not be seen as an alternative to a face-to-face discussion but more of an aid to help guide a consultation.

The fact that there are so many different questionnaires highlights the complexity of the conversations healthcare professionals have with psychosexual clients. One assessment or scale does not suit all situations.

TABLE 4.4

Common Screening Tools to Identify Sexual Dysfunction

Checklist
Male and Female Sexual Functioning Questionnaires
• Female Sexual Function Index (FSFI)
• Sexual Function Questionnaire (SFQ)
• Female Sexual Distress Scale – Revised (FSDS-R)
• Sexual Interest and Desire Inventory (SIDI)
• International Index of Erectile Function (IIEF)
• Male Sexual Health Questionnaire (MSHQ)
• Premature Ejaculation Profile (PEP)
• Index of Premature Ejaculation (IPE)
Sexual Function Questionnaires for Specific Patient Groups
• PROMIS Sexual Function and Satisfaction (PROMIS SexFS)
• UCLA Prostate Cancer Index (UCLA-PCI)
• Expanded Prostate Cancer Index Composite (EPIC)
• Sexual Activity Questionnaire
• Sexual Function – Vaginal Changes Questionnaire (SVQ)
• European Organisation for Research and Treatment of Cancer (EORTC) QLQ-C30
• Multiple Sclerosis Intimacy and Sexuality Questionnaire (MSISQ-19)
• Multiple Sclerosis – Female (SEA-MS-F)
• Pelvic Organ Prolapse Incontinence Sexual Questionnaire (PISQ) and PISQ-IR
• Spinal Cord Injury – Secondary Conditions Scale (SCI-SCS)
• Sexual Function Questionnaire – Medical Impact Scale (SFQ-MIS) for assessing impact of childbirth on sexual function
• Antipsychotics and Sexual Functioning Questionnaire (ASFQ)
• Peyronie's Disease Questionnaire (PDQ)
• Female Genital Self-Image Scale (FGSIS)
• Penile Dysmorphic Disorder Scale
Treatment Outcome and Sexual Quality-of-Life Questionnaires
• Erectile Dysfunction Inventory of Treatment and Satisfaction (EDITS)
• Treatment Satisfaction Scale (TSS)
• Psychological and Interpersonal Relationship Scale (PAIRS)
• Self-Esteem and Relationship Scale (SEAR)
• Sexual Quality of Life – Female (SQOL-F)
• Sexual Quality of Life – Male (SQOL-M)

These questionnaires really come into their own when conducting research in this field as they provide an objective measure of sexual function within a study group.

Table 4.4 shows a list of the common questionnaires and is part of the output from the International Consultation on Sexual Medicine (ICSM) 2016 (13).

Psychosexual Discussions in Practise

In all medical consultations there are two agendas at play (12). The doctor's agenda involves the identification of symptoms and signs which point to a diagnosis and treatment pathway. The patient also has their own agenda, and this is informed by their understanding of their symptoms, fears, concerns and expectations of the consultation and of you as the healthcare professional. As skilled professionals, healthcare workers are challenged with gathering information from both of these agendas in the few minutes they have with the patient. This is done by the appropriate use of questions, active listening, reflection and summary.

Listening

The greatest skill the psychosexual practitioner can develop is the ability to listen.

To do this work you have to become an expert listener and skilled in the use of silence. You are not only listening to the patient, their ideas, fears, desires and expectations; you are listening to the whole room, not only the words that are said but the way in which they are expressed, the tone of voice and the phrases used. You notice the ease with which somebody discusses their intimate life, their manner: nervous, fearful, joyful.

The patient sends out verbal and non-verbal cues which reveal how they are really feeling. The skilled practitioner recognises these and may pick up on and reflect these back to the patient, in order to access their agenda and reveal how they are really feeling about their problem.

Body language can be very revealing and you must attend to this. Notice eye contact, nervous movements, defiant postures. Note these during the consultation but also, and very importantly, during the psychosexual examination.

The examination is a very important part of the psychosexual assessment, not touched on in this chapter, and can provide a rich source of information that allows us to reveal the inner feelings of an individual.

But the listening does not end there. In working with psychosexual problems, you have to listen to your own emotions too. What feelings are being engendered in you as you consult with a patient? Attending to this will give further clues into the patient's condition and add to the wealth of information that is revealed not by talking but by listening.

To truly listen we have to be comfortable with silence; often, allowing patients to talk and truly express themselves will provide the richest material to help form a realistic and true impression of their sexual problem and the impact it is having on their internal and external world, as well as the subconscious processes that are at work to cause or exacerbate the problem. Reflecting this world back to the patient can bring therapeutic understanding and recovery.

Legal Considerations and Safeguarding

As a psychosexual practitioner it is essential to be aware of the legal framework in which you work. Earlier in the chapter the importance of confidentiality was stressed; however, there are times when the law dictates that confidentiality cannot be maintained.

The great skill of the psychosexual practitioner is to open up the patient and to try to understand their world. In doing so, elements of their life may be revealed that make you concerned about their safety or the safety of others, partners or children, that are not in the consultation room, for example, evidence of abuse or domestic violence.

It is essential to be familiar with the safeguarding policies in the institutions in which you work – to know when confidentiality has to be broken to protect others and be able to share this with the patient when necessary.

Conclusion

Sex and intimacy are important parts of life. Problems in this area are common. Despite the potential impact of these difficulties on an individual's mental health and well-being, patients often do not proactively talk about their experiences with their healthcare providers. In addition, discussions are not routinely initiated within the healthcare setting.

Healthcare practitioners need to feel comfortable about raising these issues with their patients and do all they can to facilitate these discussions. Many sexual problems can be improved greatly simply by reducing the anxiety associated with keeping a sexual issue hidden.

In the practise of psychosexual medicine, you need to feel comfortable opening a discussion and then listening to all the individual or couple brings into the consultation room, from what they say to how they feel. A joint understanding of the multiple biopsychosocial elements that underlie sexual problems can be very therapeutic.

REFERENCES

1. Mercer CH, Tanton C, Prah P et al. Changes in sexual attitudes and lifestyles in Britain through the life course and over time: Findings from the National Surveys of Sexual Attitudes and Lifestyles (Natsal). *The Lancet* 2013;382(9907):1781–1794.
2. Flynn KE, Reese JB, Jeffery DD et al. Patient experiences with communication about sex during and after treatment for cancer. *Psychooncology* 2012;21(6):594–601.
3. Laumann EO, Paik A, Glasser DB et al. A cross-national study of subjective sexual well-being among older women and men: Findings from the Global Study of Sexual Attitudes and Behaviors. *Arch Sex Behav* 2006;35(2):145–161.
4. Hordern AJ, Street AF. Communicating about patient sexuality and intimacy after cancer: Mismatched expectations and unmet needs. *Med J Aust* 2007;186:224–227.
5. Stead ML, Brown JM, Fallowfield L et al. Lack of communication between healthcare professionals and women with ovarian cancer about sexual issues. *Br J Cancer* 2003;88:666–671.
6. Alexander SC, Fortenberry JD, Pollak KI et al. Sexuality talk during adolescent health maintenance visits. *JAMA Pediatr* 2014;168(2):163–169.
7. Sobecki JN, Curin FA, Rasinski KA et al. What we don't talk about when we don't talk about sex: Results of a National Survey of U.S. obstetrician/gynecologists. *J Sex Med* 2012;9(5):1285–1294.
8. Lindau ST, Gavrilova N, Anderson D. Sexual morbidity in very long term survivors of vaginal and cervical cancer: A comparison to national norms. *Gynecol Oncol* 2007;106:413–418.
9. Schein M, Zyzanski SJ, Levine S et al. The frequency of sexual problems among family practice patients. *Fam Prac Res J* 1988;7(3):122–134.
10. Meystre-Agustoni G, Jeannin A, de Heller K et al. Talking about sexuality with the physician: Are patients receiving what they wish? *Swiss Med Wkly* 2011;141:w13178.
11. Jashim MJ. Patient-centred communication: Basic skills. *Am Fam Physician* 2017;95(1):29–34.
12. Stewart M, Roter D. *Communicating with Medical Patients*. Thousand Oaks, CA: Sage, 1989.
13. Hatzichristou D, Kirana PS, Banner L et al. Diagnosing sexual dysfunction in men and women: Sexual history taking and role of symptoms scales and questionnaires. *J Sex Med* 2016;13:1166–1182.
14. Avasthi A, Grover S, Sathyanarayana Rao TS. Clinical practice guidelines for management of sexual dysfunction. *Indian J Psychiatry* 2017;59(Suppl. 1):S91–S115.

5

Physical Aspects of the Sex Response

Ian K. Walsh

Introduction

The physical aspects underlying the sexual response are complex, but largely represent neurological, vascular and hormonal phenomena, all of which are largely under the control of higher centres in the brain and spinal cord. Many of the physical manifestations are common to both sexes, but important differences are discussed in this chapter.

Control Mechanisms

There are various physiological and homeostatic mechanisms influencing and governing the physical aspects of the sexual response, ranging from arousal to orgasm and beyond. It can be seen from Figure 5.1 that there is a wide and complex array of influences from a variety of inputs, including those from vascular, hormonal, neuronal sources and higher centres. The extent and pattern of influence vary between sexes, as well as among and within individuals in any set of given circumstances.

Facilitatory (+) influences are provided via all nerves except sympathetic nerves, which have an inhibitory (−) influence. Higher centres, hormones and neurotransmitters may have either facilitatory or inhibitory influences.

Neurovascular Anatomy

Motor Nerves

The prime neurological mover in the sexual response is the parasympathetic nervous system, actuated by pelvic splanchnic nerves derived from the anterior rami of the second to fourth sacral nerves (Figure 5.2). They enter the inferior hypogastric part of the prevertebral plexus, passing through the deep perineal pouch and perineal membrane to reach the erectile tissues (nervi eregenti). Stimulation of these nerves effects vasodilatation of the relevant arteries.

Sensory Nerves

From the sensory aspect, the dorsal nerve of the penis or clitoris (from the second sacral spinal segment) is the primary innervator (1). Dorsal nerve branches enter the glans penis or clitoris ventrolaterally, providing a rich sensory innervation, and additionally supply the frenulum in males, the latter structure receiving additional innervation from the perineal nerve (2) (Figure 5.3).

The anterior third of the scrotum and labia majora are innervated by the ilioinguinal and genital branch of the genitofemoral nerves (both from the L1 spinal segment), while the posterior two-thirds are innervated laterally by the perineal branch of the posterior femoral cutaneous nerve (from S2) and medially by scrotal and labial branches of the pudendal nerve (perineal nerve, S3).

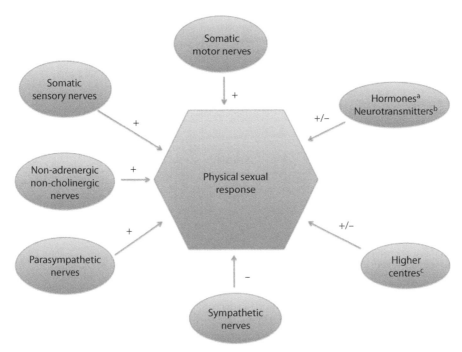

^a For example, testosterone, dihydrotestosterone, oestrogen, prolactin, vasoactive
  intestinal polypeptide, dopamine, oxytocin.

^b For example, nitric oxide, prostaglandins, cyclic guanosine monophosphate,
  calcitonin gene-related peptide.

^c For example, hypothalamus, mesolimbic pathway, prefrontal cortex, hippocampus.

FIGURE 5.1 Control mechanisms involved in physical sexual response.

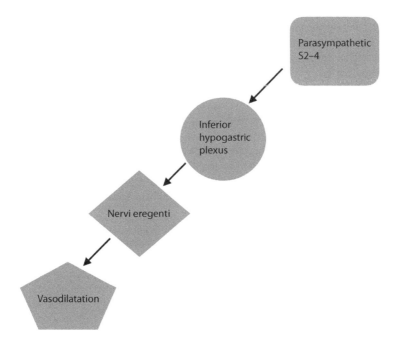

FIGURE 5.2 Motor nerves involved in the sexual response.

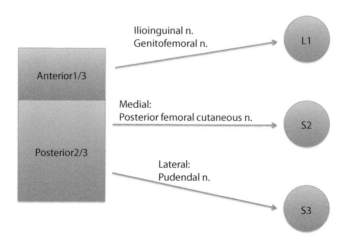

FIGURE 5.3   Sensory nerves of labia and scrotum.

Arterial Supply

The arterial blood supply of the penis and clitoris is derived from the internal iliac artery via the internal pudendal artery. Branches specifically related to sexual function include the perineal artery (giving rise to the transverse perineal and posterior scrotal/labial arteries), the artery of the bulb of the penis/vestibule, the urethral artery and both deep and dorsal arteries of the penis/clitoris.

The superficial and deep external pudendal arteries originate from the femoral artery in the thigh and supply the skin of the penis, clitoris, scrotum and labia majora.

Venous Drainage

Perineal veins generally accompany the corresponding arteries to connect via the internal pudendal veins, draining to the internal iliac vein. The deep dorsal vein of the penis/clitoris drains mainly the glans and corpora cavernosae, and travels along the midline, below the inferior pubic ramus to connect with a venous plexus surrounding the prostate in males and bladder in females.

External pudendal veins drain the anterior parts of the scrotum and labia majora and connect with the femoral vein. Superficial dorsal veins of the penis and clitoris drain the corresponding skin and pass to the external pudendal veins.

The Sexual Response Cycle

The mainstay theory of the human sexual response cycle is the four-stage model (excitement/arousal, plateau, orgasm and resolution), as described by Masters and Johnson (3) (Figure 5.4).

More recently, a broader appreciation of the sexual response cycle has been described, incorporating psychological, emotional and cognitive aspects in a triphasic neurophysiological model of desire, excitement and orgasm (4).

The incentive-motivation model moves away from a physiological construct, taking into account social and environmental influences and stimuli acting on a sensitive sexual response system. This model further explains that sexual activity itself can influence the sexual response, particularly sexual desire (5).

Specifically in relation to female sexual response, it appears that closeness and attachment may significantly augment and enhance sexual response in a circular, reinforcing manner (6).

However, some authors have reported conflicting evidence, describing female sexual response as being more aligned with the linear model typically applied to males (7).

Recent research, reinforced by brain imaging techniques, has emphasised the circular model and expanded on the influence of psychological, biological and sociocultural factors within a complex

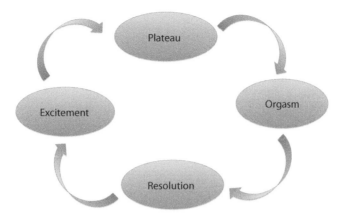

FIGURE 5.4   The four-stage model of physiological responses to sexual stimulation. (From Masters and Johnson. *Human sexual response*. New York, NY: Bantam, 1981 [1st ed., 1966]. With permission.)

network of components (8,9). This network encompasses cognitive, emotional, neuronal and motivational components, all of which should be taken into consideration during evaluation and treatment (10).

Erogenous Zones

Derived from the Greek *eros* 'love' and English *genous* 'producing', these zones are defined as body surface areas with heightened sensitivity which, when stimulated, may create a sexual response. Erogenous zones are classified as being either specific or non-specific and sensitivity depends upon the concentration of nerve endings at a given site.

Non-specific zones include areas with a high density of sensory nerves and/or hair fibres, such as the ears, neck, inner arms, mid-arm bend, thoracic sides and soles of the feet.

Specific zones associated with the sexual response include the genitals, as well as non-genital sites such as the lips, nipples and anus. A common feature of the areas such as the latter is their representation as mucocutaneous junctions, where nerve endings are closer to the surface than hair-bearing areas.

Arousal/Excitement

Sexual arousal can result from a variety of sensory stimuli, including tactile, visual and olfactory sources. Sufficient stimulation may lead to the aroused individual seeking further sexual arousal by direct stimulation of erogenous areas, such as breasts, nipples, genital or anal areas. The time for an individual to reach a fully aroused state depends on a variety of factors, including setting and circumstance. While the time to reach full arousal is very much individualistic, the average is 10 minutes and this appears to apply to both sexes (11).

Various genital and extragenital manifestations of the sexual response are exhibited by both sexes. The extent and some of the associated features are listed in Table 5.1.

In females, arousal is additionally evidenced in the genitalia by widening of the vagina, represented by expansion of its inner two-thirds, together with elevation of the cervix and uterus. With reduced libido or desire, women may report deep dyspareunia and lower abdominal pain, which can be accounted for by the cervix and uterus not elevating during penile thrusting. Increased blood flow to the labial and clitoral skin may be exhibited by a darkened colouration in these areas.

In males, accompanying genital manifestations of arousal include thickening and contraction of the dartos muscle of the scrotum, which results in elevation of the testes, as previously listed. There may be an accompanying emission of pre-ejaculatory fluid, also known as pre-seminal or Cowper's fluid (12). This is a clear, semi-viscous alkaline fluid produced mainly by the bulbourethral (Cowper's) glands and mucus-secreting (Littre's) urethral glands. The volume of emitted pre-ejaculatory fluid ranges from 0

TABLE 5.1

Genital and Extragenital Manifestations of Arousal/Excitement

Manifestation	Extent and Resultant Effects	
	Female	**Male**
Nipple erection	++	+
Corporal (cavernosum) tumescence	++	++
Lubrication	+++	0/+ (pre-ejaculatory fluid; see following)
Elevation (cervix, uterus, testes)	+	+
Pupillary dilation	++	++
Tachycardia	++	++
Blood pressure rise	+	+
Tachypnoea	+	+
Increased genital blood flow	Engorgement of labia and clitoris, and congestion of vaginal walls	Swelling of testes (increase in testicular size by 50%), engorgement of glans penis, prominence of penile veins
Flushing of chest/upper body	+/++	0/+
Tremor	0/++	0/+
Amygdala-hypothalamus activity	+	++

to 5 mL (13). This fluid assists lubrication and neutralises any acidic urine in the urethral lumen, which would otherwise be hostile to sperm in the subsequently definitive ejaculate. It should be noted that the fluid may contain viable spermatozoa, which may have contraceptive ramifications.

Extragenital manifestations are both features of, and contributors to, the arousal response. Nipple stimulation and/or erection either instigates or augments the arousal response in over 80% of females and over 50% of males (14). Approximately 50%–75% of females and 25% of males exhibit skin flushing of the chest or upper body. In females, such flushing typically begins below the breasts and may spread to the entire body, while male sexual flushing most often begins in the upper abdominal or lower chest region, spreading upwards (15). Flushing usually resolves soon after orgasm, but may persist for a matter of hours afterwards.

Lubrication

Although most lubrication during heterosexual intercourse is provided by female secretions, the male also contributes to a lesser extent by producing mucus from urethral and bulbourethral glands under parasympathetic stimulation.

Vaginal lubrication increases during ovulation and sexual arousal. The lubrication fluid consists mainly of transudate of plasma from engorged vaginal mucosa, augmented by mucus produced by the Bartholin's glands and supplemented at ovulation by cervical mucus. The fluid is typically a slightly acidic complex of water, hydrocarbons, glycols, ketones, acetic and lactic acids. Consistency, colour and odour of this fluid vary with sexual arousal and phase of the menstrual cycle, and may be further affected by diet, drugs and infection. The acidity of female lubrication fluid (typically pH 4–4.5) complements the alkalinity of the male ejaculate (pH 7–8) to produce a neutral combination which is non-hostile to spermatozoa (16).

Erection

Sexual arousal usually produces an erectile response in both sexes. While the presence and sensory experience of an erection can itself contribute to the arousal process, the primary purpose in males is to facilitate penetration.

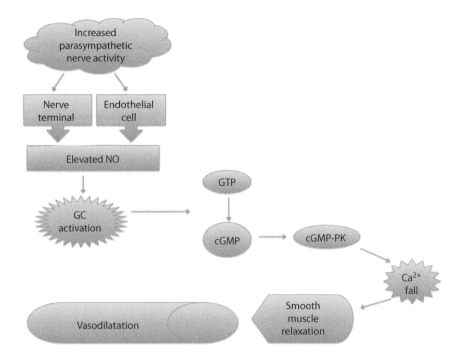

FIGURE 5.5 Neurovascular cascade underlying penile or clitoral erection.

Erection is primarily a neurovascular cascade phenomenon, with an underlying mechanism of smooth muscle relaxation in the corpus cavernosae of the penis or clitoris (see Figure 5.5). Sexual stimulation results in an increase in pelvic parasympathetic activity, with a resultant release of neurotransmitters (primarily nitric oxide [NO]) from cavernous nerve terminals and endothelial cells. The increased NO levels increase the conversion of guanosine triphosphate (GTP) to cyclic guanosine monophosphate (cGMP) via activation of a soluble enzyme (guanyl cyclase [GC]), with a resultant block in calcium channels via activation of a cGMP-dependent protein kinase. It is the subsequent fall in intracellular calcium levels within cavernosal smooth muscle cells which accounts for the smooth muscular relaxation allowing increased inflow of blood to cavernosal arteries and arterioles.

This inflow results in tumescence, primarily as a vascular expansile process of the corpora cavernosae. Tumescence is further enhanced by expansion of cavernosal sinusoids, which results in compression of the outlying venous complexes and plexi, preventing outflow of blood and effectively obliterating venous capacity during the active erectile period.

The male erection is described in further detail in the following section.

Male Erection

Traditionally, three types of male erection are recognised, although these are not mutually exclusive entities; a significant degree of overlap is evident in most erectile activity.

Reflexogenic

This is induced by direct genital stimulation, sensory signalling being carried in the pudendal and sacral parasympathetic nerves. Such erectile activity may, therefore, be preserved to some or all degrees following high (cervical or upper thoracic) levels of spinal cord injury.

Psychogenic

This results from more peripheral sensory stimulation of typically non-sexual sensory organs and includes visual, auditory and cognitive input. The motor pathway from cerebral activation is via thoracolumbar and sacral autonomic centres to lower cavernous nerves. It is for this reason that patients with low (sacral) spinal cord lesions typically have profound erectile dysfunction.

Subconscious

Also often referred to as *nocturnal*, this erectile activity usually occurs during rapid eye movement sleep. Such erections may serve to increase tissue oxygenation to the corpora cavernosae, putatively preventing corporal fibrosis, which underlies much organic erectile dysfunction (17).

Subconscious erections may also occur as the result of stimulation of sacral nerves by a full bladder; conversely, bladder overactivity is also associated with erectile dysfunction (18).

This type of erection is often still active in patients with erectile dysfunction from psychogenic or hormonal causes (e.g. androgen-reducing treatment for benign and malignant prostatic disease, pituitary tumours).

There are six recognised phases of the male erectile process (Figure 5.6):

1. *Flaccid*: The baseline, inactive, resting state. The penile blood content is largely venous in character.
2. *Latent (filling)*: This phase is evident in the early stages of arousal or pre-arousal. Some increased flow is evident in the pudendal artery. Some penile lengthening occurs.
3. *Tumescent*: With increasing stimulus and arousal, the penis expands, elongates and may pulsate.
4. *Full erection*: The penile blood content is now largely arterial in character, with intracavernosal pressure approaching systolic blood pressure.
5. *Skeletal or rigid*: This phase occurs during orgasm and ejaculation and is of short duration. The ischiocavernosus muscle contracts and intracavernous pressure may exceed systolic blood pressure.
6. *Detumescent*: This final phase occurs shortly after ejaculation, or more slowly following removal or cessation of erotic stimuli. Sympathetic nerve activity causes the contraction of smooth muscle surrounding the cavernosal sinusoids and arterioles. This phase ends with the return to the flaccid phase.

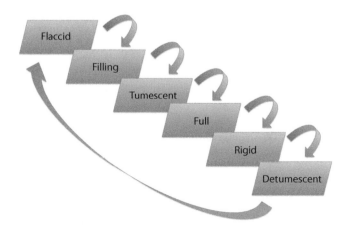

FIGURE 5.6   Phases of the male erection.

Emission and Ejaculation

Emission is the forerunner of ejaculation and is primarily mediated by the sympathetic nervous system, with outflow from twelfth thoracic to second lumbar spinal cord segments via the hypogastric and pelvic parasympathetic plexi. Contraction of the vas deferens and ampulla expels sperm into the urethra via the ejaculatory ducts. This accounts for 10% of ejaculate volume. Seminal vesical contraction expels a further 60% via these shared ejaculatory ducts, while the prostate contributes 30% via prostatic sinuses on either side of the posterior urethral lumen ducts into the urethra. In the urethral lumen, further mixing occurs with previous secretions from bulbourethral and small periurethral glands. Closure of the internal urethral sphincter, with simultaneous relaxation and opening of the external sphincter, facilitates direction of semen into the bulbar urethra.

Male Ejaculation

Male ejaculation is instigated by stretching of the posterior urethra by this emitted volume of semen, which elicits sensory nerve excitation, in turn causing reflex contraction of the ischiocavernosus and bulbocavernosus muscles, innervated by the pudendal nerve (from S2–S4). This causes rhythmic, wavelike, propulsive contractions of corporal and ductal structures, forcing semen through and from the urethra. Such expulsion is augmented by contraction of skeletal muscle of the pelvic floor, trunk and abdomen.

The ejaculate is expelled from the urethra at velocity circa 10 miles per hour (19). A typical ejaculation consists of five to ten contractions and once the first contraction has occurred, the subsequent ones follow automatically until ejaculatory completion. The first and second boluses of ejaculation are typically the largest and can account for almost half of the total ejaculatory volume of between 0.1 and 10 mL (20,21). A greater volume of ejaculate may result from either prolonged abstinence from previous ejaculation or from a longer duration of stimulus leading up to ejaculation (22). Some authors have reported a positive correlation between the volume of ejaculate and ejaculatory pleasure, while others have described an association between strength of ejaculation and heightened pleasure (23). Post-ejaculation contractions may also be experienced in some males (24).

In healthy males, ejaculation is associated with several non-genital phenomena, often considered components of the male orgasm. Such activity includes rhythmic anal sphincteric contraction, together with elevations of heart rate, ventilatory rate and blood pressure. There is debate as to whether genital and non-genital manifestations of ejaculation are all part of the complex of male orgasm, or if the latter is a distinct entity. The latter model is supported by the fact that some men can achieve multiple orgasms, yet fail to ejaculate and also that ejaculation can also occur in the absence of the full orgasmic experience (25). Orgasm per se is closely associated with the release of the neuropeptides oxytocin and prolactin from the anterior pituitary; these play an important role in regulating the acute sexual drive following orgasm in males (26).

Female Ejaculation

There are two distinct phenomena currently described as female ejaculation, one of which is 'true' female ejaculation, as distinct from the more dramatic 'female ejaculation' frequently exhibited in pornographic imagery (27).

First, the purported 'ejaculation' may, in fact, represent urinary incontinence. Such urinary loss during female orgasm may represent a variant of stress, urge or mixed urinary incontinence, or may be a specifically orgasmic phenomenon. In any event, the urinary loss can be dramatic and copious. This may be related to pre-existent lower urinary tract dysfunction, especially stress urinary incontinence. Treatment of the underlying urological issues may more significantly impact positively on quality of life on the basis of improved sexual function than would be anticipated by resolution of urinary symptoms per se (28).

'True' female ejaculation is associated with the expulsion of a small volume of whitish, viscous fluid (29,30). This fluid is thought to be produced by female urethral and/or paraurethral glands (collectively and confusingly described by some authors as 'the female prostate'), and it has been reported that the production of such fluid positively contributes to the female erotic experience (31).

Detumescence and Male Refractory Period

Penile detumescence begins almost immediately following ejaculation and is typically complete within 1–2 minutes. Detumescence usually occurs in two stages: In the first stage, the penis reduces to approximately 50% of its flaccid size, and the second stage entails penile size returning to flaccid dimensions.

Detumescence is followed by a refractory period, during which the penis remains poorly or totally unresponsive to erectogenic stimuli. This period can last from as short as a few minutes in younger males to as long as days for older males, with the average refractory period being 30 minutes. The refractory period is often accompanied by a reduction or absence of sexual desire and can also be accompanied by penile hypersensitivity, whereby further sexual stimulation may be painful (32).

The detumescent period is closely related to the release of pituitary oxytocin and prolactin during ejaculation, which inhibits dopamine, with dopamine being responsible for sexual arousal (33).

Female Orgasm

Most female orgasms result from clitoral stimulation. The distal urethra and adjacent vagina are of shared embryonic origin and, from a sexual sensory viewpoint, form a functional unit with the clitoris as the main contributor (34).

The glans clitoris has a similar density of sensory nerve endings as the glans penis, which accounts for how 70%–80% of women reach orgasm by clitoral stimulation alone. The clitoris may also be stimulated indirectly by vaginal penetration and orgasm achieved in this way. Orgasm may also be reached by stimulation of the distal vaginal roof and periurethral areas of the anterior vaginal wall, as these areas are also richly innervated, although to a lesser extent than the clitoris (35). It has been argued that the sensitivity of these areas is a result of underlying clitoral structures, rather than sensory nerve density (34).

As in males, female orgasm is under autonomic nervous system control. Similarly, the female orgasm is also associated with non-genital phenomena, such as tachycardia, tachypnea, increased depth of respiration and blood pressure elevation. Compared with males, however, the female orgasm is typically more difficult to achieve and has stronger associations with cognition and higher-level cerebral functions, together with psychosocial factors, including emotional bonding and attachment (36).

During female orgasm, the experience of intense pleasure, sometimes with an altered state of consciousness, is accompanied by involuntary rhythmic contractions of pelvic striated musculature encircling the vagina, often associated with uterine and anal smooth muscle contractions (37). The release of pituitary neuropeptides oxytocin and prolactin may contribute to such smooth muscle contraction, and oxytocin is also associated with the sense of well-being, satiety and sense of emotional bonding associated with the post-orgasmic state (38).

Female Refractory Period

In females, the post-orgasm penile hypersensitivity experienced by many males may be represented by the experience of similar clitoral hypersensitivity, which may prevent further orgasm by virtue of pain, rather than representing a prolonged refractory period per se (39).

Beyond this, the female orgasm can be multiple and repeated. In addition to the generally accepted understanding that women do not experience a true refractory period, there is some evidence to suggest that sequential and subsequent orgasms may increase in intensity with the accrual of continuing stimulation (32,39).

Summary

The physical aspects of the sexual response represent both cause and effect, with a wide variety of complex interactions between key anatomical and physiological elements. The central components of physical sexual responses are neurological and vascular, with additional contributions and influences from muscular and hormonal domains. Many of the responses are similar in both sexes, but the sexual response cycle differs between males and females, as typified by differences exhibited in realms such as recovery following orgasm.

Knowledge of the mechanisms underlying sexual response should assist in understanding some of the genesis of sexual dysfunction. The holistic practitioner should always remain mindful of the fact that all such physical responses are ultimately and continuously governed by the ultimate influence of higher centres, a subject beyond the remit of this chapter, but covered in greater detail in subsequent chapters.

REFERENCES

1. Long RM, McCartan D, Cullen I et al. A preliminary study of the sensory distribution of the penile dorsal and ventral nerves: Implications for effective penile block for circumcision. *BJU Int* 2010;105(11):1576–1578.
2. Yang CC, Bradley WE. Innervation of the human glans penis. *J Urol* 1999;161(1):97–102.
3. Masters and Johnson. *Human Sexual Response*. New York, NY: Bantam, 1981 (1st ed., 1966).
4. Kaplan HS. *Disorders of Sexual Desire*. New York, NY: Brunner/Mazel, 1979.
5. Laan E, Both S. What makes women experience desire? *Fem Psychol* 2008;18(4):505–514.
6. Basson R. Using a different model for female sexual response to address women's problematic low sexual desire. *J Sex Marital Ther* 2001;27:395–403.
7. Giles KR, McCabe MP. Conceptualizing women's sexual function: Linear vs. circular models of sexual response. *J Sex Med* 2009;6:2761–2771.
8. Basson R. Human sexual response. *Handb Clin Neurol* 2015;130:11–18.
9. Brotto L, Atallah S, Johnson-Agbakwu C et al. Psychological and interpersonal dimensions of sexual function and dysfunction. *J Sex Med* 2016;13(4):538–571.
10. Kingsberg SA, Althof S, Simon JA et al. Female sexual dysfunction–medical and psychological treatments, committee 14. *J Sex Med* 2017;14:1463–1491.
11. Rellini AH, McCall KM, Randall PK et al. The relationship between women's subjective and physiological sexual arousal. *Psychophysiology* 2005;42(1):116–124.
12. Chudnovsky A, Niederberger CS. Copious pre-ejaculation: Small glands-major headaches. *Int J Androl* 2007;28(3):374–375.
13. Zukerman Z, Weiss DB, Orvieto R. Does pre-ejaculatory penile secretion originating from Cowper's gland contain sperm? *J Assist Reprod Genet* 2003;20(4):157–159.
14. Levin R, Meston C. Nipple/breast stimulation and sexual arousal in young men and women. *J Sex Med* 2006;3:450–454.
15. Archer A, Lloyd B. *Sex and Gender*. Cambridge University Press, 2002, 85–88.
16. World Health Organization. *Laboratory Manual for the Examination of Human Semen and Sperm-Cervical Mucus Interaction* (3rd ed.). Cambridge, UK: Cambridge University Press, 1992.
17. Montorsi F, Oettel M. Testosterone and sleep-related erections: An overview. *J Sex Med* 2005;2(6):771–784.
18. Irwin DE, Milsom I, Reilly K et al. Overactive bladder is associated with erectile dysfunction and reduced sexual quality of life in men. *J Sex Med* 2008;5(12):2904–2910.
19. Marieb E. *Anatomy and Physiology*. Boston, MA: Benjamin-Cummings, 2013.
20. Rehan N, Sobrero AJ, Fertig JW. The semen of fertile men: Statistical analysis of 1300 men. *Fertil Steril* 1975;26(6):492–502.
21. Gerstenburg TC, Levin RJ, Wagner G. Erection and ejaculation in man. Assessment of the electromyographic activity of the bulbocavernosus and ischiocavernosus muscles. *Br J Urol* 1990;65(4):395–402.
22. Pound N, Javed MH, Ruberto C et al. Duration of sexual arousal predicts semen parameters for masturbatory ejaculates. *Physiol Behav* 2002;76(4–5):685–689.
23. Rosenberg, MT, Hazzard MA, Tallamn CT et al. Is the amount of physical pleasure with ejaculation related to volume or strength and force of ejaculation? *J Sex Med* 2006;3:14–69.
24. Bohlen JG, Held JP, Sanderson MO. The male orgasm: Pelvic contractions measured by anal probe. *Arch Sex Behav* 1980;9:503.
25. Wibowo E, Wassersug RJ. Multiple orgasms in men – What we know so far. *Sex Med Rev* 2016;4(2):136–148.

26. Kruger THC, Haake P, Chereath D et al. Specificity of the neuroendocrine response to orgasm during sexual arousal in men. *Eur J Endocrinol* 2003;177:57–64.

27. Pastor Z. Female ejaculation orgasm vs. coital incontinence: A systematic review. *J Sex Med* 2013;10(7):1682–1691.

28. Walsh IK, Donnellan SM, Stone AR. The effect of pubovaginal sling surgery on female sexual function. *J Urol* 2000;163(4):74.

29. Moalem S, Reidenberg JS. Does female ejaculation serve an antimicrobial purpose? *Med Hypotheses* 2009;73(6):1069–1071.

30. Rubio-Casillas A, Jannini EA. New insights from one case of female ejaculation. *J Sex Med* 2011;8(12):3500–3564.

31. Sevely JL, Bennet JW. Concerning female ejaculation and the female prostate. *J Sex Res* 2010;14(1):1978.

32. Rosenthal M. *Human Sexuality: From Cells to Society.* Boston, MA: Cengage Learning, 2012, 134–135.

33. Haake P, Exton, MS, Haverkamp J et al. Absence of orgasm-induced prolactin secretion in a healthy multi-orgasmic male subject. *Int J Impot Res* 2002;14(2):133–135.

34. O'Connell HE, Sanjeevan KV, Hutson JM. Anatomy of the clitoris. *J Urol* 2005;174(4):1189–1195.

35. Kilchevsky A, Vardi Y, Lowenstein L et al. Is the female G-spot truly a distinct anatomic entity? *J Sex Med* 2012;9(3):719–726.

36. Wallen K, Lloyd EA. Female sexual arousal: Genital anatomy and orgasm in intercourse. *Horm Behav* 2011;59(5):780–792.

37. Mestin CM, Levin RJ, Sipski ML et al. Women's orgasm. *Annu Rev Sex Res* 2004;15:173–257.

38. Georgiadis JR, Kringelbach ML. The human sexual response cycle: Brain imaging evidence linking sex to other pleasures. *Prog Neurobiol* 2012;98:49–81.

39. Rathus SA, Nevid A, Jeffrey S et al. *Human Sexuality in a World of Diversity* (2nd ed.). Boston, MA: Allyn and Bacon, 1995.

6

Psychological Background to Psychosexual Medicine

Caroline Hunter

Introduction

In Chapter 5, we heard about the physiology of the human sexual response. Clearly, sex is not just about physiology (or anatomy), but psychology also plays a part. In other words, our sexual response is as much to do with our thoughts and feelings as our physical sensations. It might even be argued that one can hardly envisage one without the other. We could ask the question 'Can a purely physical sexual response take place without any accompanying emotional or cognitive input?'

When I was a medical student, the following happened:

> My group of students was sent along to a gynaecology operating theatre, the main purpose being for us to practise vaginal examinations on anaesthetised patients. The woman was having a minor procedure. I've no idea what for; this was no concern of ours. I queued up, scrubbed and gloved hands held in front of me, ready to take my turn. The girl before me carried out a rather vigorous bimanual examination. The patient began to twitch and convulse. 'Oohoo she enjoyed that', said the consultant. This was the point when I realised she was having an orgasm, asleep and at the hands of a medical student she didn't know existed. I was fascinated and appalled in equal measure. I blushed scarlet under my surgical mask, hoping the nonchalant boys waiting their turn wouldn't notice. (I should say that this was many years ago, and a similar scenario would be very unlikely to occur today. I would like to think we treat our patients with more respect.)

Perhaps this is the closest we can get to the idea of a purely physiological response. But even then, I have sometimes wondered: Did she experience pleasure at the time of the orgasm? Did she feel a release of sexual tension afterwards? If not, can we even refer to what went on as a sexual response?

I have frequently heard people use the expression 'It was just sex, it meant nothing, just scratching an itch' or words to that effect. Can this really be true? If so, why did they even need to point that out? The very act of making that statement implies that there might be more to sex than just the scratching of the itch. It would be hard to imagine a dog making that statement. 'It was just sex'. Of course it was. Although if the dog can talk, we might begin to imagine he might also experience sex in a more meaningful way.

In other words, it is almost impossible to think about the human sexual response without taking into account both physical and psychological aspects.

Institute of Psychosexual Medicine (IPM) practitioners attend to both, and it is our job to wonder what is going on in the minds and bodies of all our patients. Because physical investigations and treatments are more readily available within medical settings, IPM training focuses primarily on the psychology of our patients. In this chapter I outline different approaches to treatment of psychosexual dysfunction, including a brief summary of cognitive behavioural therapy (CBT). I then look in some detail at the principles underlying our own psychodynamic approach.

Different Approaches to Treatment

In order to have a clear understanding of psychosexual medicine, it would seem helpful also to understand what it is not. This is of benefit to clinicians and patients alike.

When teaching, I like to invite my audience to consider every human activity as having three different components: the physical, the thinking, and the emotional. I point out that as clinicians, we are very comfortable dealing with the body, examining, carrying out investigations and providing physical treatments. We are also quite good at managing the thinking, cognitive/behavioural side. We spend time explaining, giving information, getting consent and encouraging behavioural change which will improve the health of our patients. But my audience will generally agree that the emotional world of our patients is less well attended to. We may be sensitive doctors, nurses or physiotherapists, using our empathy to find the right words, tone of voice, or level of touch in an examination, but we do not usually take time to think about this and use it for the benefit of our patients. This empathic level, the attention to what it is like to be our patients, and to be with them, why they feel the way they do, and how to use this, is what psychodynamic psychotherapy is all about.

The physical approaches to the treatment of psychosexual dysfunction are not the concern of this chapter, but we do well to remember that medicine is not averse to using physical treatments to help sexual difficulties that are exclusively of psychological origin. If we refer our patients to hospital doctors, such as gynaecologists, urologists or dermatologists, the chances are that they will be offered pharmacological or surgical solutions. Or if we refer for physiotherapy they will receive exercises or massages to help release muscle tension. It is therefore essential that those working in psychosexual medicine have a basic knowledge of the physical treatments available, in order to provide information to their patients and ensure informed consent when considering referral.

Cognitive Behavioural Approaches

In the same way, it is my opinion that those using the IPM approach should have a basic understanding of CBT, which is a well-established and widely offered approach to the treatment of psychosexual dysfunction. It is my intention to give a brief outline of CBT as sex therapy, and to highlight the differences between the two approaches.

This is only a brief outline, and further information can be found on the College of Sexual and Relationship Therapists (COSRT) website (www.COSRT.org.uk).

The CBT/COSRT approach can be summarised as follows:

- It is problem orientated.
- The therapist takes an 'expert role'.
- Specific aims are established.
- 'Homework' is set.
- There is a strong preference for both partners to attend.

Therapy as described by a Relate psychosexual therapist (personal communication) takes the following form:

- I. Initial interview, 1 hour, couple
- II. History taking, 2 hours each, individually
- III. Formulation: Round-table couple
- IV. Treatment, chosen from the following:
  - Sensate focus, with intercourse ban
  - Self-focus
  - Relaxation exercises
  - Other exercises, such as fantasy training, erotic exposure, communication training, cognitive restructuring

Sensate Focus

A summary of sensate focus is as follows:

- Patient develops heightened awareness of sensations rather than focussing on performance
- Immediately achievable goals set – to 'enjoy touching' rather than to 'achieve penetration'
- Explicit instructions given 'non-genital pleasuring', 'genital pleasuring', 'containment without thrusting'

Ground rules are as follows:

- Choose a time and place acceptable for both of you, where you will not be disturbed.
- Make the surroundings as pleasant as possible, choosing music, lighting and aromas to suit you.
- Turn off the phone and, if necessary, lock the door.
- Take turns giving and receiving touch, allowing equal time for each of you.
- When it is your turn to touch, take plenty of time to explore the other person's body. Experiment with different sensations and types of touch. Take pleasure in experiencing the texture, form and temperature of the other person's body.
- When it is your turn to be touched, make sure you let the other person know what you like and what you do not like.
- The goal is enjoyment and pleasure. Enjoy the journey rather aiming towards any specific destination.
- Take as long as you want over each phase. Often, the slower you take it, the more you will get out of it.
- Only move from one stage to the next when both partners agree.

A minimum number of sessions is required and is usually agreed upon at the start of therapy. Underlying the couples' work is an attention to the relationship as reported by the clients and as witnessed in the room by the therapist. I have heard it said that in this work the 'couple' is the client – in other words, what is created between them is studied, rather than the psychology of each individual.

The IPM approach is different in many ways, as summarised in Table 6.1.

IPM practitioners may also sometimes use cognitive behavioural approaches. For example, it is not unusual to suggest that a woman practises self-examination at home. This could be viewed as 'homework'. Likewise, many COSRT therapists have experience of psychodynamic approaches, and will use these as part of their work with couples.

TABLE 6.1

Stages in Different Professional Approaches

	Relate/COSRT	**IPM**
Specialist referral	Always	Clinicians use skills within own practice in addition to specialist clinics
Couples	Strong preference for couples to attend	Based on individual psychotherapy and partner not encouraged to attend (or actively discouraged from attending)
Homework set in the form of exercises	An essential component of the therapy	No, the work takes place in the room between clinician and patient
Genital examination	No, most therapists are not clinicians and it is not a part of the process	One of the main tools of IPM work; clinicians are expected to be able to perform genital examinations and consider it in every case

Psychodynamic Psychotherapy

The IPM approach to the treatment of psychosexual dysfunction is the main theme of this book and is discussed and explained in many ways by many different authors. It is my intention here to provide some of the theoretical psychological background to the way we work.

The IPM prospectus states the IPM 'offers a type of brief therapy, based on psychoanalytic skills introduced by Drs Michael Balint and Tom Main and developed by Institute Members' (1).

I have picked out three psychoanalytic principles that I consider to be of particular importance in our work, and I look at each of them in turn.

Psychoanalytic principles are as follows:

- The unconscious
- Defence mechanisms
- Therapeutic relationship, transference and countertransference, and parallel process

The Unconscious

Unconscious processes are as follows:

- 'Referring to mental processes of which the subject is not aware' (2).
- 'Aspects of ourselves that so disturb us that they give rise to anxiety or psychic pain may be consciously rejected and become more or less unconscious' (3).

The above definitions make reference to things that are 'more or less unconscious' and 'of which the subject is not aware'. The idea of something that is completely unconscious can be difficult to comprehend, and probably of limited use in brief interpretive psychotherapy. Something that is 'more or less unconscious' however, is not completely forgotten, but is never or rarely thought about.

EXAMPLE 6.1

A patient who had a traumatic childbirth 5 years ago and has not been interested in sex ever since may be surprised that her doctor is inviting her to talk in detail about it. In doing so she may notice that she still remembers the experience as if it was yesterday, and begin to wonder if this and her loss of libido might be connected.

EXAMPLE 6.2

The young man with erectile dysfunction is asked by the nurse what makes him angry. He says nothing, he never gets angry. But when he talks about his ex-girlfriend who cheated on him the nurse points out that he sounds a bit angry. He begins to realise that his failure to get an erection in his current relationship may be related to this unexpressed anger at the betrayal by his ex.

In both of these cases there is a need to recover something that has been repressed in order to make sense of the present. This is not so much the actual memory of the events as of the emotions that were not fully experienced at the time.

The clinician who remembers that her patients have an 'unconscious', that they are not so much keeping things from others as from themselves, will be better equipped to help them remember what they have put away and forgotten, and thus begin to make sense of their physical symptoms.

Psychological Defence Mechanisms

- Tactics developed by the ego to protect against anxiety
- Thought to safeguard the mind against feelings and thoughts that are too difficult for the conscious mind to cope with
- In some instances, are thought to keep inappropriate or unwanted thoughts and impulses from entering the conscious mind

The concept of the defence mechanism is fairly easy to grasp. I think it is helpful to understand defences in terms of a patient's early development: Growing up, we learn ways to manage our emotions, particularly the ones we are encouraged to believe are unacceptable. These would tend to be those with negative associations such as anger, envy, jealousy, shame and embarrassment. But we should remind ourselves children may also be discouraged from showing some of the more joyful emotions: pleasure, excitement and humour.

A child faced with a strong feeling he or she does not know what to do with may cope in a number of ways:

- Ignore it (avoidance)
- Pretend it is not happening (denial)
- Blame someone else (projection)
- Behave in a babyish way (regression)
- Make excuses for it (rationalisation)
- Try and explain it in a grown-up way (intellectualisation)
- Go too far the other way (reaction formation)
- Stop feeling it (repression)
- Develop a physical symptom (somatisation)

These coping mechanisms are entirely appropriate as children, and I explain to my patients that this is what got them through difficult times. The problem starts in adulthood when they persist and are beyond our conscious control.

If we consider one of our common presentations, that of a woman with primary non-consummation, we might notice a number of possible defences in operation preventing her from getting help for her problem:

- *Avoidance*: She never thinks about it. Does not go near the doctor in case she tells her to get a smear. Does not visit her friend with the new baby.
- *Denial*: Says it does not bother her (with tears in her eyes).
- *Projection*: Blames the mother-in-law. It is all her fault, she is so nosy.
- *Regression*: Fills her bedroom with soft toys and has lots of cuddles with her husband.
- *Rationalisation*: She has just been too busy. Once the house is finished they will get around to having sex.
- *Intellectualisation*: Some people are born with vaginal openings that are small. She has read about it on the Internet.
- *Repression*: She has not had sex yet, and she feels she should, but it genuinely does not bother her.
- *Reaction formation*: She is the first to talk about sex with her friends and tell a dirty joke.
- *Somatisation*: Sex is too painful. In fact, her vagina has started to burn all the time. There must be a treatment that will take the pain away.

An awareness of the concept of psychological defences can help a clinician in the following ways:

- An understanding of defences can help make sense of what is going on in the consultation, and what is at the root of the patient's problem.

- An observation of defences can point to areas of difficulty: The more powerful the defence, the more painful the emotion it is protecting.
- Instead of trying to 'batter down' a defence we can 'pay tribute' to it: 'This seems very difficult to talk about'. 'That's a very painful story but I notice you are still smiling.'

Transference and Countertransference (the Doctor-Patient Relationship)

Transference

- 'The experiences of feelings, drives, attitudes, fantasies and defences towards a person in the present, which do not befit that person but are a repetition of reactions originating in regard to significant persons of early childhood, unconsciously displaced onto figures in the present' (4)

Countertransference

1. Therapist-derived:
   - 'The therapist contaminates the field with his own feelings from elsewhere' (3).
2. Patient-derived:
   - 'What the doctor feels is part of the patient's illness' (4).
   - 'The analyst must use his emotional response as a key to the patient's unconscious' (5).
   - 'The analyst's emotional response to his patient within the analytic situation represents one of the most important tools for his work' (6).

These concepts of transference and countertransference seem the most difficult for my students to grasp. However, I feel they are so fundamental to our work that it is worth taking the time to understand them.

Put simply, all of our adult interactions are to some extent influenced by the way we have been treated growing up.

This is particularly the case when we are in situations where we feel vulnerable and out of control:

- If we have had a positive experience of being parented we are likely to respond warmly to our doctor, teacher, or therapist.
- If we have been misunderstood we may feel misunderstood over and over again, and despair of anyone ever being able to understand us.
- If we had a competitive relationship with a sibling we may find ourselves competing with our partner.
- If we were not handled sensitively as babies we may find the physical intimacy of adult sexual relationships overwhelming.

Transference often results in two people describing the same encounter different ways:

Example: Susan and James

Susan, who had a difficult relationship with her mother, comes out of the Relate initial interview feeling small and stupid. She complains to James, 'That woman was looking down on us'. James, who lost his mother when he was a baby, looks surprised and slightly hurt, 'I thought she was lovely; I think she is the answer to all our problems'.

Our expectations of sex are to some degree shaped, often unconsciously, by our experiences of intimacy when we were younger:

Susan dreaded having sex with James from the moment they first became a couple. She was convinced he would find her repulsive and could not bear the thought of showing her body to him. The fact that her father was always telling her to lose weight and trying to stop her from eating had led her (unconsciously) to assume that all men would feel like that about her.

> James thought finding Susan was the most wonderful experience of his life. But when it came to sexual intimacy he found he became very anxious. The thought that Susan would leave him would come into his head at inconvenient moments and he would lose his erections. He had no memory of losing his mother, and would say, 'It didn't affect me, I was too young to know anything about it'.

There is a component to countertransference that comes from the therapist's own past. In this way it is simply her own 'transference' but occurring in a therapeutic relationship:

> When the therapist met Susan and James for the first time she felt very warm towards James. He reminded her of her much-loved younger brother, who even had the same name. She noticed this and put that thought on one side.

Some of what is felt in the therapeutic relationship has as much to do with the patient's internal world as that of the therapist. This is a more difficult concept, and has to be experienced and put into practice before it can be fully accepted:

> The therapist liked Susan as well, they seemed a lovely couple. But she found herself feeling inexplicably sad as she sat and listened to them. She wondered if underneath their cheerful exterior they were actually hiding a deep sadness, both from her, and maybe also from each other. She also noticed herself feeling a bit critical towards Susan. The thought came into her head, 'Poor man, he's lovely; it must be awful for him not to have sex'.
>
> Having some experience in psychodynamic therapy, she reflected on this after they had left the room. During the round-table discussion, she found a way to make use of both these feelings. She said to them, 'It must be very sad for you to be so fond of each other and not be able to have sex' and to Susan, 'It seems that you are expecting me to blame you. I wonder if maybe you are blaming yourself a lot'.

How does an understanding of transference and countertransference help in practice?
This is a question that I hear quite often from students of psychosexual medicine. My answer would be that while I very rarely use the actual words except when making formal presentations, having a name for what is going on helps me to organise my thoughts and remember to take it into consideration.

Here are some more examples where these concepts can be applied in clinical practice.

CASE 1: TRANSFERENCE – SARAH

Sarah attends her genitourinary medicine (GUM) clinic having made the appointment herself. She is very anxious about attending as she is going to tell someone about her sexual difficulty. When she arrives the receptionist cannot find her name on the list. Sarah feels panicky, but instead of showing this she becomes rude. The receptionist is polite at first but (understandably) loses her patience and snaps at her, 'I'm doing my best; the computer has been playing up'. This causes Sarah to panic even further, she thinks, 'Why does this always happen to me?' She starts to raise her voice. The receptionist finds her name and tells her through gritted teeth to sit down.

The nurse has heard the disturbance and asks the receptionist what is going on. The receptionist explains that Sarah was very rude to her. The nurse, who does not like the receptionist to be treated badly, feels very annoyed. When she calls Sarah in, she is a little abrupt and not her usual warm smiling self. Sarah's anxiety reaches new heights. She feels like crying but covers it up by being brief almost to the point of rudeness. The nurse has had enough of her. She has no idea what Sarah is actually looking for today. 'I'll see if the doctor can see you, but she is very busy.'

The doctor is indeed very busy, and has also heard a bit of the disturbance in the waiting room. She can tell from the nurse's face that Sarah has not made a good impression. She is tempted to say she can't see her, but reluctantly agrees. While the doctor is waiting for Sarah to come in, she takes a moment to think about some teaching she received the night before. She was reminded that we respond to our patients in different ways, and this can cause a spiral of negativity that stops them from getting the help they need. Maybe Sarah interprets helpful, or at least neutral, responses as hostile and rejecting, which results in her getting the very response she is expecting.

So, when Sarah comes into the room she puts on her usual welcoming smile. She says, 'I'm so sorry we are having trouble with our computer today. Coming to this clinic is difficult enough without having to go through that'. Sarah hesitates; for a moment she thinks the doctor is just being sarcastic, but she really doesn't seem to be. She bursts into tears. The whole story of the sexual difficulty pours out. The doctor groans inwardly but a part of her is delighted that her new understanding of transference has allowed Sarah to begin to get the help she needs.

CASE 2: COUNTERTRANSFERENCE – MICHAEL

Michael is suffering from erectile dysfunction. He has an appointment with the physiotherapist for some pelvic floor exercises, which his doctor feels might help. He feels fine about going, anything that helps; his partner Matthew is beginning to get impatient. The physiotherapist notices that Michael seems to be expressing no emotion at all. She wonders why this might be, since most men who come to see her with this problem are at least a little embarrassed and sometimes downright annoyed. As she is examining him she chats about his relationship. 'How long have you been together? Where did you meet him?' Michael chats back, tells the story of the romantic meeting, the first date, when they moved in together. The physiotherapist responds in the same tone, but finds herself feeling increasingly anxious. Michael says something seemingly innocuous about Matthew, that he is a clean freak. He even checks the cutlery after Michael has put it away in the drawer. Michael is laughing, but the physiotherapist finds herself feeling furious. She checks herself, what might be making her feel so strongly about this? Nothing in her own experience could account for the fury she is now feeling. She formulates the idea that perhaps Michael is repressing his anger and she is feeling it for him. This might even account in part for his sexual difficulty. She knows repressed anger can sometimes make intimacy very difficult. She waits until they have sat down, and says very gently, 'I can't help wondering if you might be a bit annoyed with Matthew'. Michael hesitates, he begins to deny it. The physiotherapist smiles at him. He stops mid-sentence. 'You know that's what Michael says. He's always telling me I repress my anger. Passive aggressive he calls me'. The physiotherapist says, 'That sounds a bit annoying. Nobody likes to be called that'.

This is the beginning of working with Michael to understand that his sexual difficulty might be attributed in part to his unacknowledged anger. The physiotherapist's understanding of countertransference, that some of what she is feeling may be coming from the patient's unconscious, has enabled her to make a very gentle interpretation which has allowed Michael to get effective help for his problem.

Parallel Process

- 'The supervisor's emotion is a reflection of something which has been going on in the therapist-patient relationship, and, in the final analysis, in the patient' (7).
- 'Parallel process re-enactments…are a rich source of information about the underlying dynamics which do not come across in the conscious and verbal descriptions and narratives' (8).

The term *parallel process* describes the way in which unacknowledged thoughts and feelings can be passed from one situation to another through the unconscious of those involved. This is an essential component of psychosexual medicine in practice; in fact, it is difficult to imagine how we would do our job if this did not occur.

'Coming from the Patient'

There is an expression much used in psychosexual medicine: An emotion, or even an idea, may be described as 'coming from the patient'.

When the clinician has been in direct contact with the patient we could call this 'therapist-derived countertransference'. In other words, something in the patient's unconscious has found its way into the therapist's conscious experience. But it can also happen at more removed levels, in which case the term *parallel process* comes into play.

CASE 3: PARALLEL PROCESS – LAURA

Laura has lost her libido. She is talking to the nurse about it, and the subject comes up of her mother who is living in her house. 'She cares so much. She wants to know everything about me. It's such a comfort to know she is in the next room'.

The nurse is not so sure. She thinks, 'That mother sounds very intrusive'. She tries to suggest this to Laura who gets angry and defensive.

When the nurse presents the case to her seminar group she forgets how she felt at the time, and describes the relationship between Laura and her mother exactly as Laura would have done. She is shocked and rather annoyed at their response: 'How awful! How can they have sex with that mother in the next room!' She insists that the mother is not a problem at all. A member of the group points out that their sex life was fine before the mother moved in. The nurse starts to make excuses. 'It was nothing to do with that. It was just a coincidence'. The atmosphere in the group becomes uncomfortable. The seminar leader invites the group to think about what might be happening. Someone says, 'Maybe this is coming from the patient'. The nurse smiles sheepishly. She remembers, 'Actually I said something similar to Laura about her mother and she became very cross'.

The next time the nurse meets Laura she holds this in mind. When Laura starts chattering on about her mother she tries a more reflective approach. 'It would be difficult for anyone having their Mummy in the next room. It must be particularly hard for you, since you have such a good relationship with her'. Laura looks suspicious for a moment then starts to cry, 'I feel so guilty. She's done so much for us. My husband is always complaining about her and we end up arguing. I just wish sometimes she would be a little less interested in everything we are doing'.

This parallel process re-enactment has given the group an opportunity to experience the unconscious operating in the here and now of the seminar. It has also helped the nurse to understand the dynamics of the consultation with her patient, and make a more appropriate intervention.

Parallel process (Figure 6.1) occurs at several levels in psychosexual medicine so that when the seminar leader brings the group to her own supervision, that of the leaders' workshop, it can still be in play.

The leader presents the case of Laura and her intrusive mother to the leaders' workshop. The group discusses it with interest, and starts asking a lot of questions. The leader feels uncomfortable, thinking, 'Don't they think I can manage my own group?' The workshop leader notices the atmosphere and says, 'I wonder if the seminar leader feels a bit like Laura, and is experiencing this group as an intrusive mother'. The workshop leader, who is highly experienced in group dynamics, also thinks to herself, 'Any minute now they might turn on me and experience me as interfering'. However, possibly because she has allowed herself to think consciously about parallel process and remember it can happen at every level, it does not happen on this occasion, and the group settles down and gets on with the afternoon's work.

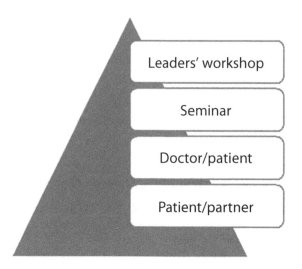

FIGURE 6.1   Parallel process in the IPM.

Psychoanalytic Theory and the Institute of Psychosexual Medicine

It has not been a tradition in the IPM to teach this psychological background to our work, nor has it been a requirement of trainees that they know anything of the psychoanalytic principles underlying it. In fact, there has been a tendency to go the other way and look on 'theory' as something unnecessary and perhaps even undesirable. There are arguments on both sides.

Should We Use the Language of Psychoanalysis?

Yes:

- It gives structure to our thinking.
- We can communicate clearly what we mean.
- It may expand our understanding.
- It will keep us focussed on the unconscious.
- It connects us with a shared psychotherapeutic community.

No:

- It complicates our communications.
- It takes us away from the here and now of consultations.
- It is an avoidance of painful feelings.
- It is in conflict with our stance of 'not knowing'.

It is clear that too much attention to theory can be a defence against difficult emotions (remember intellectualisation as a defence mechanism). But it is surely possible to think and feel at the same time. We can be both knowing and unknowing, to empathise with our patients' painful stories and still be able to notice the defences against intimacy and the reactivation of past relationships which are contributing to their current difficulties. By bringing these ideas into the forefront of our attention, I assert that we can be of greater use to our patients and can justifiably say, as our prospectus claims, that we practise a therapy 'based on psychoanalytic skills'.

REFERENCES

1. Prospectus of the Institute of Psychosexual Medicine. Update 21 March 2014, Available from: www. IPM.org.uk
2. Rycroft C. *A Critical Dictionary of Psychoanalysis*. London: Penguin Books, 1995.
3. Bateman A, Brown D, Pedder J. *Introduction to Psychotherapy*. London: Routledge, 2000.
4. Greenson RR. The working alliance and the transference neurosis. *Psychoanal Q* 1965;34:155–181.
5. Balint M, Balint E. *Psychotherapeutic Techniques in Medicine*. London: Tavistock, 1961.
6. Heimann P. On counter-transference. *Int J Psychother* 1950;31:81–84.
7. Searles HF. The informational value of the supervisor's emotional experience. *Psychiatry* 1955;18: 135–146.
8. Benson J. *Working More Creatively with Groups*. London: Routledge, 2001.

7

Interaction of Mind and Body in Psychosexual Medicine

Caroline Hunter

> Demons in all traditions are often shown gnawing viscera. This is because of the primordial understanding that consciousness and memory are not stored in the brain alone, but in the whole body. Things we have done that we would rather not confront – painful and undigested experiences – are stored in the viscera. (1)

Introduction

The interaction of mind and body is what psychosexual medicine is all about. It is practised by doctors and allied health professionals who carry out investigations, examination and treatments in their day-to-day work. The Institute of Psychosexual Medicine (IPM) practitioner learns to observe the part that the mind plays in physical symptoms, and to develop the skill of using these observations to help patients understand themselves better.

This is not an easy thing to grapple with. We are faced with questions such as: 'To what extent are the mind and body separate?', 'Which comes first, mind or body?', 'Is consciousness merely a product of brain activity?' and particularly relevant to our work, 'If the psyche can produce somatic symptoms, how does this happen?'

These questions have been asked as far as back as the time of the philosopher Plato and are not within the scope of this book. It is enough to acknowledge that centuries of philosophical debate have failed to come up with answers with which everyone agrees. Fortunately for us, we are clinicians, and need only concern ourselves with the mind-body problem as it presents in our work, and as pragmatists, find ways of giving explanations to our patients that are helpful and make them feel better.

In this chapter I develop the ideas of Chapter 6, concentrating on the concept of somatisation, the psychological defence mechanism that is responsible for the psychosexual problems with which we deal.

Somatisation

Somatisation has many different definitions but the one I find most useful, and use when teaching about mind-body interaction, is this:

> An emotional response to a stress is converted into a physical symptom which symbolises the conflict. (2)

I particularly like the phrase 'which symbolises the conflict'. Psychosomatic symptoms are not random; Lady Macbeth did not wake up in the small hours of the morning with an urge to go to the toilet. Where would have been the poetry in that? As can be seen throughout this book, our patients produce physical symptoms that are highly symbolic of the unconscious conflict.

We use this symbolic language to describe our emotions in everyday life: 'My heart was broken', 'he was a pain in the neck', 'that was a weight off my shoulders', 'I was sick to my stomach'. We do not mean to suggest our hearts are actually broken, or that there was a real weight on our shoulders. We might go so far as to say, 'My eyes were *literally* popping out of my head' but we still do not expect anyone to actually think this is what has happened.

In thinking about somatisation and the development of psychosomatic symptoms, I find it helpful to consider the process occurring at different levels, which might be seen as degrees to which the individual is consciously connected with what is happening:

1. The level of fully conscious awareness. It could be said that we 'somatise' almost continually, in that we experience emotions in our bodies as well as in our heads. It is difficult to imagine an emotional response without its physical equivalent. Can I really feel angry in my head alone? I think I am angry, but how can I be sure?

2. The physical symptom is experienced as separate from the emotion, but the connection is still apparent:

    • If I wake up in the morning with my stomach churning, this may be the first thing I notice, but if I stop to remember that today is the day I re-sit my driving test, I soon realise it isn't what I ate the night before that is making me feel unwell.

    • If I have to deliver a lecture to 100 potentially critical colleagues, my mouth will be dry, my palms sweaty and my face flushed. I might wish to think that I have a virus which will get me out of having to deliver the talk, but in my heart of hearts I know it is only pre-performance nerves that is doing this to my body.

3. Sometimes the connection between the physical symptom and the underlying emotion is lost, or possibly has never been consciously experienced. In this case we will understandably assume that what we are experiencing is a result of a physical problem rather than a psychological one.

If the patient cannot experience a connection between his symptoms and his feelings he is likely to seek medical help for them.

EXAMPLE 7.1

Mr Brown has been suffering from chest pain for years. He has had extensive investigations that have not demonstrated any pathological cause for his symptoms. He is not reassured and returns to his doctor on a regular basis, convinced there must be something wrong. His wife has noticed that his symptoms get worse every time his mother comes to visit. She points this out to him. He has no idea what she is talking about; he is totally fine with his mother's visits.

Alexithymia

There is a group of people, thought to represent some 10% of the population, who find it difficult to express and/or consciously feel their emotions. These people are described as having alexithymia. Alexithymia, which literally means having no words for emotions, was first described by Peter Sifneos in 1972 as follows: 'The ability not only to recognise and express emotions but also to verbalise them is significant. Some patients experience a difficulty in this area. When they are asked to talk about how they feel they mention repetitively and endlessly only somatic sensations, without being able to relate them to any accompanying thoughts, fantasies or conflicts' (3).

Alexithymia is not a disorder so much as a tendency. As such it seems reasonable to think that it is the result of a combination of nature and nurture.

Nature plays its part in that some people are naturally in touch with their emotions and find it easy to notice and put into words what they are feeling. For others, this comes less easily.

In addition to this innate ability, or its absence, the role of upbringing is also important. If a child grows up in an environment where emotions are readily expressed and made sense of, she is likely to learn to be able to do the same for herself. If she is brought up in a home where feelings are never talked about, she may struggle with her own emotional world.

One of the important roles of parenting is to help a child make sense of her emotional world. Observe a naturally empathic mother and you will see her providing a commentary for her toddler: 'That's exciting/scary/horrible/sad', 'Dolly is lonely/happy/confused/jealous'. The child whose mother does not do this will be unlikely to notice something is missing, nor will anyone else think anything is amiss. As long as a child's physical, and perhaps also educational, needs are met, the failure to teach the child the language of emotions will probably pass unnoticed.

Alexithymia and Somatisation in Clinical Practice

Referring to the concepts of alexithymia and somatisation may be helpful when dealing with patients with psychosexual problems, particularly when trying to manage difficult ideas around mind-body interactions. Understanding that a patient has difficulty either experiencing emotions, or putting those emotions into words, can be a very helpful starting point. Likewise noting a patient's general tendency to somatise, and to seek medical help for the symptoms, can be the beginning of understanding the underlying cause of their psychosexual dysfunction.

Consider two patients with similar experiences but different levels at which they are experiencing the interaction of mind and body.

CASE 1: CLAIRE

Claire had an abnormal smear last year. She was quite upset when she got the phone call from the colposcopy clinic. She spoke to her friend about it and after a long chat felt a bit better. She told her boyfriend she could not think about having sex with him until after this was all sorted. The whole idea just made her feel too anxious. After the colposcopy she received the all clear in a letter from the hospital. She was hugely relieved. She told her boyfriend she was still feeling a bit upset by the whole experience, but thought they might try having sex again. The first time they had sex she noticed memories of the abnormal smear popping into her head but she soon got carried away by the pleasure of the experience and was able to dismiss the thoughts.

CASE 2: CATHY

Cathy also had an abnormal smear requiring colposcopy. When the phone call came through she was overwhelmed by a feeling of dread and horror. She found herself crying inconsolably. Her flatmate asked her what was wrong. She said, 'I don't know. I've had this appointment for the hospital, but I shouldn't be feeling so upset'. She woke the next morning with a sharp pain in her lower abdomen. The first thought that came into her head was 'I've got cancer'. She started crying again. When she met her boyfriend that evening she could hardly speak to him. Eventually she managed to say, 'I think I've got cancer'. Her boyfriend did not react as might be expected but instead looked a little bored. This was not the first time Cathy was convinced she had a serious illness. She could hardly eat or sleep, her abdominal pain kept her off work, she was in such a state that by the time she attended the colposcopy, she could barely allow the gynaecologist to examine her. When she got the letter saying everything was fine she hardly reacted at all. She had been reading about all the women who had died of cervical cancer despite having had a normal smear, and she knew her abdominal pain must be the sign of something very serious. Eventually she tried to have sex with her boyfriend. She was so tense that attempts at penetration were impossible and very painful. She was now convinced there was something seriously wrong. She went back to her general practitioner (GP). The GP knew her well and suspected that she was presenting emotional pain as physical symptoms. She asked her gently what was happening when the pain started. Cathy replied that she could not remember, nothing much, everything was fine. There followed a series of visits to gynaecology, genitourinary medicine, private specialists, but nothing helped, and Cathy's sex life became non-existent.

Cathy's presentation is all too familiar to those working in psychosexual medicine. Until someone could find a way to help Cathy see that her difficulty understanding her emotional world, in other words her alexithymia, resulted in her producing physical symptoms for which she sought medical help, in other words somatising, she would continue to seek reassurance from the medical profession, and continue to fail to find it.

Working with Mind and Body in Clinical Practice

It is not easy to communicate to our patients the idea that the mind and body interact at a deep and often unconscious level. We fear offending them – 'Are you saying it is all in my head doctor?' – or strengthening their defensive positions – 'There is absolutely nothing wrong in my life. I am completely happy and always have been'.

The skill of psychosexual medicine is to pick up clues about what might be unconsciously at the root of the problem, and find ways of putting these into words that are helpful and allow the patient to come to an understanding of their problem.

CASE 3: TOM

Tom comes to his doctor complaining of an inability to get an erection. He cannot even masturbate anymore and his early morning erections are half-hearted. He asks the doctor for Viagra as he is certain the problem must be a physical one. The doctor asks a few questions, and notices that Tom is displaying very little emotion when talking about his sexual difficulty. She imagines the development of erectile dysfunction in a young man in his 20s might be at least a little distressing, but there is no sign of this in Tom. She begins to wonder whether this problem may be more to do with his mind than any actual pathology. After taking a medical history and examining him, she is becoming more of the opinion that Tom may be somatising. She organises some basic investigations but notices herself becoming anxious. She feels she owes it to Tom to discuss the possibility of a psychosexual component to his difficulty, but is not sure how to go about it. She does not want to offend him. She does not want to be wrong, and 'accuse' him of it all being in his head when he actually has some serious underlying medical condition. She cannot face trying to explain to him that the mind and body do indeed interact, especially as she is not entirely sure how this happens.

Patients with psychosexual dysfunction present their inability to express emotions in different ways. In Cathy's case, she was aware of feeling something, but was unable to put into words what was wrong. The more overwhelmed she became by her emotions the worse her physical symptoms became. In Tom's case, he was so far removed from his emotional world that his only symptom was a physical one.

Each patient needs to be met and communicated with at their own level, and an understanding of how alexithymia can take on different forms may help the clinician negotiate the difficult path to finding the words to help each individual.

In order to begin to help Cathy the doctor will need to find a way to calm her. As long as she is overwhelmed by her emotional experience she will not be able to consider the idea of mind-body interaction. Calming a patient is not the end point, but the start of a process that will result in her being able to understand herself better.

For example, a physiotherapist may try simple breathing exercises, or trigger point massage when she first meets Cathy. She is aware that this in itself will not be enough to put an end to Cathy's painful symptoms. Once she has established a rapport, and shown Cathy that she can start to feel better simply by being in a calmer environment, she can begin to explore Cathy's world with her, and understand why the abnormal smear had such a devastating effect.

Tom does not need to be calmed down. He is not troubled by his emotions at all. But the doctor has sensed that if she is not careful in what she says she risks provoking unacknowledged anger in Tom which might alienate him and make it difficult for her to use her skills to help him. She needs to introduce her ideas in a way that will make sense to Tom.

She might decide on the first occasion to say very little, and limit herself to one comment. She may say something along the lines of:

> It must have been difficult for you to come and speak about this with me. I'm so glad you felt you were able to ask for help. Let's see what the tests show and if they are all fine, which I expect they will be, we might think next time about what else might be at the root of your difficulty.

This may not seem to be very much, but the doctor is subtly introducing Tom to the idea that she is not only interested in his physical symptoms, but in the whole of him, mind, body, and emotions.

Origins of Somatisation

It is apparent that many of our psychosexual patients are 'Somatisers'. By this I mean that they have a tendency to produce physical symptoms not just in their sexual life, but in other areas as well. Observing this pattern may help patients to see the connection between their physical problems and their emotional world, and allow them to accept the psychosomatic roots to their sexual dysfunction.

CASE 4: JOAN

Joan, a woman in her early 50s, presented to the practice nurse for a smear. She had three children, all normal deliveries, and had been married for 25 years. She was well known to the nurse as she previously had several episodes of distressing symptoms, which thankfully had never amounted to anything serious. The most recent one happened at work. Joan was overcome by a difficulty in breathing. She was rushed to hospital, but all was found to be well. She also had a history of severe migraines, which had not troubled her so much recently. The nurse was pleased to see Joan. She was a pleasant woman who never dwelt on her troubles, which had been considerable, culminating in a short prison sentence for her husband for small-scale embezzlement. However, when the nurse tried to pass the speculum for the smear she was unable to insert it far enough to visualise her cervix.

The nurse was surprised but noticed that there appeared to be something on Joan's mind. She took a moment to think about this and then said, 'It seems you weren't as surprised by this as I was'. Joan hesitated. 'My husband and I haven't been able to have sex for years. It's too painful'. The nurse noticed that Joan did not cry, but she had stopped smiling. She invited Joan to sit down, and explained to her about vaginismus, how the mind can cause the vagina to effectively shut everything out.

Joan went on to receive several sessions of psychosexual therapy from a local specialist. During these sessions she began to realise how stressful her adult life had been, and how the only time she sought help, or allowed herself to be taken care of, was when there was something physically wrong with her. On one occasion she was talking about her early life. She described her mother: 'She wasn't very warm, she never hugged us. We were expected to get on with it'. She paused. 'Except when we were ill. She was lovely then. Made us feel so special and cared for'. The therapist did not speak. She just looked at Joan and raised her eyebrows slightly. Joan looked confused for a moment and then her face cleared. 'You think that's what I still do to myself'. This was the final piece of the puzzle for Joan. Her tendency to produce physical symptoms at times of emotional stress at last made sense to her, and gradually she learnt to take better care of herself, both mind and body.

Some psychosexual patients display negative views of their bodies that may present in other ways. For example, it is not uncommon to hear stories of eating disorders, such as anorexia nervosa, in women who subsequently present with sexual dysfunction. There may also be stories of self-harm, or abuse of drugs or alcohol. Such women will often express a dislike of their whole bodies, not just the sexual parts. These women may find the genital examination particularly difficult, and go to great lengths to avoid it.

CASE 5: MARIA

Maria found a doctor specialising in psychosexual medicine on the Internet, and referred herself. She had never been able to allow her husband to penetrate her, and there had been no sexual contact for over a year. She had an eating disorder as a teenager and still struggled to feed herself properly. She also had a period of depression that caused her to leave her job and remain off work for 6 months. She was feeling a little better and wanted to try and sort her problem out. She was desperate for a baby, even though she was only 26. She blamed herself entirely for her sexual difficulty. Her husband had no problem with his erections and was very understanding. She was very close to her mother, who knew all about her problem. The doctor found herself wincing at the suggestion of the mother who knew all about Maria's private life, but put the thought to one side. Working with Maria was difficult. She was unable to understand the cause of her sexual difficulty, although she readily accepted that it was all in her head. She said repeatedly how pathetic she was and that it did not surprise her that she had done this to herself. The doctor tried to find some clues in Maria's upbringing, but none were forthcoming. Maria began to resent the doctor's perceived intrusion into her childhood, which had been so happy. The doctor noticed this, and wondered if this was a clue that Maria was harbouring an unconscious resentment of her intrusive mother, but could find no way of using this. Eventually Maria agreed to be examined. She dreaded exposing herself in this way and did not think it would help. She was convinced the doctor would find her disgusting and probably need to hurt her to examine her.

When Maria got up on the couch she was visibly shaking. She was unable to part her legs, and kept apologising. She looked almost child-like cowering on the couch. The doctor remembered an idea she had heard that examining our female patients might invoke memories of being handled as a baby, and more particularly the experience of nappy-changing. After all she had told Maria to undress from the waist down, lie on a table, and then attempted to touch her genital area. She wondered if there might be a way to use this to help Maria understand her difficult relationship with her body. She took the time while Maria was getting dressed to think about how to do this.

When Maria sat down the doctor shared her thoughts that maybe her mother had been going through some stress when Maria was very small, and that it had left Maria with some negative feelings about her body. Maria's first response was to resist this idea and leap to the defence of her mother. The doctor explained that she was not blaming her mother, but that perhaps Maria could agree that the emotional world of a mother might have an effect on the baby, and particularly how she might feel about her body.

To the doctor's surprise Maria burst into tears. She told the doctor that her own mother had been sexually abused as a child. She felt so guilty that nothing like that had happened to her, yet she still had all these problems. The doctor listened to the whole story, and then gently suggested that maybe some of her mother's distress at how she herself was treated might have been transmitted to the tiny Maria. They had such a close bond after all.

Maria struggled with any suggestion of holding her mother responsible, but eventually agreed to broach the subject with her. She was astonished by her mother's response, when she in turn burst into tears and told Maria that she had always feared Maria's problems were her fault. She confessed that Maria's naked little body had filled her with feelings of shame and dread, which made her feel so guilty she could hardly bear to bathe her or change her nappy.

This was a very difficult time for both Maria and her mother, but their relationship was indeed as close as Maria believed it to be and they gradually worked their way through it. Maria's mother had coped with her own emotional pain by trying to ignore it. She became a practical woman who met her children's physical needs exceptionally well. She was always kind and put her children first. This left Maria feeling anxious and self-critical; she knew something was wrong but was unable to voice what it was. She blamed herself for feeling bad, especially when her mother had done everything for her. The understanding that neither of them was to blame, and the real guilty party was the man who abused Maria's mother, enabled Maria to start to feel better about herself. She still noticed herself producing physical symptoms at times of stress, and still found penetration difficult, but being able to put words to what had been going on in their lives was the beginning of a healing process for both Maria and her mother.

Maria's mind-body problems were at least to some extent the result of her relationship with her mother when she was too small to make any sense of it. It is not possible to go back in time and watch how the mother handled her baby, and even if we were able to, the communications might be too subtle to be noticeable to an observer. Maria was fortunate in that her mother had been open with her about her own abuse, and was able to accept responsibility for Maria's experience of her own body. It is not difficult to see that similar mechanisms might be operating in many of our patients who have poor relationships with their bodies and find it difficult to tolerate physical intimacy.

Conclusion

Alexithymia and *somatisation* are just words, and it is possible to work effectively in psychosexual medicine without having formally been introduced to these concepts. However, psychosexual patients bring their physical symptoms to the consultation and expect to get physical treatments for them. These patients have difficulty putting their emotions into words, and part of our job is to give them names for what it is that troubles them. Being able to put words to what we can see so clearly in front of our eyes may help us to find ways of communicating more effectively with our patients. As we are reminded in the tale of Rumpelstiltskin, naming something gives us power over that thing. By being able to name to themselves and others what has been going on for them, how the mind and body have connected to produce their symptoms, they can start to find words for their emotions, and begin to gain more power over their own lives.

REFERENCES

1. Black J. *The Secret History of the World*. London: Quercus, 2010.
2. Psychodynamic Psychotherapy. Available from: https://blogs.ncl.ac.uk/mbbspsychiatry/files/2010/03/dynamic.pdf
3. Sifneos PE. *Emotional Crisis*. Cambridge, MA: Harvard University Press, 1972.

8

Physical Treatments for Sexual Problems

Nicola Carter

Introduction

Institute of Psychosexual Medicine (IPM) training is appropriate for clinicians who examine patients and as such are well placed to address the interplay of emotional, psychosocial and physical aspects of sexual problems.

However, our individual healthcare training and experiences are as unique as our patients' stories. Thus, the knowledge and experience of physical aspects and treatments will vary widely between healthcare practitioners (HCPs). A pelvic floor physiotherapist will have a different range of experience from an erectile dysfunction nurse specialist; a consultant psychiatrist's very different from an obstetrician's range of experience.

Hence this chapter will aim to provide a broad overview of what is available, not a replacement for an individual's deeper understanding of their specialism, or with sufficient detail to provide professional development in a new discipline.

The relevance of physical treatments will vary with clinical setting, but the advantage of IPM training is that it allows observation and use of the HCP-patient relationship throughout a seemingly 'physical' consultation so that management may be as holistic as possible. At times, physical treatments will be the most significant, at others they may be used as an adjunct, a negotiation tool, or part of a temporary collusion around a physical aspect on a journey towards acknowledgement and understanding of deeper issues.

Physical Treatments for Male Sexual Problems

Erectile Dysfunction

Erectile dysfunction (ED) is probably the sexual problem to which physical treatments are the most relevant. There may be several reasons for this. As we saw in Chapter 5, the ability to achieve and sustain an erection is a complex process and hence vulnerable to dysfunction. It is difficult for a man to achieve sexual pleasure without some erection, and full penetrative sex requires a greater and sustained firmness. This has resulted in a long-standing demand for effective physical solutions.

It is worth emphasising at this point that before considering any treatments for ED that full consideration should be given to the physical conditions that ED may be symptomatic of. In some cases screening for diabetes and cardiovascular risk factors such as hyperlipidaemia, obesity, hypertension and family history should be undertaken as well as an assessment of exercise tolerance. It is important to know that the additional exercise of sexual intercourse is not likely to precipitate angina or another cardiovascular event.

This section aims to provide an introduction to treatment types including:

1. Phosphodiesterase type 5 inhibitors (PDE5s)
2. Alprostadil
3. Vacuum pump devices and rings
4. Penile prostheses

TABLE 8.1

Phosphodiesterase Type 5 inhibitors (PDE5s)

Name	Dosage	Affected by Food	Use with α-Blockers
Avanafil	50–200 mg as required 15–30 minutes before sex. Max one dose per day.	Action delayed if taken with food	Use 50 mg initially rather than 100 mg
Sildenafil	25–100 mg as required approximately 1 hour before sex. Max one dose per day.	Action delayed if taken with food	Use 25 mg initially rather than 50 mg and take the α-blocker 4 hours after the sildenafil
Vardenafil	5–20 mg as required 25–60 minutes before sex. Max one dose per day.	Action delayed if taken with food	Use 5 mg initially rather than 10 mg
Tadalafil	10–20 mg as required.[a] At least 30 minutes before sex.[b]	Not affected by food	Avoid use with α-blockers

Source: This table is compiled from *British National Formulary 72*, September–March 2017. London: BMJ Group and Pharmaceutical Press, 2016, 735–739 (1).

[a] N.B. Max dose of tadalafil is 20 mg per day but not recommended as daily dosing. Use 2.5–5 mg as daily dose.
[b] Tadalafil may persist in the system for more than 24 hours – clinical experience suggests 36 hours average.

Phosphodiesterase Type 5 Inhibitors

The introduction of sildenafil in the late 1990s heralded a revolution in treatment for men with a physical cause of ED. Doctors working in psychosexual medicine at the time will have been aware of men for whom IPM and other psychologically based interventions were not working. PDE5s were viewed initially with some scepticism – surely, they would detract from looking at the underlying issues? In fact, they have been positive life-changers for many men and their partners, and the ability for an IPM-trained doctor to be able to safely prescribe, as well as address the inevitable feelings of distress in the room, proved to be a real benefit for the majority. They must not be used by men taking nitrates of any type.

An overview of the four available PDE5s is given in Table 8.1.

There are obviously differences between the medications but there is no objective answer to the most common question men ask, 'Which one is the best?' It is possible to say that they will not work for about 20% of men and 40% of men with diabetes, and that they do not work at all unless there is sufficient arousal. None of them can be taken by men also using nitrates as this may lead to severe hypotension. Anxiety and fatigue may stop the medications from working, and they may never result in the firmness of erection that the man aspires to, albeit sufficient for penetrative intercourse.

There is hence a degree of trial and error involved in finding the 'best' medication and dose for an individual and explaining this at the beginning is helpful to manage the real concern that ensues when there is not instant success. It is worth explaining that a drug should not be considered to have failed until it has been used at the highest dose tolerated on a number of occasions with sufficient arousal. It is important to emphasise that the longer a man has been without an erection, the longer it can take to be restored with PDE5s and that no matter how supportive his partner, trying by himself initially during masturbation can feel less pressured, if he is comfortable with self-pleasure. Once established on a suitable medication, it is often possible to reduce the dose. Physiologically, an erection becomes easier to achieve, and there is the additional impact of decreasing performance anxiety and increasing confidence over time.

It will be noticed that tadalafil 5 and 2.5 mg are licenced for daily dosing, and this is often more convenient when the patient is taking a plethora of other medication. It may also ease the problem of planning for sex that some men or their partners find insurmountable and allows for intercourse to happen more frequently.

This overview applies to general usage of PDE5s, and sensitive consulting and the reassurance of a regular prescription may be sufficient for men with predominantly organic aetiologies. For IPM prescribers however, it can be useful to use the oral treatments even when the aetiology appears mixed or mainly psychological.

Others may feel so pressured to 'perform' or unable to 'work' psychologically within an IPM setting, that progress is extremely limited without concurrent prescribing. Two vignettes may help to demonstrate this.

CASE 1

JB is a 29-year-old club doorman who had been using sildenafil without a prescription for 10 years. He did not have ED prior to starting to use the medication but describes peer pressure to use it recreationally. He is part of a 'gym culture' that encourages anabolic steroid use and strongly identified with an image of masculinity that is dependent on achieving long-lasting erections during sexual encounters with women at the end of 'nights out'. He had not experienced sex within a relationship. A number of health issues led him to stop steroids and try achieving erections without a tablet.

He discovered this was not possible and became extremely distressed and depressed; this persisted after his natural testosterone levels had re-established. Consultations allowed him to look at past issues that contributed to his beliefs about 'real men', understand more about what women meant to him, and look at how he met women and how that might change in the future.

He had used medication for so long that he found it difficult to move forward despite making progress in insight. A combined approach of support and decreasing doses of sildenafil – 100 mg down to 12.5 mg over 12 months – allowed him to enter a relationship which became a satisfactory sexual one.

CASE 2

MD is a 50-year-old office worker with chronic scrotal pain following a vasectomy 10 years ago. He was on a cocktail of opioid analgesia and gabapentin. Although he continued to work, his activity levels had dropped, he had gained weight and intercourse had become painful. He had developed ED during the past 5 years.

His ED was clearly multifactorial, but during the consultation it was clear that he was also acting as carer for his wife, and that sexual intercourse would probably not be achievable for her. She came to the consultation and made it clear that she did not really want to resume penetrative sex.

During the examination he became upset. I wondered if it was due to pain but in fact, his concern was that going to work and going out had become so stressful because he could not handle his penis well enough to pass urine without significant leakage. The penis was mostly embedded in suprapubic fat and he felt it had gradually shrunk.

There was undoubted psychological distress although it was not entirely focussed on ED. It was felt that a course of daily dosing with tadalafil may be beneficial on a number of counts. It had the benefit of increasing resting penile 'tone', so that he could successfully pass urine in public. This greatly improved his confidence and he felt able to look at weight loss. He became able to masturbate by himself, and they were able to resume a sex life, without penetration, that brought them both pleasure and an increased sense of intimacy.

Alprostadil

As suggested above, there is a significant proportion of men for whom oral treatment does not work adequately or at all. Once the issues of arousal and testosterone levels have been addressed as possible explanations, the man may wish to consider non-oral options.

Alprostadil is a prostaglandin analogue which acts locally on the penile spongy tissue to produce an erection without the need for arousal or specific testosterone levels. It is self-administered after initiation and training by a HCP on an as-required basis.

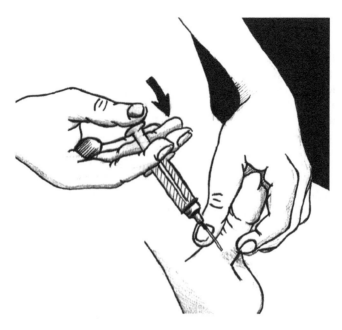

FIGURE 8.1   Injection technique. (Courtesy of Sidonie AR Brough, from prescribing information courtesy of Pfizer.)

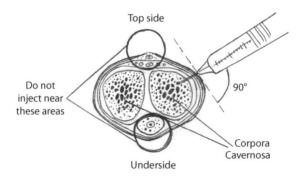

FIGURE 8.2   Cross-sectional penile anatomy involved in an injection. (Courtesy of Sidonie AR Brough, from prescribing information courtesy of Pfizer.)

Intracavernosal Injection

This is the most commonly used and effective method, and for many men with ED, the only method that can achieve a 10:10 hardness score (2). For some this outweighs the prospect of learning how to administer it, even if oral treatment works for them.

The disadvantage is the commitment involved and the potential intrusion on lovemaking.

A supportive partner is a real advantage here. Initiating the method is usually done in a specialist clinic during which titration up to an appropriate dose is carried out. Advice is also given about priapism because although still rare, it is more common than with oral methods. Men are advised to attend the accident and emergency department if they have an erection lasting more than four hours, for treatment with aspiration and lavage of the corpora. If this fails, sympathomimetics can be used although they are unlicenced (3). The injections can be used up to three times per week with at least 24 hours between each injection (Figures 8.1 and 8.2).

Urethral Application

This avoids the use of injection if this is an issue for the man and can be used seven times per week with a maximum of two doses per 24 hours. It may not produce such consistent erection hardness as the injection,

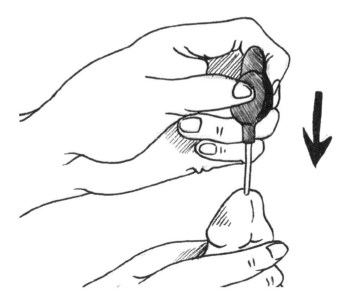

FIGURE 8.3 Intraurethral alprostadil. (Courtesy of Sidonie AR Brough.)

and the tissues can expand unevenly. It also involves titration to an appropriate dose and training to allow the man to successfully introduce the small dissolvable pellet (prescribed as a 'stick') into the urethral meatus. Some men also notice marked stinging of the meatal skin after introducing the pellet (Figure 8.3).

Topical Application

This is used as a cream containing 3 mg/g alprostadil and is a more recent addition to treatment options. It is prescribed in an applicator so that 300 micrograms can be delivered and massaged into the tip of the penis 5–30 minutes before planned intercourse. This can be used two to three times per week with a maximum of one dose per 24 hours. It is a less 'invasive' feeling option but lacks the same success rates as the previous two methods. However, some men will definitely benefit from a trial, and it may also be used as an adjunct to other treatment regimes (4).

Vacuum Pump Devices and Rings

The basic principle of these devices is that an erection is produced without the need for arterial flow. The penis is placed within the device and a vacuum is created by manually pumping air out from around the penis. The negative pressure causes the spongy tissues to expand, and this expansion is maintained by the use of a penile constriction ring fed over the device and onto the base of the penis before the device is removed.

Again, this device requires training and commitment from the man and partner; some men find it unacceptable because the erection is cold, having been produced without arterial blood. However, it does not have any pharmacological side effects and is not arousal dependent.

It is also useful as an adjunct to other therapies and frequently used as 'physio' for the penis after surgery or prolonged periods of time without an erection (5). Regular mechanical expansion of the tissue does help the achievement of an erection with arterial blood.

Some men who have a venous 'leak' of blood from the penis may also use the ring alone to help maintain the erection. They are prescribable separately from the devices (Figure 8.4).

Penile Prosthesis

Surgically implanted prostheses are an option for men for whom none of the above options have worked or for whom injectables or vacuum pumps are unacceptable. This may include men who have had diabetes for many years and men with significant Peyronie's disease who may need corrective surgery concurrently (Figure 8.5).

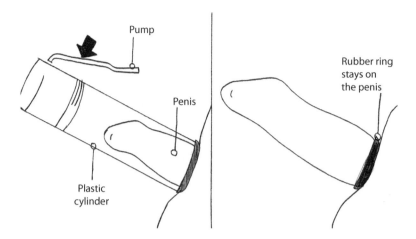

FIGURE 8.4   Use of a pump and/or ring. (Courtesy of Sidonie AR Brough.)

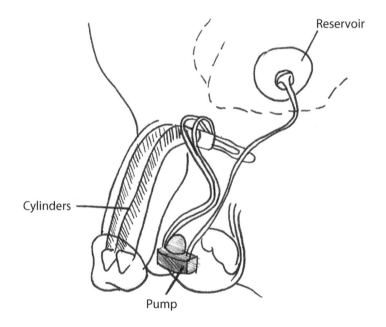

FIGURE 8.5   Implanted prostheses. (Courtesy of Sidonie AR Brough.)

There are two basic types:

   a. Malleable – in which two semi-rigid rods are inserted into the corpora and produce a permanent semi-hard erection. The disadvantage of this is that it may be difficult to conceal or uncomfortable when not being used in a sexual setting.

   b. Inflatable – in which two rods are inserted and connected to a fluid-filled chamber which can then be externally pumped and deflated by the user. This has the advantage of not having the permanent hardness but needs the man's input to inflate and deflate appropriately.

Both types obviously have the disadvantage of surgical insertion, and the most common problem resulting in removal is infection, especially in diabetic men. However, they are a useful addition for those with significant medical conditions for whom sexual intercourse is important. It is therefore helpful to inform men that this is an option where appropriate and to be aware of the nearest available services.

National Health Service Funding for Erectile Dysfunction Treatments

At the time of writing, it is only sildenafil as a generic drug that is able to be prescribed for ED without restriction in the National Health Service (NHS). The other PDE5 inhibitors and all formulations of alprostadil are subject to restrictions. Only those men who meet the criteria listed in Part XVIIIB of the Drug Tariff (Part XIB of the Northern Ireland Drug Tariff, Part 12 of the Scottish Drug Tariff) can receive NHS prescriptions for the above drugs, and the script must be endorsed 'SLS' (special licenced substance).

One of the criteria is that the man's ED must be causing him 'severe psychological distress', and in this case a locally agreed 'specialist' may prescribe on the NHS as mentioned. An IPM prescriber is in a good position to function as that specialist.

The position regarding vacuum pump devices will vary depending on region, and it will be necessary to know what the local funding arrangements are. These can also be purchased privately by the patient, as can the penile rings.

Ejaculatory Disorders

Retarded Ejaculation

This is generally thought of as a psychological sexual problem but in cases where it results from spinal cord injury or neuropathy, low-intensity shock wave therapy may be tried to produce ejaculation (6). This has been available for some years but is currently being developed further. It may be helpful for men who wish to ejaculate themselves in respect of trying to achieve a pregnancy with their partner.

Oral medications have not been found to be of proven benefit.

Premature Ejaculation

Physical treatments for premature ejaculation (PE) have a place when symptoms are extreme and long-standing, and where psychological interventions have had no impact and the distress remains. As with ED, sometimes a combined approach of therapy and prescribing can be helpful in the medium term with physical treatments being gradually used less as confidence and insight increase.

Most physical treatments for PE are unlicenced in the United Kingdom. There is one licenced oral medication:

Dapoxetine

This is a short-acting selective serotonin re-uptake inhibitor (SSRI) that can be used on an as-required basis taken orally 1–3 hours before intercourse is planned. It is usually started at 30 mg and increased up to 60 mg if required and providing there are no other medical or pharmacological reasons that restrict use of the higher dose. It can be used once in 24 hours, although most regions will have guidelines that commonly suggest its use once or twice per week.

Prescribing is also restricted to men who fit agreed criteria:

- Poor control over ejaculation
- A history of PE over the last 6 months
- Marked distress or interpersonal difficulty as a consequence of PE
- Intravaginal ejaculatory latency time (IELT) of less than 2 minutes

There can be up to a three- to fourfold increase in IELT which may be of enormous benefit for men for whom PE is moderate and severe, i.e. IELT less than 60 seconds and lifelong. It can boost confidence and may then facilitate greater engagement with behavioural and psychodynamic therapies. Although side effects with SSRIs are common, they are less troublesome for many men with this short-acting preparation (7).

Review of treatment is advised regularly in order to assess continuing need, particularly in view of the fact that for most men PE is psychological in origin and best managed by psychosexual therapy.

Selective Serotonin Re-Uptake Inhibitors (SSRIs)

Unlicenced medications have been available for longer and the most commonly used are the SSRIs that have been used as daily oral preparations for many years for the treatment of depression and anxiety, as it was noticed that they could affect sexual function, especially delaying or preventing ejaculation in men. The effect appeared to be dose related and to resolve when medication was stopped.

This side effect has been used to help men with PE, and is particularly useful when there are concurrent mental health problems (which may be related to the PE as cause or effect), but also purely as treatment for PE alone. The difficulty has been in finding a universally agreed regime of type of SSRI, dose (including titration up and down) and duration of treatment.

Many men are also uncomfortable using daily preparations with an increased risk of side effects, and also a medication that is more commonly used for mental health problems. The individual clinician therefore has to decide, based on their familiarity with and confidence in SSRIs, whether to discuss their use for patients they see who have PE.

Cost issues mean that in some local guidelines, therapy and standard SSRIs are suggested before use of dapoxetine, but prescribers must always be comfortable with their own 'out-of-licence' prescribing decisions.

Topical Anaesthetic Preparations

Topical lidocaine or prilocaine preparations are helpful for some men alone or as an adjunct to other modalities. They are unlicenced for PE and there is no helpful evidence for or against their effectiveness (8). The gel or cream needs to be applied to the tip of the penis and a condom is needed if the partner wishes to avoid numbness. The loss of sensation may make it difficult for the man to maintain his arousal and erection.

Other Unlicenced Preparations for ED and PE

Clinicians may come across many preparations that are said to work for male sexual dysfunction and some of these suggestions will come from patients themselves.

Some of these may be prescribable medications such as tramadol, which is only licenced as analgesia, or privately available treatments such as ginseng.

It is beyond the scope of this chapter to deal with this area and clinicians may research individual treatment as appropriate.

The aforementioned unlicenced treatments for PE are included because they are acknowledged as acceptable practice.

CASE 3

TB is a 35-year-old lecturer with long-standing severe PE. He had previously tried behavioural therapy and that had helped to a degree. He felt the PE contributed to the end of a long-term relationship. He then received brief psychodynamic psychosexual counselling which helped clarify how childhood events may have contributed to his current problems. He became significantly depressed and received SSRI medication which he found helpful both for mood and for PE during masturbation.

He felt confident enough to stop the SSRI and enter a new relationship. The PE was still present, but not as severe or as great an issue with this partner. However, when they decided to try for a pregnancy and she had a miscarriage and then seemed unable to conceive again quickly, his PE worsened.

Although acknowledging the impact of the additional stress, he did not feel his mental health was the problem it had been in the past. He did not want to take a daily SSRI again and met both NHS and local prescribing criteria for initiating dapoxetine.

He used this on an as-required basis until his partner achieved a further pregnancy which resulted in a healthy infant, after which he was able to stop the medication.

Loss of Sexual Desire

This is a complex area and the relevance of physical treatment, namely testosterone (T), is dependent on appropriate and accurate diagnosis in symptomatic men. The basis of diagnosis is a persistently lowered free testosterone level in samples taken in the morning, usually before 10 a.m. In order to obtain the free levels most laboratories will provide a SHBG (sex hormone-binding globulin) level and, if relevant from results and clinical details, will also run prolactin, luteinizing hormone, follicle-stimulating hormone and thyroid function tests. It is useful to know the local testing laboratory's 'normal range' and also local endocrinology guidelines on testosterone replacement therapy. This is especially true for late-onset hypogonadism which has a wide range of sexual and non-sexual symptoms and for which many specialists are now moving away from replacement therapy. Lifestyle modification is likely to be especially important for those men with borderline results, for whom obesity and insulin resistance are significant, and may be thought of as first-line therapy by many endocrine specialists.

There are four approaches to testosterone replacement therapy (TRT). The transdermal approach is currently the most commonly used:

1. *Oral:* Testosterone undecanoate is absorbed via the hepatic lymphatic system and then to the systemic circulation. Since this is dependent on lipid content of ingested food, it results in a very variable testosterone level over 24 hours.
2. *Transbuccal:* This is delivered via a sustained release muco-adhesive buccal testosterone tablet that needs to be applied and removed every 12 hours since it is not fully dissolvable.
3. *Transdermal:* These are used daily and give more uniform testosterone levels throughout a 24-hour period. They are available as patches and gels, and the latter give less skin reaction and normalized testosterone levels although caution must be taken with regard to partner transfer within the first 12 hours after application.
4. *Injectable:* These vary in half-life from weekly to 12 weekly preparations, the latter being safer, more acceptable and better able to produce levels within a normal range.

Follow-up protocols may vary, but after stabilisation most teams would follow up at least annually. Prostate-specific antigen (PSA), digital rectal examination (DRE) and haematocrit are the most crucial investigations. Consideration of PSA trends and DRE will inform the need for prostatic biopsy (9). Treatments of thyroid and prolactin disorders are not within the scope of this chapter but should be recognised as potential causes of loss of desire as well as other sexual dysfunctions.

Physical Treatments for Female Sexual Problems

Vaginismus

Consideration here needs to be given to the meaning of physical treatment. The majority of male disorder treatments are pharmacological, and most are well-established. This is not the case for partial or complete vaginismus. However, in the same way that vacuum pump devices are useful for ED, the use of vaginal trainers/dilators may also have a place. These are a set of low-friction hollow plastic tubes that are graded in size from approximately index finger size to the largest, which is equivalent to a larger-than-average erect penis. They are used with lubricant and either held by the fingers or an applicator that accompanies most makers' sets. They are prescribable on the NHS in the United Kingdom which is an indicator of their establishment in the treatment of female sexual disorders.

The latter are never likely to be the sole treatment modality for vaginismus; the psychosexual element is likely to be of greater importance. However, for some women the dilators at least allow a tangible way of initiating discussion around perceptions of vaginal and penile size and can facilitate a gradual understanding of the true flexibility of the vaginal muscles and walls. They may be used alongside or following other behavioural therapies such as self-examination and Kegel's pelvic floor exercises, named after an American gynaecologist who first developed these exercises in 1948. They are helpful and used within the psychosomatic examination so that learning about their use and the individual woman's vagina can be shared.

Botulinum toxin is sometimes used although this is not well-established as a sole treatment. There is evidence that it may work better in cultures in which virginity is prized. It may be that in these cases it is the phobia about the loss of virginity rather than penetration that is the main problem (10).

Painful Intercourse

There is overlap between vaginismus and dyspareunia in aetiology and management, and vaginal trainers/dilators may have their place for some women experiencing painful intercourse.

Again, treatments are not just pharmacological, and it is interesting that there are a considerable number of options to facilitate women to have penetrative sex, perhaps mirroring the considerable treatment options to allow men to achieve an erection sufficient enough to also achieve penetration. Historically this is the area of lovemaking to have received the most attention and arguably still does.

Physical treatments will largely be dictated by the diagnosis category. There may be overlap of diagnoses, and psychosexual support is crucial even when the pain is established to be of a predominantly physical aetiology.

1. *Topical Treatments and Lubricants:* These may be useful when a specific skin/vulval condition has been recognised as either the sole cause of pain or one aetiological factor among many. From a psychosexual perspective, it is also helpful to encourage the woman to explore her feelings around touching the vulval area in order to apply or insert specific treatments.

    a. *Lignocaine gel/cream:* These are licenced to be used topically in the vulval area and some women may benefit from their use 5 minutes prior to self-examination, use of trainers or before penetrative sex. Ideally, the underlying cause for pain should be clarified and working towards withdrawing their use the main aim.

    b. *Soap substitutes:* These can be useful longer term or intermittently where pain is secondary to irritation caused by dryness in association with other skin conditions like eczema, post-menopausal atrophy or reactions to other treatments such as anti-fungals. The most commonly used are mixtures of benzalkonium chloride, chlorhexidine, isopropyl myristate and liquid paraffin.

    c. *Dermatitis treatment creams:* Emollients and topical steroids can both be used in specific vulval skin conditions to ease pain and irritation. Again, diagnosis is crucial, often requiring skin biopsy, so treatment is often initiated in secondary care, ideally at multidisciplinary vulval clinics where input from dermatology and gynaecology is available.

    d. *Candidal vaginal and external topical treatments:* It is worth considering these both as a cause for some women with superficial dyspareunia as well as a treatment for others who may not have had their fungal infection treated adequately. The former sometimes have pain because of a local reaction to their topical treatment and may do better with oral anti-fungals. The latter may feel their persistent pain with penetration is due to a different cause but in fact when they are re-examined, there still a florid vulvovaginitis requiring a longer treatment programme.

e. *Lubricants and vaginal moisturisers:* There are many commercial products available and some are NHS prescribable. There is evidence that polyacrylic acid vaginal moisturiser can be as effective as topical oestrogen for some women (11). However, it is important that the woman finds a product that is suitable for her needs and that she finds easy to access and use.

2. *Injectables:* Injection with botulinum locally has not been shown to have consistent benefit above placebo.

3. *Oral Analgesia:* The commonly used medications are the tricyclic anti-depressants (TCAs) amitriptyline and nortriptyline, and the anti-convulsants gabapentin and pregabalin. This group is used widely for many chronic pain syndromes and is part of a multidisciplinary approach to the treatment of pelvic pain and vulvodynia. There are no universally agreed treatment regimens, but it is usual to start at a low dose of the treatment and titrate up according to response and side effects. If an effective well-tolerated dose is achieved then treatment may continue for several months or years before withdrawal of medication again over a period of time can be achieved.

4. *Hormone Replacement Therapy:* Hormone replacement therapy (HRT) is available in oral, transdermal and topical preparations, and the replacement of oestrogen can have a significant benefit for women suffering dyspareunia as a result of changes in lubrication and thinning of vulval and vaginal tissues. Obviously, women may have other troublesome issues as a result of the climacteric and may therefore choose oral or transdermal HRT. However, for women with dyspareunia, topical HRT is the most appropriate, and with modern low-dose pessary preparations the impact on the endometrium is minimal and monitoring biopsy or the addition of a progestogen is not required. In addition, low-dose topical oestrogen may be suitable for women with a past history of breast cancer. In this situation it is necessary to liaise with the women's oncologist before initiating any therapy and obviously only if she is comfortable with the idea of hormone treatment.

5. *Physical Therapy:* This could be thought of as an extension of the psychosomatic examination. There is opportunity to discuss pelvic floor muscles, and explore the woman's ability to be aware of and contract and relax these as part of the 'teacher-patient' aspect of the examination. A continuation of this may be self-exploration and a more formal approach to Kegel's pelvic floor exercises and relaxation techniques. For some women, taking things further with electromyography biofeedback sessions and deep massage of the pelvic floor by specialist physiotherapists may also be helpful (12).

6. *Other Therapies:* Other treatment modalities are explored within pain, vulval and pelvic pain clinics. Some specialists have used spinal block to treat severe cases. Laser therapy is said to help with pain (as well as incontinence and vaginal sensation) but is not available on the NHS at this time. Fat implants are also being looked at for vulval pain secondary to severe cases of lichen sclerosus.

CASE 4

VR is a 30-year-old doctor who had always had problems with painful penetrative sex. It had been a mixture of deep and superficial and she had had normal scans in the past. She had seen a sexual therapist and received cognitive behavioural therapy, which she said was useful in a general way but did not help with the sexual issues. She was taking amitriptyline for chronic headache and low back pain, had seen physiotherapists with regard to the latter and practised yoga regularly.

Examination was useful in a number of ways. There was evidence of fissuring and inflammation that suggested skin problems and she did feel that the discomfort had been more superficial of late. It also allowed discussion about what she felt about her vagina – her fantasies as opposed to her logical medical knowledge – and allowed introduction of the idea of self-examination once the external skin issues were resolved.

She was seen at a local specialist vulval clinic and the changes were felt to be due to candidiasis. She was treated for this as well as being prescribed soap substitutes and emollients. They also gave her some lignocaine cream to use before intercourse and asked the pelvic floor physiotherapist to see her regarding the pain. She had two sessions of pelvic floor massage.

When she came back to clinic, she recognised that externally the skin felt better and that her low back pain had improved with the massage. She felt unable to try intercourse at this point and I reflected that a lot had been done 'to' her rather than her own involvement with that part of her. She agreed, and we continued with a joint self- and psychosomatic examination. The tenderness externally had definitely improved and she was able to explore her own vagina and muscles and dispel the fantasies.

She requested and was able to use the vaginal trainers and gradually give herself the confidence to resume trying intercourse. During the sessions it also became clear that her long-term partner was controlling emotionally and that sexual sessions were dominated by his demands.

Eventually their relationship ended and she is now in a new relationship and able to enjoy a pain-free and pleasurable sex life.

Problems with Female Orgasm

There are no UK-licenced pharmacological agents to treat difficulty with clitoral or vaginal orgasm. If there is an issue with strength of physical arousal as part of aetiology, then devices such as vibrators used internally or externally may help. There is also a device that can be fitted onto the women's finger that has a stippled surface said to increase sensation and some women find the clitoral suction cup useful as it increases blood flow to the external part of the clitoris. These physical devices are not prescribable but reasonably costed.

In the case of spinal cord injury, the implantation of a sacral nerve stimulator may help.

Sexual Arousal Disorders

Vibrators and clitoral suction devices may be used, and lubricants can also be important. Where arousal is affected by a hormonal decrease in lubrication then HRT may be considered as part of management of arousal problems, and there is also hormone precursor replacement therapy being developed that may be useful in the future.

The PDE5s did not prove useful in initial trials looking at female arousal problems. Their use has been recommended off licence in specific patients with neurological disorders. Other agents such as alprostadil, levodopa and apomorphine have not been shown to be effective enough for further exploration or licencing (13).

Persistent Genital Arousal Syndrome

Although poorly understood and thankfully rare, persistent genital arousal syndrome is worth mentioning here. The SSRIs that might have side effects of suppressed arousal and are used for male premature ejaculation seem to have an unpredictable effect on this condition. There is some evidence that the SNRIs (serotonin and noradrenaline re-uptake inhibitors) such as duloxetine and venlafaxine may help, as can the anti-epileptic and mood-stabilising medication valproic acid. Topical anesthetics and ice can be tried although these are unlikely to be of lasting relief (14).

Loss of Sexual Desire

Again, there are no physical treatments licenced in the United Kingdom for this problem. Testosterone therapy is not licenced here nor in the United States and the 300 microgram patch remains licenced in Europe for surgical menopause only. The implant is still available and licenced as HRT. It is available privately off licence but its long-term effects on breast cancer and insulin resistance in women are not known (15). Levels should be monitored and oestrogen therapy given alongside in order to avoid creating an increased androgen:oestrogen ratio such as that found in polycystic ovarian syndrome where it is linked to an increased cardiovascular disease risk.

The problem seems to be that although some studies showed an improvement in desire measured by rating questionnaires, the mechanism of action of testosterone in women remains poorly understood, especially in relation to sexual function. Many years of use of the combined oral contraceptive, for instance, has not demonstrated an increase in sexual desire in women using pills with a more androgenic progestogen component and studies do not seem to show increased sexual function in women with PCOS.

Tibolone similarly is not licenced for the treatment of loss of desire and should be used considering the same risk:benefit ratio as HRT for an individual woman.

Flibanserin is a centrally-acting agent licenced in the United States 2 years ago for the treatment of female sexual interest/arousal disorder (FSIAD) in pre-menopausal women. More recent studies have also shown some evidence for efficacy in treating hypoactive sexual desire disorder in post-menopausal women (16). However, studies into this and other newer agents such as bremelanotide are sponsored by the pharmaceutical industry, and there has been controversy in the United States about the awarding of the US Food and Drug Administration licence.

Summary

This overview of physical treatments for sexual problems will hopefully have provided an insight into a significant field of management. As stated at the beginning, it can only be used as an introduction and clinicians will develop their understanding of some of these approaches dependent on the specialism and environment in which they work.

As holistic healthcare professionals with training and experience in psychodynamic approaches as well as clinical patient experience, we are perhaps best placed to allow people to understand the treatment options available to them. The cases in this chapter hopefully give a few examples of the value to our patients of using appropriate physical treatments in conjunction with IPM approaches to managing complex problems.

REFERENCES

1. *British National Formulary 72*. London: BMJ Group and Pharmaceutical Press, 2016, 735–739.
2. Porst H, Buvat J, Meuleman E et al. Intracavernous Alprostadil Alfadex – An effective and well tolerated treatment for erectile dysfunction. Results of a long-term European study. *Int J Impot Res* 1998;10:225–231.
3. Porst H. Erectile dysfunction. In Y Reisman, H Porst, L Lowenstein, F Tripodi, PS Kirana (Eds.), *The European Society of Sexual Medicine (ESSM) Manual of Sexual Medicine* (2nd updated ed.). Amsterdam: MEDIX, 2015, 48644.
4. Porst H. Erectile dysfunction. In Y Reisman, H Porst, L Lowenstein, F Tripodi, PS Kirana (Eds.), *ESSM Manual of Sexual Medicine* (2nd updated ed.). Amsterdam: MEDIX, 2015, 293.
5. Pahlajani G, Raina R, Jones S et al. Vacuum devices revisited: Early penile rehabilitation following prostate cancer therapy. *J Sex Med* 2012;9(4):1182–1189.
6. Kamischeke A, Nieschlag E. Update on medical treatment of ejaculatory disorders. *Int J Androl* 2002;25:333–344.
7. McMahon CG, Althof SE, Kaufman JM et al. Efficacy and safety of dapoxetine for the treatment of premature ejaculation. *J Sex Med* 2011;8:524–539.
8. Dinsmore WW, Hackett G, Goldmeier D et al. Topical eutectic mixture for premature ejaculation (TEMPE): A novel aerosol delivery form of lidocaine-prilocaine for treating premature ejaculation. *Br J Urol Int* 2007;99:369–375.
9. Corona G, Maggi M. Hormonal disorders and male sexual dysfunction. In Y Reisman, H Porst, L Lowenstein, F Tripodi, PS Kirana (Eds.), *ESSM Manual of Sexual Medicine* (2nd updated ed.). Amsterdam: MEDIX, 2015, 373–375.

10. Ghazizadeh S, Nikzad M. Botulinum toxin in the treatment of refractory vaginismus. *Obstet Gynaecol* 2004;104:722–725.
11. Fernandes T, Costa-Paiva LH, Pinto-Neto AM. Efficacy of vaginally applied estrogen, testosterone or polyacrylic acid on sexual function in post-menopausal women; a randomized controlled trial. *J Sex Med* 2014;11:1262–1270.
12. Peterson CD. Sexual pain disorders. In Y Reisman, H Porst, L Lowenstein, F Tripodi, PS Kirana (Eds.), *ESSM Manual of Sexual Medicine* (2nd updated ed.). Amsterdam: MEDIX, 2015, 911.
13. Brotto L, Bitzer J, Laan E et al. Women's sexual desire and arousal disorders. *J Sex Med* 2010;7(1):586–614.
14. Paraskevi-Sofia K. Sexual desire and arousal disorders in women. In Y Reiman, H Porst, L Lowenstein, F Tripodi, PS Kirana (Eds.), *ESSM Manual of Sexual Medicine* (2nd updated ed.). Amsterdam: MEDIX, 2015, 887.
15. Kingsberg S. Testosterone treatment for hypoactive sexual desire disorder in post-menopausal women. *J Sex Med* 2007;4:227–234.
16. Portman DJ, Brown L, Yuan J et al. Flibanserin in post-menopausal women with hypoactive sexual desire disorder: Results of the PLUMERIA study. *J Sex Med* 2017;14(6):834–842.

9

Sex and Disability

Nichola Chater

Introduction

This chapter draws on several years' experience of applying the Institute of Psychosexual Medicine (IPM) approach in a neurorehabilitation setting, currently at Walkergate Park in Newcastle-upon-Tyne, and previously in both a community service and a brain injury rehabilitation unit in Liverpool. The type of work means that some understanding of other therapeutic models is important and sometimes used in practice; this is illustrated. It is not uncommon for a patient and their partner to attend clinic together, and this is explored. Although one chapter cannot act as a manual for understanding and managing sexual problems related to disability, some factual and practical information is included, and further resources are suggested.

Attitudes and Expectations

As in all aspects of psychosexual medicine it is important to be aware of one's own expectations and beliefs, and consider whether these may factor in a particular consultation. For example, working in a neurorehabilitation setting I have found a common belief that sexual problems are too complicated to address without the right experience or training. This leads to a feeling of inadequacy and avoidance. The IPM approach encourages making therapeutic use of such insights; for example, if a trained health professional can feel overwhelmed and inadequate, might not a patient have similar anxieties and questions? Could avoidance also be a part of a patient's response to sexual function, or their partner's?

CASE 1

Norah, recovering from a stroke, described how her husband changed the subject, or replied 'Well let's worry about that later', every time she tried to speak to him about having sex. She believed this was because he no longer found her attractive, and she was anxious he might find her disability too much in the longer term. She asked if her husband could also attend and the doctor agreed. At the second appointment with her husband Norah eventually shared these feelings; her husband responded that she was right, he did avoid the subject, but because he had no idea whether sex would be possible, and he was frightened that he might cause her harm.

Part of a therapeutic approach may be helping a person to identify where the expectations or beliefs of others might be a factor in the clinical picture. Arguably, it is particularly important to consider this with regard to disability and sex. Writing in a blog Keith R. Murfee-DeConcini (1) describes how other people's views on disability impact on relationships. He cites examples of how people with disabilities may be judged differently from others in terms of forming a relationship; also assumptions may be made that a partner would be a caregiver, and expectations that difficulty in a relationship would be due to disability. There is research evidence to support this, for example a qualitative study on attitudes towards disability and sexuality from Alberta (2) found a dominant view that people with disability were asexual; they highlight the risk that such a view might be internalised, with potentially damaging implications for self-esteem and sexuality.

Much connected with disability can become 'medicalised', with powerful experts giving diagnoses and treatments and offering prognosis. Life can fill up with the need for equipment, adaptations, appointments, examinations, treatments and forms to be completed – for some this comes as a shock with an acquired illness or injury in adult life, for others it has been part of their growth and development since childhood. It may be difficult in this context to develop or maintain sexuality. Sometimes an appropriate role for a clinician in psychosexual medicine is to draw attention to this, or to give permission for sexuality to be talked about.

CASE 2

Paul was recovering from a multiple sclerosis (MS) relapse: 'I can't get an erection all the time, and sometimes I can't use it. Can you fix it? Is there a pill or something you can do?' This consultation could have been managed as erectile dysfunction, perhaps discussing a trial of a prescription for phosphodiesterase type 5 inhibitor. 'Sex feels very important to you', the doctor observed. 'Yes, it is, before I was ill we used to have a really active and varied sex life, now it feels as if there's nothing'. The doctor sensed the sadness, 'You feel you have lost a lot?' The patient was quiet, and his partner spoke, 'I think he's afraid he might lose me, that I won't stay with him; I miss the sex too, but part of me doesn't want to try anything. I'm so tired, life is so busy, and I'm scared about how he'll feel if we try and it fails'. The doctor was quiet as the couple spoke to each other, eventually agreeing they could make time do some things they thought were fun together, and for now just cuddle.

While considering the possible effect of 'medicalisation' on sexuality, it is worth mentioning the question of assessment. There are a number of clinical and electrophysiological well-validated assessment methods that might be used, as advocated by Courtois et al. (3) for patients with neurological problems. As yet these have not been used in the clinic at Walkergate Park Neurorehabilitation Centre.

The reasons for this are: clinical work allowing therapeutic change has been reported by patients without the use of formal measures; a concern of the clinicians to avoid the possibility of the assessment tool dictating the agenda; possible 'distancing' of the clinician or the patient from emotions, and the therapeutic use of these, especially if physiological/electrophysiological assessments are used. It is an area for re-consideration and there is ongoing discussion.

Therapeutic Approach

The brief consideration of attitudes and expectations should demonstrate that there is no single therapeutic approach which can be appropriately used in every circumstance. This section outlines some models which can be used, and drawn on when appropriate, alongside the skills developed through IPM training.

Some clinicians have found a conceptual scheme for behavioural management of sexual problems called the PLISSIT model (4), helpful when working in the field of disability. It describes a range of interventions of increasing complexity: permission, limited information, specific suggestion, intensive therapy. The model has been used in neurorehabilitation settings to encourage all staff to appreciate their therapeutic contribution to ensuring sexuality can be addressed in patient care (5); all staff may signal permission to discuss sexuality, for example using open-ended questions, or more focussed comments such as 'some people have found this medication has affected their sex drive'. Certain staff may give limited information or make specific suggestions, for example how to manage a catheter during sex. It is likely that very few will offer 'intensive therapy', but all staff should be able to connect a patient with an appropriate person who can. The model was further developed in 2007 by Taylor and Davis (6), as the expanded PLISSIT (ex-PLISSIT) because they observed that health professionals tended to signal permission mainly by leaving around leaflets, which they felt was more part of the second stage, limited information, and they wanted to promote reflection as an integral part of each stage, by both the patient and the practitioner. In this respect, it might be seen to have some overlap with IPM work. Taylor and Davis encouraged the understanding that sexuality could be a part of every aspect of care, and that sexuality may change.

Guidelines for interdisciplinary practice in addressing sexuality after stroke (7) were produced in response to evidence for the importance of sexuality on quality of life after stroke and evidence that it was often not addressed in practice. People from different clinical disciplines were asked to consider how their professional code of practice was relevant to supporting the sexuality of their patients. The final document summarises each code of practice, lists potential issues impacting on sexuality and the possible role of clinicians from the different disciplines. It shows that sexuality can be considered in clinical care by most professional groups working with stroke patients, and in that regard, it helpfully overlaps with ex-PLISSIT. It is likely that the guidelines will be relevant also to other clinical areas.

A model from MS practice by Foley and Werner (8) can be useful for providing a structure to consider possible causes for sexual problems related to MS which might then be addressed. The model divides the potential issues into primary (direct damage or impact on sexual pathways or organs); secondary (indirect effect on sexual function, e.g. pain, fatigue, continence, spasticity, depression, medication); and tertiary (psychosocial issues). The division should not be taken as indicating a hierarchy of importance or relevance, or as an order for structuring a clinical consultation; this depends on what the patient brings, and when. But the framework can be helpful for reflection, or as a prompt to what could be important, and again, may be useful in clinical practice wider than MS Foley and Werner also advocate the use of modified sensate focus as part of treatment. This is an adaptation of Masters and Johnson's behavioural techniques (9), described as 'body-mapping'. It can be helpful in encouraging or re-gaining intimacy, and in identifying particular areas of the body where touch is experienced as pain secondary to neurological changes; this can then be taken into account during sexual activity.

Addressing sexual problems in the context of neurological disorder not uncommonly requires management of bowel and bladder function, spasticity, or giving attention to other physiological disorders of function. For some clinicians, this may be part of their knowledge and skill set, but for others the role may be enabling the patient to talk about sexual problems, identifying how particular disorders of function are impacting on this, and then ensuring that appropriate referral to a colleague is achieved. The psychosexual clinician should continue to review the patient while specific problems are addressed by others, thus protecting time for observing and reflecting on feelings.

It is probably appropriate that clinicians offering sexual counselling in the context of disability should be able to talk to their patients about how a particular disorder may affect sexual function using their knowledge of anatomy and physiology of sexual response, and also be able to offer some practical suggestions. For example, things like positioning, lubrication, reviewing medication for potential impact, or considering the use of possible sex aids (e.g. high-frequency vibrators can be tried to augment diminished sensation). This is further explored in the section 'The clinician as a teacher'. It is important to be honest about not knowing or having all the answers, and commit to finding out what might be helpful; this shared un-knowing and learning together can be empowering for patients, who often obtain a lot of information from a range of sources and may value being able to discuss it.

The Clinician as a Teacher

An interactive website developed for women in India (www.sexualityanddisability.org) (10) describes itself as 'constructed as a bunch of questions a woman with a disability might have – about her body, about the mechanics and dynamics of having sex, about the complexities of being in an intimate relationship or having children, about unvoiced fears or experiences of encountering abuse in some form'. All such issues have been raised, at different times, and by men as well as women, in the sex and relationships clinic at Walkergate Park Neurorehabilitation Centre. Giving information about altered function and the possible impact on sexuality has been a significant part of the work, and sometimes has needed to be offered in small amounts over a prolonged period. It is not uncommon for a patient to ask for the same information to be offered to their partner. While it is important to consider how the anatomy and physiology might be relevant, it is also important to avoid assumptions and generalisations. There are particular considerations if a patient has brain injury; this is discussed further under issues for particular groups.

Training with the IPM encourages understanding of the interplay of mind and body in sexuality, and places a particular emphasis on the therapeutic use of physical examination. In the neurorehabilitation context, physical examination has sometimes been requested by patients, like Sam, whose concern was, 'Am I normal down there?' Sometimes guided self-examination has been valuable as a teaching resource, although more commonly drawings, diagrams and models have been used to teach both general anatomy and physiology related to sexual function, and how a particular diagnosis might affect this. Rarely do patients come asking for such help; usually they have been referred because of a problem with some physical aspect of having sexual intercourse.

CASE 3

Sue was referred for 'problems with sex'. In the clinic Sue explained she had never attempted sexual activity before, but now had a partner. She enjoyed kissing her partner, but 'went rigid' when her partner attempted to caress her. Sue said she 'wanted to have sex because that was what everyone did with a partner'. Then after a pause she said, 'But I don't know anything about it'. She described 'a great sense of relief' at being able to ask what she thought were 'stupid questions', she said she'd had some sex education at school but not really understood it, and all the time found it difficult to concentrate because she wanted to ask, 'But what about me, am I the same as everyone else?' (Sue has spina bifida.)

Matters of General Concern

A number of practical concerns about sexual function may be common to people across diagnostic groups; it is not possible to address all such issues within this brief overview.

Catheters

Common questions from clinicians and patients concern catheters. A supra-pubic catheter should have little impact on penetrative sexual intercourse; similarly, if intermittent self-catheterisation is practised the bladder can be drained just before sexual intercourse to help reduce urine leakage. If an indwelling urethral catheter is present the urologist might advise whether the catheter can be temporarily spigoted, or in some cases, a patient taught to remove and re-insert a catheter. Breaks in the integrity of the system, and frequent removal and re-insertion do, however, increase the risk of urinary tract infection. If the catheter is left in place women can fold the catheter back out of the way, perhaps taping it to the lower abdomen, and men can fold back the catheter along the erect penis, sometimes using a condom rather than tape to hold the catheter in place. Lubrication is helpful, and water-based lubricants should be used, rather than petroleum jelly type, to avoid damaging the catheter. The risk of urinary tract infections should be minimised by attention to hygiene before sexual activity.

Some patients may find a catheter challenges their perceptions of sexual attractiveness, it is appropriate that this is addressed in the psychosexual consultation.

Medication Affecting Sexual Function

Another common concern is medication use. Several drugs used in cardiology, neurology or mental health, among other disciplines, can have adverse effects on sexual function as dealt with elsewhere in this book. It may be possible to consider an alternative medication, or to consider the timing of the doses in relation to sexual activity. Sometimes a temporary 'medication holiday' may be possible; discussing this with a pharmacist could be helpful.

Spasticity

This can impact significantly on sexual function. A simple approach is to first consider whether there are any factors provoking spasticity, such as an infection or unmanaged pain. The timing of sexual activity in relation to any medications to manage spasticity may be important, for example if sexual activity is attempted in the morning it could be helpful to wait until about half an hour after anti-spasticity medication has been taken. Sometimes changing the body position using supportive cushions or pillows can be very effective, and I have worked with a physiotherapy colleague to look at bespoke positioning systems to reduce spasticity. Sexual excitement itself can provoke spasticity and, if painful or intrusive, an increase in medication dose to cover this can be helpful. If tight spasms affect particular muscles important in sexual activity, for example spasms of the thigh adductor muscles, then focal treatment to relax these muscles with botulinum toxin may be very helpful.

Fatigue

Other examples of general issues include: sex and fatigue, positioning and possible sex aids. Fatigue is a common problem with many neurological disorders, and particularly in MS but also following a stroke or head injury. It is likely patients with such conditions will have access to advice on fatigue management as part of managing their condition. What may not be appreciated is the impact of fatigue on sexual drive. Fatigue and apparent lack of interest in sex can be misunderstood by sexual partners. This might be explored in sexual counselling; also useful is identifying times when fatigue is less of a problem, and thinking about the timing of sexual activity in relation to this.

General Resources

There are some helpful resources available; one such is a book about sex written for people who live with chronic pain, disabilities or illness (11). It is wide ranging and may be useful also to partners, and supporting clinicians. As well as general topics some more detailed information for specific conditions is included. Also available is a succinct book written by doctors working in sexuality and reproductive healthcare with practical advice to clinicians (12).

A lot of information can be found from particular specialist societies, often under a diagnosis, and it is worthwhile looking on websites for whether a society provides leaflets related to sexual function. Much is available without charge, and membership of the society may not be required to access these resources. An occupational therapist working with the MS Society of Western Australia has compiled an extensive summary of sex aids, including assisting with positioning, which are 'More Accessible' products; the products are not necessarily designed with disability in mind but she has particularly considered this in her review (13).

Particular Issues: Brain Injury and Spinal Cord Injury

Brain Injury

When a patient has brain damage or developmental delay of any form, including learning disability, it is important to take account of their cognitive function. For example, can they concentrate, and for how long? Are they better able to understand and remember if information is presented in a particular way? What understanding do they have and what words do they use? Can they conceptualise abstract ideas? Is the brain injury affecting behaviour, personality or mood, and how might that impact on a relationship or their capacity to consent to sexual activity and their ability to understand and assess or manage their risk?

A range of work may be necessary to address issues such as those in the following sections.

Potential Interventions – Brain Injuries

- Help a person, their family and partner to understand the effects of brain injury
- Provide support to re-learn (or learn) and practise general social skills
- Provide support or counselling for a person with an acquired brain injury, and their partner to come to terms with what has happened
- Encourage re-learning (or learning) and re-engaging in sexual activity, perhaps using a modified Masters and Johnson approach to encourage communication, turn taking, intimate contact and eventually consider penetrative sexual intercourse

Depending on the local setup some of this work might be addressed in groups, and with other colleagues (e.g. psychologist, occupational therapist, nurse) during a general rehabilitation or social skills programme, but some will be better done with individuals and their partners, if they have partners. As might be appreciated, this can take time, sometimes brief work over a prolonged period is better to allow for fatigue and cognitive ability. Use of teaching materials, as mentioned above, can be helpful. Aloni and Katz (14) have produced a training manual derived from clinical practice and research evidence, and although written for work in the context of acquired brain injury some of the material is relevant to people with learning disability.

Spinal Injuries

Men and women with spinal cord injury can experience problems with sexual function such as erectile and ejaculatory dysfunction and fertility concerns in men, and in women problems with arousal and orgasm. The neurology of sexual arousal is complex and the type of problems experienced will vary depending on the level of the spinal cord injury (15). Erectile dysfunction can be managed with the same treatments offered to men without a spinal cord injury, including trial of phosphodiesterase-5 inhibitors, vacuum devices, intracavernosal injections and penile prostheses (see Chapter 8). Depending on the level of the spinal cord injury there will be diminished or altered sensation for both men and women, and women may have reduced vaginal lubrication. Managing the physiological changes may well be part of the care offered from a spinal injuries centre.

A key role of the psychosexual physician could be in these potential interventions

Potential Interventions – Spinal Injuries

- Helping patients to understand the reasons for physiological changes
- Exploring emotions
- Discussing and identifying altered physical sensations, perhaps helping a person to recognise the changes happening within their body that can indicate sexual arousal
- Supporting the patient in adapting sexual techniques, behaviours, beliefs and expectations, possibly working on modified sensate focus, as noted previously

Some patients will ask if their partner can/should attend; if this is offered it is probably best to have some shared appointments, while maintaining other appointments with the patient only, to ensure opportunity within the safety of a consultation to explore feelings, some of which may be difficult to express/share with a partner present. Ongoing relationship counselling is beyond the remit of psychosexual therapy, but helping a couple to identify a need for it may be.

CASE 4

Jane came to the clinic referred by her general practitioner for advice about sexual function after a spinal injury 18 months previously. Jane was very well dressed and had neat hair and makeup. She smiled, and sounded very cheerful as she asked for some 'pointers about managing my spasms if we have sex and some ideas about being a bit dry'. As the doctor took some information about Jane, her spinal injury and the medications she was using to manage spasticity, Jane commented, 'I'm managing very well, you know, everyone says so'. 'That's an interesting comment', the doctor observed. 'Well I am', she said, 'I mean I don't get angry, or at least I don't show it, and I'm not sad'. 'You say you don't show being angry', repeated the doctor, 'but you've felt angry?' Jane paused, looked away, and fiddled with her wedding ring, the doctor was quiet. 'I did feel angry, very angry... I found my husband had been watching porn, he never did before; at least I don't think he did. I felt like he'd hit me, and now I don't know what to do. I can't say anything'. Jane paused crying a little, and trying not to show it, she went on, 'I can't be angry, can I, because it's my fault, he wouldn't need to watch the porn if I wasn't like this'. The doctor noticed a feeling of being overwhelmed, and confused, uncertain about how to help the patient, and shared it with the patient, then asked, 'I wonder if that might be how you feel?' 'It is, I don't know what to do, there is a counsellor at the practice, and I've thought about going, maybe I will'.

Particular Aspects of Physiology of Sexual Response in Spinal Cord Injury

The role of the autonomic nervous system in sexual arousal and orgasm is complex, with involvement of the sympathetic and parasympathetic pathways, their associated nerves and plexuses connecting to the brain via the spinal cord. Additionally, animal models and human studies using functional magnetic resonance have shown involvement of the brainstem medulla, which links to the vagus nerve and other brain areas from the medulla (16). This is important because it is a non-spinal pathway, and women with complete spinal cord injury have reported experiencing sensations of menstrual pain, cervical and vaginal stimulation and orgasm. Awareness of the potential for sexual stimulation via this root may be helpful for women with spinal injury. Komisaruk et al. (17) researching in this field, believe there is potential for patients to use real-time brain imaging and self-stimulation as a biofeedback tool to improve sexual function.

One clinical concern in spinal injury is autonomic dysreflexia/hyper-reflexia (AD). This is the loss of regulation, and loss of co-ordination of the complementary roles of the sympathetic and autonomic nervous systems. It is associated with spinal injury, particularly at levels of injury above T6, but can sometimes occur in other neurological conditions such as MS, Guillain–Barré syndrome and brain injury. AD can lead to cardiovascular emergencies (e.g. stroke, myocardial infarction), retinal haemorrhages or pulmonary oedema. Sexual activity, particularly ejaculation, can provoke AD. One part of management is the use of an antihypertensive (e.g. nifedipine or glyceryl trinitrate [GTN]) sometimes as a prophylaxis. If this is the case then patients should not use phosphodiesterase type-5 as part of management of sexual dysfunction because of the risk of an excessive drop in blood pressure. For a patient seeking help with sexual dysfunction who has been diagnosed with AD, it would be wise to liaise with the team who first diagnosed and managed their AD.

Courtois et al. (18), researching the phenomenon of orgasm, postulate that it involves autonomic dysreflexia, but in the absence of neurological damage an immediate and powerful supra-spinal inhibition acts to rapidly lower blood pressure to normal within 2 minutes, and quickly restore normal function. A degree of AD may be tolerated by some patients with neurological damage and is not clinically harmful. Courtois et al. suggest that this can be useful to help patients with spinal injury recognise arousal and orgasm; it might include for example cardiovascular signs (e.g. altered heart rate, flushing); other autonomic features (e.g. desire to void, bowel changes, sweating, goose pimples); and muscular changes (e.g. contractions, or increased spasms/spasticity).

Fertility

Fertility may be a concern. In general, spinal cord injury does not impact on a woman's fertility after an initial phase of recovery, which might include several months of amenorrhoea. Men may have problems with ejaculation and reduced quality of sperm. Management will be by a specialist centre, with a potential collaboration of urology, fertility specialists and spinal injury services. Such a centre may have psychology or specialist counselling, if not, the psychosexual clinician might support the patient and their partner. It may be helpful to have some understanding of how sperm can be collected so as to appreciate how any negative feelings may have arisen, or alternatively, how feelings may have necessarily been suppressed. This is outlined in the following text; more complete information is referenced (19).

The first line of treatment may be with a medical vibrator, in a clinic or hospital environment (although sometimes patients purchase and trial their own high-frequency vibrators at home). The aim is to stimulate the dorsal nerve of the penis by applying the vibrator to the glans penis; sometimes if an enhanced effect is needed a vibrator is used which 'sandwiches' the penis. Careful monitoring for possible AD will be maintained throughout, including continuous blood pressure monitoring. With spinal cord injuries above T10 most men will achieve an ejaculation, however it is much less likely with lower injuries because of the loss of an intact sympathetic ejaculatory pathway. For lower-level lesions, or when penile vibratory stimulation fails, electroejaculation may be offered. This uses electrical stimulation via the rectum, delivered with the patient lying on their side, sometimes using sedation, sperm collected by another clinician milking the urethra. If retrograde ejaculation, rather than anterograde ejaculation, is thought to be likely the patient may be catheterised first, with a sperm washing buffer instilled in the bladder just before the procedure, and urine then collected and centrifuged. For a small number of men surgical sperm retrieval may be necessary, and there are different ways of achieving this.

Multiple Sclerosis

This is the most common neurological disorder in the United Kingdom; it has an unpredictable course, affects a wide age span, affects both genders and can involve both the brain and the spinal cord. In terms of sexual function much that has been said in this chapter can be relevant. The classification of sexual problems by Foley and Werner (8) into primary, secondary and tertiary illustrates the wide range of problems which may occur. To expand on this a little, common primary disorders include lack of sensation in the perineum, reduced lubrication, difficulty achieving orgasm in both, and problems with erectile dysfunction in men. Secondary factors such as neuropathic pain may mean light touch may be experienced as an unpleasant burning pain. Medication may help this, including a consideration of topical anaesthetic creams, such as lignocaine based. Fatigue is very common and often severe, but may be better or worse at particular times of the day. The timing of sexual activity can be adjusted to allow for this. Spasticity is often present, managed as discussed previously. As a good rule of thumb if patients are experiencing mobility problems it is likely that they may also have problems with bladder, bowel and sexual function, but may not volunteer this. Bowel and bladder problems can result in continence concerns. Other secondary concerns may involve the brain such as cognitive problems, or mood disorders. One of the hardest things for patients, which can impact on their mood or their partner's, is that the disease course cannot be predicted making it difficult for people to adapt. Psychosocial issues indirectly affecting sexual function can be many; for example a need for carers and lack of privacy, transport and access problems restricting social outlets and activities; financial worries; and negative perceptions of disability and body image. In all aspects of disability it is difficult for people to be spontaneous when considering social and leisure activities.

Summary

The IPM approach can contribute to addressing sexual problems related to disability. It is likely that a range of other therapeutic approaches may be required and some of these have been discussed. The clinician may have an important teaching role; some factual and practical information has been discussed and some further resources have been suggested. Work with partners is often appropriate. Work may need several sessions over a prolonged period. Some concerns may be common to a range of conditions, and there are particular issues related to brain injury and spinal cord injury, which have been outlined.

REFERENCES

1. Murfee-DeConcini Keith. Dating with Disabilities. Available from: https://www.yai.org/blog/dating-disabilities Blog date: 15 August 2014. Accessed 12 November 2018.
2. Esmail S, Darry K, Walter A et al. Attitudes and perceptions towards disability and sexuality. *J Disabil Rehabil* 2010;32:1148–1155.
3. Courtois F, Gerard M, Charvier K et al. Assessment of sexual function in women with neurological disorders: A review. *Ann Phys Rehabil Med* 2018;61(4):235–244.
4. Annon JS. *The Behavioural Treatment of Sexual Problems: Brief Therapy*. New York, NY: Harper and Row, 1976.
5. Chandler BJ. Sex and relationships in neurological disability. In RJ Greenwood, MP Barnes, TM McMillan, CD Ward (Eds.), *Handbook of Neurological Rehabilitation* (2nd ed.). Hove, UK: Psychology Press, 2003, 299–312.
6. Taylor B, Davis S. The extended PLISSIT model for addressing the sexual wellbeing of individuals with an acquired disability or chronic illness. *Sex Disabil* 2007;25(3):135–139.
7. Barrett C, White C. *Sexuality After Stroke: SOX Guidelines for Interdisciplinary Practice*. Melbourne: La Trobe University, Australian Research Centre in Sex, Health and Society and The Victorian Stroke Clinical Network, 2014.
8. Foley FW, Werner MA. How MS affects sexuality and intimacy. In R Kalb (Ed.), *Multiple Sclerosis* (5th ed.). New York, NY: Demos Medical, 2012, 147–180.
9. Weiner L, Avery-Clark C. Sensate focus: Clarifying the Masters and Johnson's model. *Sex Relat Ther* 2014;29(3):307–319.
10. Sexuality and disability. Available from: www.sexualityanddisability.org
11. Kaufman M, Silverberg C, Odette F. *The Ultimate Guide to Sex and Disability*. San Francisco, CA: Cleis Press, 2003.
12. Cooper E, Guillebaud J. *Sexuality and Disability A Guide for Everyday Practice*. Oxford, UK: Radcliffe Medical Press, 1999.
13. Higson N. *The MA + Guide. A Guide to More Accessible Sexuality-Related Assistive Technology*. Wilson, WA: The Multiple Sclerosis Society of Western Australia, 2012.
14. Aloni R, Katz S. *Sexual Difficulties After Traumatic Brain Injury and Ways to Deal with It*. Springfield, IL: Thomas Books, 2003.
15. Steadman C, Hubscher C. Sexual function after spinal cord injury: Innervation, assessment, and treatment. *Curr Sex Health Rep* 2016;8:106–115.
16. Komisaruk BR, Gerdes CA, Whipple B. Complete spinal cord injury does not block perceptual responses to genital self-stimulation in women. *Arch Neurol* 1997;54(12):1513–1520.
17. Komisaruk BR, Beyer-Flores C, Whipple B. *The Science of Orgasm*. Baltimore, MD: Johns Hopkins University Press, 2006.
18. Courtois F, Charvier K, Vezina J-G et al. Assessing and conceptualizing orgasm after a spinal cord injury. *BJU Int* 2011;108(10):1624–1633.
19. Ibrahim E, Lynne CM, Brackett NL. Male fertility following spinal cord injury: An update. *Andrology* 2016;4(1):13–26.

10

Basic Communication Skills: The Here and Now/There and Then

Gillian Vanhegan

KEY POINTS

- Understand that the practitioner is the unknowing clinician
- Allow the patient to lead the consultation
- Notice the patient's demeanour, dress, attitude and unconscious projections
- Observe and absorb any information about the patient prior to and during the consultation
- Actively listen to the patient
- Give timely reflections and interpretations, which the patient can use

---

The Consultation

The medical consultation with a patient, whether it takes place in general practice, a hospital clinic or a community clinic is usually fairly formulaic. In our training as clinicians we are taught how to greet the patient, confirm their identity and ask the necessary questions to find out what their complaint is. In some settings there are structured templates to complete. When doctors and allied health professionals start to see patients with psychosexual complaints, it is often difficult to move away from this conventional approach. The psychosexual problem might be presented in a direct and overt way by the patient and in this case the clinician would ask some questions to clarify what exactly the patient means, the length of time the problem has been present and related issues. The consultation should always be 'free floating', with the clinician observing what is happening, noting the thoughts and feelings in the room and allowing the patient to lead the discussion.

These consultations can be difficult, as the clinician may not feel comfortable about addressing sexual issues. There are often time constraints in clinics and surgeries and the practitioner is afraid of running behind or of opening a 'Pandora's Box', that he or she does not feel competent to deal with. This perceived lack of ability can make the practitioner feel unskilled or on the back foot and embarrassment can arise in the consultation. It is important to remember that the patient has chosen this healthcare professional at this moment to ask for help, this needs to be acknowledged and the patient's problem should not be dismissed or ignored.

The patient will often have chosen the clinician by testing them out, with previous visits for different issues. They might ask questions, such as 'Have you seen anyone with this problem before?' and 'Am I normal?' They have a deep need to have their problem addressed and not to feel that the problem is too much for the practitioner. Under these circumstances, even if the practitioner feels inadequate, he or she should listen to the patient and reflect back what he or she is hearing; this will facilitate the patient to think more clearly about the difficulty and open up about the problem.

The Practitioner's Defences

The practitioner needs to be aware of the patient's feelings and his or her own feelings, so that the two do not become confused. There is 'transference' (1) of the patient's feelings on to the practitioner, these can often be of impotence or anger, in return there is 'countertransference' from the practitioner. He or she may not work well, if the patient reminds them of a disliked teacher, from their past or a bullying elder sibling, acknowledge the feelings and then the consultation can continue. It is very important that the practitioner knows what is coming from their own feelings (2), and what is coming from the patient. Sometimes the health professional can feel they are inhibited or 'walking on eggshells', because of something that the patient has said, such as the angry patient, who has seen another healthcare professional, whom the patient has reported to the authorities for perceived malpractice. The young woman, who is very defended and unable to consummate her sexual relationship, often has power over her partner and the clinician (3), who is trying to help her, and if she has reported the previous practitioner, the current one is very inhibited.

The practitioner can experience other events in his or her own life, such as the loss of a partner, when a patient gives a similar history about their own partner, the clinician needs to be aware of and remain separated from their own feelings and not pre-judge the situation, but listen to the patient's feelings.

The Patient's Defences

The patient who makes phone calls to change the appointment several times before the visit is often hiding extreme anxiety about the consultation. The practitioner can feel annoyed by the patient, who seems to be hiding in the corner of the waiting room, behind a pillar or on their phone and does not leap up when his or her name is called. All of these scenarios and many more are examples of how the patient tries to hide their anxiety and delay what they perceive as potential exposure to a stressful interaction.

Examples

A few years ago, I was waiting for a patient, who had a 30-minute appointment at 11 a.m., and she arrived at 11:25 a.m. with a hot takeaway cup of coffee. She had obviously waited for a hot cup of coffee, although she knew that she was running late. I felt angry about her wasting my time, but I stood back and looked at what was happening. I said to her 'I do not think that you want to be here', it was the best thing I could have said, in the remaining 5 minutes she poured out her story of how her husband had made the appointment for her. She was finding him an increasingly tyrannical and controlling man, who reminded her of her stepfather, who had come into her life after the death of her father and had presumed that he could always tell her what to do. In the few minutes available to us, we could both see why her husband was complaining about her lack of libido over the recent months. Another appointment was made so that we could look closely at her feelings and think about actions she could take to improve the situation.

Sometimes a patient will bring someone else into the consultation with him or her, a classic defence is a mother with her baby. The mother will bring the baby to the clinic or surgery often complaining about a problem, which she perceives the baby has, but really, she is showing her defence about revealing her own problem. In one consultation a mother was winding her baby with blows to his back, which became increasingly strong as she told me about her lack of orgasm since his delivery. I had to point this out to her, so that she could relax and not continue this angry action, but look at her feelings about the changes in her body since delivery and her change in role from a 'lover' to a 'mother'.

CASE 1

A city worker in a smart black suit with a large briefcase presented for a consultation. The patient's chair is at the side of my desk, she picked it up and moved it to the far side of my desk and then a couple of feet backwards away from the desk. This created a barrier between us and I commented, 'You do not seem to want to be near me', and she replied, 'This is more business like', and she sat down and placed her briefcase on her lap as a further defence. She had come for a cervical smear test and remained stiff and awkward as I asked the usual questions about pregnancies, periods and her last smear test. Although she was 28 she had never had a test and had never had sex with her fiancé. I pointed out, that if she was a virgin she did not need to have a smear test yet, at which point she looked distressed and said 'I used to have sex with no problem at all, I had a boyfriend when I was at university, but then I was called for a smear test when I was 25 and have never been able to have sex since then', she felt something had happened and her fiancé could not enter her, because it was too painful.

I suggested that I examine her to find out what the problem could be. She went behind the screen and took a while to take off her underwear, there was obviously anxiety about agreeing to this examination. I found myself saying that I would be very gentle and wondered what she was worrying about. This seemed to free her up to talk about her terrible experience with the first smear attempt. She said that the nurse had tried to do the smear and then said, 'The neck of your womb is not in the right place, I must call the doctor to do this smear'. The patient said that the nurse left her lying there with no cover over her, so that she felt very exposed and the doctor took a long time to come to see her. When he arrived, she said that she knew immediately that the nurse should not have called him, as he seemed in a rush, he said 'Relax, relax' and hurt her a lot. She said that the more he persisted in examining her, the more tense she became and, in the end, he said, 'I am unable to take this smear, you must come back in 3 months'. She had never returned to that clinic.

As a doctor, I was horrified by the behaviour of these healthcare professionals, but these were my feelings, so I said to her 'I wonder how you felt' and to my surprise she said, 'I felt awful, my body had let me down'. It was terrible to realise that she had taken all this as her fault and did not blame the doctor and nurse at all. She let me examine her and her cervix was not difficult to find. After I had taken the cervical smear test, she examined herself and felt reassured about her normality. I asked her if she wanted any vaginal trainers to give her confidence about her own anatomical normality and she said, 'No thank you, I am going home to use the real thing!' We both laughed and there was such a change of atmosphere in the room; all the tension at the beginning of the consultation had disappeared.

Previous Experiences

Historical events from the patient's past, that have occurred in the 'There and Then' can become vivid to the patient in the 'Here and Now' of the consultation.

Experiences, such as poor or insensitive medical treatment, sexual assault, physical abuse, surgery, childbirth, termination of pregnancy and many other human experiences can produce secondary vaginismus in women, such as in this case. Each consultation is different, and the practitioner needs to observe the body language, actions and words of the patient to understand their individual experience and effect. The psychosomatic examination of the genital area in both sexes is often a 'Moment of truth', when the patient feels freed up to talk about their deep anxieties. Men also can experience assault, abuse and traumatic loss, such as, a job loss or separation from a partner, which can lead to problems with obtaining or maintaining an erection. This may be due to their subconscious anxiety or loss of confidence.

The Patient's Defence of Religion or Culture

Sometimes patients hide behind culture or religion. In the consultation the patient, with a sexual difficulty, might say 'This is because I am a good Catholic/Muslim/Jew/Jehovah's Witness, you must understand'. The practitioner rather than agreeing that they understand, comments to the patient 'I wonder what your religion means to you'. In this way the patient has an invitation to expose their true feelings and not use religion as an excuse for their erectile problems or vaginismus.

The patient might quote the religious teaching of 'No sex before marriage', but then talk about their siblings or friends, who are happily living with sexual partners. They see the different way, in which they are behaving and gradually realise that this is something to do with their inner world and not necessarily to do with a religion.

I have seen many patients suffering from vaginismus, which is a profound involuntary spasm of the vaginal muscles, which stops penetration by the patient's partner or the vaginal examination by a practitioner. This spasm is psychogenic and occurs because of a deep-seated need to avoid having a part of another person inside them. This is can be due to fantasies, such as the vagina being too small, the presence of a thick impenetrable barrier, the genitalia opening up into the bladder and guts and many more frightening ideas. It is easier to help a patient, who is aware of her fantasies and able to share them with the clinician, but other patients will, unknowingly, hide behind the defence of 'not knowing'. This puts up a wall between patient and clinician, which has to be gently removed brick by brick or like peeling the layers off an onion.

Tears

Tears can be another very strong defence on the part of the patient. As healthcare professionals we have a deep need to help people and to stop the tears, but it is important to look behind the tears. They can be sobbing and childlike, in the case of a patient, who is having difficulties with growing up and leaving their childhood behind them and will then engender protective and motherly/fatherly feelings in the practitioner. There can be tears of anger as well as sadness, in patients, who perceive that someone has treated them unfairly in some way. They may feel that they have an unthinking partner or that someone has treated them badly sexually in the past. Tears can be so overwhelming that they prevent the patient from speaking, which of course is the ultimate defence.

It is best to reflect on the tears with the patient and look at why they have occurred at this stage in the consultation, what initiated the feelings of hopelessness, anger, childishness or other feelings. This helps them to see how something from the past is affecting how they behave and communicate in the present.

The Patient's Appearance

The consultation is a brief encounter in the 'here and now', which can often tell us a lot about the 'there and then' of the patient's past.

CASE 2

A 26-year-old woman attended a sexual health clinic and complained that sex was very painful and not enjoyable with her boyfriend. She appeared much younger than her age and was dressed in an inappropriate dress, which would have suited a 12- to 13-year-old girl. She had her hair held back by an Alice band with a flower on it, rather like those worn by children and she spoke in a little girl voice. She seemed to be in a good relationship with a kind partner and I wondered what was causing the pain with sex, as she had no complaints about him. I assumed that this had always been a problem for her, but when I suggested this she said, 'Oh no, the first time I had sex it was wonderful'. I was very surprised by this comment and I asked her to tell me about her first experience. She said that she had been very young, about 15 years old, and had gone to a music festival with friends. Her whole group had fancied a certain older boy, who was about 16 or 17, but she was very proud to have been the one to catch his eye. She said they went off to a field and had wonderful sex, lying in the grass, she had been ecstatic about it.

I commented that she sounded happy about this experience and she said that she had been, until she realised that he had given her chlamydia. She talked about how dirty and awful she felt and she began to see how she could not relax about sex with her current boyfriend and was constantly punishing herself for what had happened when she was so young, leading to the pain that she was now feeling. In the consultation, she realised how the 'then and there' was affecting her life in the 'here and now' and we worked on strategies for her to forgive herself and learn to use her body as an adult woman to enjoy sex on her own terms.

The clothing that was not appropriate for her age seemed to show her need to remain a child. Her experience of having sex and joining the adult world had had unexpectedly bad results. The outcome of the consultation was to give her insights into how she could allow herself to become an adult.

The Practitioner and Patient Relationship

In this chapter we are looking at communication between the practitioner and patient and how the presentation, past feelings, examination, defences of both practitioner and patient all affect the consultation and bring the patient's unconscious feelings into the here and now. Although these consultations are patient led, the practitioner is playing an active part, by constantly observing the feelings and dynamics of what is happening and reflecting this back to the patient at appropriate moments. This different kind of consultation was studied by Michael Balint several decades ago, he said that it was 'The study of the doctor as the drug' (4), in other words how we give of ourselves in this precious and delicate interaction.

The patient will often treat us in a different way from our other patients and we need to observe and study this. Some patients will want us to see them as equals and try to blind us with their scientific knowledge, in this case we need to help them to look behind generalisations and theories and to accept themselves as an individual, possibly vulnerable human being.

As a female doctor, I am aware of the woman, who is not in a comfortable relationship with her male partner and will make comments such as 'You know what men are like'. This is the moment not to agree with her, but to find out what she feels men are like and not to be pulled into generalisations. I am sure the same occurs with men and male practitioners and the patient's attitude to the opposite sex.

CASE 3

A well-dressed man in his early 30s attended for a consultation in a specialist psychosexual referral clinic. He worked in the city and was obviously successful and well off financially, I discovered all this detail from the first 5 minutes of the consultation, when he talked without me needing to say anything. I began to think about this interaction and what was being communicated and I realised that he wanted me to see him as a big, successful man and I wondered why he was in the clinic.

He proceeded to tell me about his beautiful model-type girlfriend, who was perfect in every way, I was waiting to hear the problem in his 'fairy-tale life'. As he was in the psychosexual clinic, I nudged him towards his reason for being there, and his whole persona changed. The big square shoulders and firm jaw line both sagged noticeably, he let out a huge sigh and almost cried as he said that he was suddenly unable to get an erection, when he was in bed with his girlfriend. He was able to masturbate and had early morning erections, when he woke, so I realised that he did not have a physical cause for his problem.

The patient maintained that he adored his girlfriend and could not think of a reason for this happening. We could both sense the sadness and loss in the room and I suggested that I examine him, as he had no more ideas on the subject. From the point of view of a physical examination all appeared normal, but as a psychosomatic event it gave him a chance to reflect. When he had dressed and was sitting back in the chair, he looked at me and seemed to feel able to open up and tell me his story. He said that one night he was out with friends, he had run out of cash about midnight, he had left his friends and gone to a cash machine. While he was turned towards the machine a group of boys had come up behind him and demanded the money, which he gave to them. He said, 'I was not enough of a man, I did not stand up to them', both these feelings express his loss of potency and sexual ability and following this event he had been unable to achieve an erection.

When we talked about this traumatic experience he said that he was angry with himself for being so pathetic and parting with the money. In fact, there had been four boys and at least one had been carrying a knife, I pointed out to him, that what he had done was in fact sensible as one man cannot stand up to an armed gang. Being able to communicate his feelings about this event seemed to give him a better feeling about himself and he squared his shoulders again and walked out of the consulting room with a positive gait.

The Unspoken Word

As we have reflected, communication is not just about words, but as a health professional in an interaction with a patient we are looking for silent clues or unconscious feelings in the room.

Examples

A patient was very chatty and trying to get me on side, when she came for her cervical smear test, she was practising some avoidance as she talked about her job and the journey to the clinic. When I looked at her more closely there were large 'sweat rings' appearing under her arms and across her chest under her bra, her anxiety was palpable. I reflected this back – saying, 'This seems to be really very difficult for you'. Only then could she talk about the pain that she was experiencing with sex and her fear of a painful smear test.

A young man rushed in to my consulting room and happily poured out a lot about how kind the reception staff had been and how lovely everyone was. He was not addressing his issues and I noticed deep nail marks on the palms of his hands as he pressed his hands together to try to hide his anxiety about his premature ejaculation.

Other patients will try to keep you in a very medical consultation, although you are aware that they have a psychosexual issue and you can feel the tension in the room as they try so hard to avoid facing up to their problem. Sometimes our consulting rooms are filled with palpable sadness or unexpressed anger, all these unconscious feelings need to be reflected back to the patient, so that she or he can own their feelings.

Covert Presentations

Some patients will openly tell you about their sexual difficulty in the consultation, but others find this too difficult and their presentation of the problem is hidden or covert. General practitioners (GPs) are particularly aware of patients, who are repeat attenders at the surgery, often presenting headaches, backaches, stomach cramps and many other medically unexplained symptoms. It can take many visits before the doctor is able to facilitate the patient in revealing his or her actual problem, which is often of an emotional or psychosexual nature.

Examples

A woman went to see her GP many times complaining of very heavy and frequent periods, she brought him charts of when she bled and for how many days. He did all the relevant investigations and surprisingly the patient had an excellent level of haemoglobin and no sign of anaemia, also the pelvic scan did not show any problems. The patient was referred to a gynaecologist, who also performed an examination and did thorough investigations. Eventually the gynaecologist referred the patient back to the GP saying that although the woman complained bitterly about her perceived symptoms there was no clinical evidence of menorrhagia and the woman would not accept any treatment to reduce her bleeding.

The GP decided to examine the patient again and as he did so he explained how the tests were not showing any effects of this heavy bleeding. She lay on the bed sobbing and so distressed that the doctor was anxious that he had done something awful. The patient spoke between sobs to say that as a child she had slept in the room next to her parents' bedroom, through the wall she had heard the terrible sounds of her drunken father forcing himself on her mother. Although the patient had been married for 4 years she had never had sex and her husband left her alone because of the 'heavy bleeding'.

In this example the patient was hiding behind periods in order to avoid the issue of having an intimate relationship with her partner. The doctor was able to help her to work through her feelings once he had found out the nature of her problem. The sensitive examination by the doctor had helped the patient to reveal how the 'here and now' had allowed her to speak about the 'there and then'.

Healthcare professionals who work in sexual health clinics are also aware of clients, who are repeat attenders, always expressing dissatisfaction with their method of contraception. One young woman complained that whatever method she tried, it did not suit her, and eventually she said that the contraceptive pill was putting her off having sex with her partner. Finally, she revealed that she had only had sex once since her termination of pregnancy and that had been extremely painful. The doctor examined the young woman and found no pain on vaginal examination, the patient expressed her relief and said that she had been afraid that the scissors had been left inside her. She had a very painful fantasy that scissors had been used to 'cut out the baby', the doctor was able to help her to work with this fantasy until she was able to dismiss it and resume comfortable intercourse with her boyfriend.

Staff in sexual health screening clinics (many are integrated now) will be aware of attendees, who have endless negative tests which is often the client's covert presentation of a psychosexual problem. A middle-aged man had been attending for several months and complaining bitterly of constant urethral discharge, which was making his penis sore. He gave a history of having one long-term partner, so his risk of contracting an infection was very low. One day a nurse had more time than usual to talk to the man, his real problem was erectile dysfunction, which had started a few months previously, following a work meeting in another town. After the meeting he had gone with colleagues to a 'lap-dancing club', he had allowed one of the girls to sit on his lap, while he was fully clothed, absolutely nothing of a sexual nature had happened. This man's extreme feelings of guilt and shame had led to his erection problems. The nurse was able to help him with his fantasies about sexually transmitted infections, so that he was eventually able to resume his sex life with his wife.

CASE 4

A well-dressed, attractive woman in her early 30s saw her GP to complain of an irritating vaginal discharge, after several months of anti-fungal treatment she was still complaining, although the swab did not grow any Candida. At this point the GP referred her on to the sexual health clinic where, after a few visits, her symptoms changed to pain around the vulva, so she was sent to see the gynaecology department in the hospital. She had stopped having sex because of the pain and after several months of treatment she was sent to my psychosexual clinic.

The patient told me that sex had been great between her and her partner, but this had stopped more than a year before our meeting, when she had developed the irritation and then pain around the vulva. In the consultation she was pleasant but seemed a bit formal and stiff as if she was holding tightly on to something. When I examined her and inserted the speculum she asked if I could see anything that might cause bleeding on the neck of her womb. I was looking at a healthy looking cervix and was surprised by her question, so I enquired why she thought that she might bleed. She came to sit back in the chair and explained that she had needed a colposcopy more than a year ago and had been told not to have sex for a couple of weeks afterwards. The first time they had had sex she had bled a lot and when she went into the bathroom she had passed a horrible 'slug-like' thing that she had wrapped in tissue and shown her partner. After this event she had been too afraid to have sex so had used discharge and pain as her defence.

She talked about the colposcopy and expressed a great deal of anger about how she had gone to appointments on her own and felt very unsupported by her partner, she was frightened by the procedure and said that now whenever she parted her legs she could just see the doctor with binoculars looking at her vagina. During several visits to the psychosexual clinic she worked through her pain, anger and disappointment with her partner and began to take back ownership of her genital area from the doctor in the hospital, who had done the colposcopy. At her last visit she was a more relaxed and happy woman and sex had returned to something that was really great for both her and her partner.

Medical History

We have seen that it is not only past traumatic sexual events that can cause sexual difficulties in the present, but often medical interventions, such as smear tests and colposcopies. Men and women can need medical examinations, tests or surgery, which might seem straightforward to health professionals, but can lead to fantasies and deeper unconscious disturbances. The urethra is close to the genital area in both sexes and often bladder investigations can lead to sexual difficulties. Female patients can develop a fantasy of a small vagina, after experiencing a painful cystoscopy, bringing the 'there and then' into the 'here and now'.

Patients with fertility issues often go through a lot of interventions and find it difficult to dissociate from these, when they return to their own private sexual lives. Surgery, such as mastectomy, hysterectomy, vulvectomy or prostatectomy can leave the patient with an altered body image, which interferes with their sexual feelings. Cancer or fear of cancer acts similarly.

Women might experience pregnancy, termination, miscarriage, childbirth, menopause, all of which can be critical in influencing their inner sexual selves. Male patients can react similarly, both to their own surgery and also to surgery done to their partners. For example, the occasional man develops erectile problems after his partner's hysterectomy, as he has a fantasy about her anatomy after the operation.

Conclusion

Sometimes our patients have no idea, where their sexual problems originated, the patient does not mean to mislead the health professional, but they themselves are unaware of where their feelings are coming from. The clinician needs to look at what is happening in the consultation and give interpretations to the patient so that he or she can look within themselves and speak about the fantasies that are blocking their ability to have a happy sex life. We are seeing them in the here and now, but often the problem stems from things in the past that they have been unable to process and leave behind. Our role is to facilitate our patients in releasing their deeply held, often unconscious, feelings. As this chapter demonstrates, this facilitation is performed by a close study of the practitioner-patient interaction and by interpreting this back to the patient, so that the patient can see how they behave in relationships. The careful psychosomatic examination of the genital area is also part of the process of helping the patient to look at how the 'there and then' is affecting the 'here and now'. The process is completed by the practitioner understanding their own and the patient's defences and being aware of the unspoken feelings in the consulting room.

REFERENCES

1. Main T. *The Ailment and Other Psychoanalytic Essays*. London: Free Association Books, 1989, 238.
2. Skrine R. *Blocks and Freedoms in Sexual Life*. Oxon, UK: Radcliffe, 1997, 30.
3. Skrine R. *Blocks and Freedoms in Sexual Life*. Oxon, UK: Radcliffe, 1997, 33.
4. Balint M. *The Doctor, His Patient and the Illness* (2nd ed.). London: Pitman Medical, 1973, 4.

11

Defences in the Consultation: Developing Interpretative Skills

Andrew Stainer-Smith

> We must become the change we want to see.
>
> **Mahatma Gandhi**

Defences

Defences are barriers that act to protect. Barriers are erected when one is under threat or perceives this to be the case. They bring safety in a disturbed world fulfilling basic human needs. Once physiological needs for warmth, food and water are met we seek security warding off things that stand in the way. We construct defences against perceived threats to our well-being (1).

One assumes that patients seek professional help for psychosexual problems to fulfil their needs for happiness and self-fulfilment. How is it that in this process a person in need of help acts to make delivering that help difficult? The word *defence* comes from the language of conflict and fighting yet the aspiration of psychosexual work is a million miles away from wanting to battle. Likewise, no professional wants their own practice to stand in the way of a patient being helped. So why are we left with the reality of defences from this world of warring factions?

Patients' Defences

Patients in distress are battling within themselves. They are suffering with the effects of conflicts understood or not understood. Patients become the victims of their own conscious and unconscious conflicts. Unless we recognise this for what it is and address it honestly we do them a disservice. The distress of a failed relationship can be both consciously understood and unconsciously demonstrated in psychosomatic symptoms (see Chapter 7). We are all limited in the amount of emotional pain we can endure before unavoidable psychosomatic symptoms emerge. Nobody is immune. Once we reach our limit we are likely to resist someone delving into our private world. This is the origin of most of the defences we encounter.

A defended patient is likely either to deny a difficulty or represent the problem as coming from another source. Winnicott explained that for the infant, when rationalisation is impossible, these processes result in either burying pain away (introjection) or blaming an external source (projection) (2). So a child will become either withdrawn or hit out defending himself from an assumed foe. There is something of the child in all of us, and we cannot avoid using our instinctive strategies to deal with pain when the pain is too great. As Freud summarised, the child truly is 'the father of the man' (3).

Helping a defended patient is a challenge. One has to use all one's available skills to enable useful communication. Adults, like children, handle problems similarly either burying away unhappiness or in some form exhibiting it to others (projection). A professional trying to help will use enabling phrases that they have found helpful before. Perhaps what was found useful in the past may work again. Without information it is tempting to guess about what may be causing the sexual problem, but this is unwise. The maxim that common things occur commonly is valid in the sense that, for example, patients are frequently nervous or shy talking about sex. So a professional may make an enabling opening explaining that everything is confidential and that they will not be shocked. But a defended patient will counter that with a curt rejection. What does one do when genuine offers of help are rebuffed?

EXAMPLE 11.1: A DEFENDED PATIENT – RECOGNISING THE RELATIONSHIP AND USING IT

An angry man left the surgery waiting room complaining that his general practitioner (GP) should 'bloody well be on time'. Two weeks later he booked in again and the receptionist warned the female doctor that he may be 'difficult'. After a back injury instructing in hazardous adventure training he had become unable to ejaculate. The orthopaedic surgeon told him that with two severely worn lumbar discs he had to expect problems with sex from his damaged spinal nerves. The ED clinic offered sildenafil but he did not want that. The GP sympathised with how awful he must feel but was rebuffed with 'No, you don't know how it feels'. The GP did not feel threatened and wanted to understand this agitated man. She leant forward, stilling his restless hand that was strumming on the desk. Feeling lost to know what to say she offered 'I'm worried that whatever I say you're going to push me away'. He responded 'So?...' She replied 'I wonder if you are pushing other people away? Those closest to you?' He paused and started to talk about his wife. Their wedding was the week after the back injury and they had to postpone the honeymoon. During that week she told him that she wanted him to stop adventure training. He was gutted. He had escaped a damaging childhood after being offered an outward bound charity expedition and had set his heart on helping youngsters. Having to give this up coincided with the start of his impotence. The GP began to understand and over a period this man began to accept that his wife was trying to care for his welfare. Sex improved.

This man could not progress until the GP understood the importance of this man's burning desire to help others. When she understood how this man rejected genuine offers, she could reflect that he may be doing this to his wife.

When encountering defences the answer is first to listen with all your senses to understand the atmosphere developing in the room. Use that evidence to consider why this unique patient has encountered their particular difficulty. 'Listen' to your emotional response. Try to identify the defence, honour it with genuine respect and hope to find a way of putting it to bed – what Tom Main, army psychiatrist, described as to 'Bury it with full military honours'. This is the golden road to progress (4 p. 27). It requires emotional work to be done by both the patient and the professional utilising the professional's diacritic thinking and synaesthetic skills (see later in chapter).

Some defences manifest as discontent with someone who is not really to blame.

EXAMPLE 11.2: DEFENCE BY PROJECTION ONTO THE PROFESSIONAL

A young woman was repeatedly keen to portray her sexual partner as bullying and domineering. The nurse felt unsure and explored how accurate this was. It is a professional's job to assist a patient in taking control of their life. This woman had not realised that although being a victim gave her some control, it prevented her standing up to her partner and looking at her sexual problem. She had learnt since childhood that the only way to survive domineering parents was to buckle under and suffer in silence. The therapist wondered if this was affecting the atmosphere of the consultation. Whenever something painful was being discussed the patient retreated into silence reluctant to explain how she felt. The professional identified her own feeling that at times this young woman made her think she was being too direct or even bullying. It was important for the nurse to recognise this as evidence about how this patient works inside and use it to enable the patient to understand herself.

How the patient makes the professional feel can be indicative of what goes on in the other relationships in that patient's life. In this example the nurse was being cast by the patient in the same domineering mould as the patient's parents. The nurse felt she was being forced to tread on eggshells. Whatever the nurse said could be seen as domineering and behind the scenes lurked the family. The therapist felt the discomfort. Analytical language calls this process *projective identification* but we do not need that language to understand the unalterable fact that how the patient made the nurse feel is indicative of what goes on in other relationships in the patient's life.

This defence stood in the way of progress. The therapist's knowledge from experience is that a patient who is prepared to think more broadly about their partner may discover that what they had thought domineering may contain a real element of caring. This patient had unintentionally likened the professional to individuals in her earlier life and reacted in the only way she knew. The patient struggled with the professional, at first being certain that their partner was the whole problem. The moment of truth was when the nurse understood that the patient's repressed anger was not directed at her but an anger towards the parents spilling over into the consulting room. The nurse commented on how intense the feelings were that this patient was still having to live with. There was a silence of mutual agreement that allowed the patient to move on. Defences need to be recognised, honoured and put to bed.

The professional's ability to intervene, based on the evidence found in the here and now in the consulting room led to the patient seeing herself in a different light and newly empowered. The real victim in this case had been the relationship of the patient with her partner.

The Professional's Defences

Individual practitioners have their own history, know their particular skills, are aware of their vulnerabilities and over time notice patterns in their own behaviour. Seminar training is designed to open these areas for group discussion in a safe environment without straying into personal disclosure (see Chapter 27). As with a patient's need to feel safe before exposing matters close to their heart, a professional needs to feel safe before offering his personal interpretation of what seems to be the problem.

A professional finding himself uncomfortable in the consultation may feel a need to retreat to safer ground. So from being a listening, sharing partner in the room he may begin to teach and become an expert. It can be more comfortable giving answers and making diagnoses than admitting ignorance and acknowledging that the two parties are not clear about what the problem is.

In a similar fashion the professional's normal behaviour may change from being even-handed in assessing responsibility. It can be easier to collude with the patient, blaming an absent partner or focussing on unhappy past events. There may be occasions when identifying damaging experiences is based on evidence but one must be very cautious, especially when a strained atmosphere suddenly lightens and the patient seems unusually pleased.

EXAMPLE 11.3: A DOCTOR DRAWN INTO COLLUSION

A young, very neatly dressed mother consulted repeatedly in the year after her first child was born. Tearfully she described how sex was now too painful to allow penetration. She described her partner expecting more than she could manage of domestic tasks and rough in bed. The male doctor examined her gently during which she said 'If he were gentle like you that would be lovely'. The doctor and the chaperone both smiled and the chaperone quietly commented 'men…'. The doctor first felt that giving her confidence to stand up to her partner was all the patient required and wound up the consultation offering follow-up later if desired. Over a year later she came again saying sex was still impossible with a new boyfriend, a sensitive fellow whom the doctor had known for years. The patient smiled saying 'I know you'll tell him what he needs to do'. The doctor felt uncomfortable and realised he was being charmed. He wanted to be fair, re-examined her again finding no pain and asked what it was she found most difficult in making relationships last? She became heated stating 'Nothing is difficult for me. It's men that have the problems. They're so messy and unreliable'.

Over a period she admitted to mild obsessively compulsive traits and with extra help from a counsellor did manage sex again. She agreed it was not really pain but the 'mess' she found too difficult.

During consultations one may realise that a sticking point or moment of increased tension may not have arisen from the patient's issues but rather the professional encountering a defence in himself that he recognises as his responsibility and that needs to be acknowledged.

EXAMPLE 11.4: A PRACTITIONER RECOGNISING HIS OWN DEFENCE

An elderly cleric had lost his erections and was asking for sildenafil. The doctor noticed that descriptions of difficulties making the appointment and asking his wife to accompany him were made with comments of 'but I understand that their lives are more difficult than mine'. The doctor felt annoyed and frustrated but realised that the patient must also be annoyed and frustrated. So the doctor reflected, 'I see you seem to stay calm when your life is made difficult. You must be angry at times?' The man responded, 'There isn't time in this world to be angry'. The doctor's first reaction was a desire to go no further. He recognised his own defence in circumstances that he had previously found difficult.

However he managed to pause, to realise that it was unacknowledged pain that had made this man impotent. He knew that the patient was always expected to give to others in his public life so interpreted. 'It may help others if you stay calm but something has troubled you enough to spoil your erections'. This enabled progress. Later in seminar discussion the doctor raised the issue of difficulties when professionals stereotype patients (such as religious believers) as behaving similarly.

Over time the professional can tackle his own defences and learn.

There are always limitations to what real people can offer. We have to cope with limited time, resources and subtle pressures from employers who want to see results fitting their framework of values. Professionals usually value kindness, empathy and patient satisfaction above achieving increased patient throughput and cutting costs. When these external pressures conflict with a desire to give more, a professional needs to recognise his limits. Within the relationship must come an agreement that only so much time can be given or that one may need to refer to another agency.

Defence as a Concept: Critiques Discussed

A professional may feel secure in the belief that a patient is exhibiting a defence but immediately this raises a question – what right does a professional have to label matters that are found awkward with his patient's behavior, as in need of correcting? Is not such an approach authoritarian and patriarchal? Sigmund Freud's use of the word *resistance* which was caricatured as indicating inflexibility in the therapist was disliked. Persisting criticism of psychoanalytic work is that analytic workers are blinkered and use the concept of a defence to describe anything coming from the patient indicating disagreement with the professional's construct or theories.

Similarly, critics of psychoanalytical work may see psychoanalysts as determined to apply theory over evidence. Behaviourists will cite 'evidence' that their patients can be made to change their ways of thinking by cognitive processes, without needing to examine the past and that they will become more content. Certainly after behavioural therapies patients may score better short term on levels of contentment. Psychosexual medicine professionals aspire to a higher level of patient satisfaction. We desire to help patients understand that what has been holding them back:

- Is within themselves
- Has come from their past
- Is under their control and amenable to a different interpretation

Reaching a detailed understanding can set them up for the rest of their sexual life. To achieve this the professional must be prepared to analyse the nature and origin of defences. One must look at the difficulty and recognise patterns of human behaviour.

Psychosexual medicine addresses the criticism of those who question the importance of psychoanalytic theory. From beginning in the 1970s the technique of seminar training professionals, examination qualification and continuing case discussion has been shown to be effective. The training produces measurable change in the skills of professionals (5). It is consistently shown that treatment offered is cost effective being brief. Studies typically show a maximum of four or five consultations (6).

Effectiveness of the treatment is consistent across a range of conditions, for example non-consummation (7), with varied cultural groups (8) and within modern integrated sexual health services (9). We are on sound ground knowing that provided professionals are within a continuing supervised environment, services offered are fit for purpose. We maintain that assisting patients with painful issues in their lives can be supportive, enabling and cost effective.

To summarise, the technique of psychosexual medicine has been shown to work.

How Interpretative Skills Are Acquired During Training: Understanding Defences

Appreciating the Practitioner's Difficulty

At the start practitioners may struggle to understand the welter of feelings that come from a consultation.

EXAMPLE 11.5: A DIFFICULT CONSULTATION EARLY IN TRAINING AND HOW IT MAY BE ADDRESSED

Defences not Understood

A policeman bereaved 2 years ago had a new girlfriend who was keen on sex and intimate touching. He had climaxed once with her but not since and was asking for help to get his orgasms back. He enjoyed pleasuring her. He reported intermittent blood in his semen. A recent set of urological tests was normal. The nurse wondered whether any feelings around the loss of his wife could be preventing him from letting go. The nurse asked how he was coping with the loss but was met with a defensive statement that he was coping well. There had been no problems in his marriage. They did not need a lot of sex and the bereavement was not the cause. Silenced for a while the nurse then asked whether he could climax normally on masturbation. Again she received a closed reply that he never did that and would not consider it. She was suspicious about his denial of masturbation otherwise how had he managed to observe the blood in his semen? All he seemed keen to talk about was his new hip joint and his success at bowls. The nurse felt at a loss.

In seminar discussion it was noted that the nurse asked this man questions rather than making enabling comments. Seminar members suggested the value of comments such as 'It must be very difficult adjusting to a partner with different needs' or 'I see it is uncomfortable airing such private things with a stranger'. These are reflective comments. The group appreciated the relevance of the maxim that if one asks questions one will only get answers.

Professional training needs to be efficient and to produce practitioners who deliver appropriate, measurable patient benefit. Medical, nursing and other educational courses teach the value of gaining information quickly. This is usually in the form of questions that give yes/no answers. Sometimes this is done face-to-face but increasingly it can be done electronically or by questionnaire. A patient coming for assessment of haematuria is unlikely to spend more than a few minutes with the professional who will look inside their bladder. Consequently the patient is very unlikely to raise a psychosexual problem. This suits the needs of quick, efficient, tick-box healthcare. It does not fit the needs of a distressed patient who imagines that perhaps their haematuria has resulted from an unwise sexual encounter.

When a patient is in emotional pain a practitioner may be moved to try to lessen it by reassurance saying that in time the pain will pass or that concentrating on the positive will ease distress. But what is going on in these circumstances? The truth is that the practitioner is finding the pain difficult and wants to avoid it. A more fruitful, though difficult, approach is to acknowledge the nature of the pain, try to understand how it feels for the patient and to share it. It takes confidence for a practitioner to hold on to the emotions in the room walking alongside the patient in their grief.

Appreciating the Elements of the Professional-Patient Relationship

The Interplay of Transference and Countertransference

Two core skills are needed to understand and use the professional-patient relationship:

- To develop skills observing patients with all the senses and reflect what one has learnt from the evidence available. This involves recognising what the patient brings to the professional in the consultation and is called *transference*. Using this evidence is the process of reflection. Reflection can bring insight into the true nature of the sexual problem.

- To remain continuously aware of one's own internal reactions to what is going on. The professional must question why he responds as he does, recognising where his own life experience has brought him insight and when such insight can be interpreted in the context of the patient's sexual difficulty. He must recognise that the patient can make him respond emotionally. This is called *countertransference* and is the basis of interpretative skills; we do not only observe and listen, we bring our own psyche into the room as a resource.

The terms *transference* and *countertransference* come from psychoanalysts. They are interesting and useful to some therapists. In the development of the Institute of Psychosexual Medicine (IPM) it has not been thought essential to label interactions in everyday practice but more to appreciate the effects of both in the dynamic process of the evolving professional-patient relationship.

Psychosexual medicine developed from psychoanalysts offering assistance to doctors. Michael Balint, psychoanalyst, developed the seminar training technique for general practitioners. Psychiatrist Tom Main broadened the method to a wider range establishing the IPM in 1974. The IPM became self-sustaining and later extended its brief to offer training to other allied health professionals. Many skills learnt in IPM seminars are also found in other forms of counselling, therapy, psychodynamic, humanistic and mindfulness techniques. Unique to IPM training is combining work on the professional-patient relationship with use of the psychosomatic genital examination. At the core is the importance of analysing the atmosphere developing between patient and professional, the professional-patient relationship. Main described this as 'more than the sum of two peoples transference and counter-transference. It is a dynamic whole, built mutually and is inevitable in any human relationship. The word 'atmosphere' is vague – but I can't do better and it means something' (4 p. 238).

Psychosexual work requires a degree of openness, honesty and professional vulnerability unique to this style of medicine. These features are shared with psychoanalysis and some other psychodynamic therapies. Unique to our work is the requirement that the professional is prepared to recognise the effect that a patient has on their own emotional milieu and to use that understanding. This is the basis of the interpretative process.

Essential Cooperation in Training Groups

Practitioners in seminar training acquire skills from interacting with patients, their peers and a group leader. The group leader acts as a facilitator not making any hierarchical assumptions of superior knowledge but being a first among equals (*primus inter pares*). This style is andragogy derived from pedagogy (10). It is a direct evolution from Socratic learning focussing on developing self-understanding, skills and personal attributes that do not lend themselves to direct measurement. It is distinct from curriculum theory that sets measurable task-centred goals.

Quality traditional medicine and nursing requires validated knowledge – that a procedure is evidence-based. Learning a skill is the hierarchical process of a junior learning from master often referred to as watch one, do one, teach one. This apprentice method of learning works for the purpose for which it is intended.

Psychosexual medicine is different. What is needed is not to learn facts but to understand.

In training groups primary and secondary care professionals work together. This highlights differences in approach. Training in hospital practice is predominantly task- and disease-oriented with efforts judged by patient survival and throughput. Factual knowledge underpins this work. In primary care doctors, nurses and others are trained from the outset in consultation skills. Patient satisfaction is a special marker of good practice. Hospital practitioners may find it difficult at first concentrating in detail on the dynamics of consultations. Primary care professionals may lack knowledge of how to balance the risks and benefits of one form of treatment with another. In an IPM seminar group the two are mixed together inevitably sharing and learning from each other. In the process certain core skills become recognised as useful to understanding and managing psychosexual complaints.

The Listening Skills

Synaesthetic Awareness Combined with Diacritic Thinking

Synaesthetic skills are not widely understood. Synaesthesia is the state of blurring of perceptions from all the senses. In the pathological condition the boundaries of vision, hearing, pain perception and emotional distress become thinned to the point where a person cannot be sure what they are perceiving. Sounds may become associated with colours and visual hallucinations. Smells evoke profound emotional responses. Seeing an everyday object may become terrifying (11). In ordinary life we all experience this to some degree. Smells trigger childhood experiences. We may see a person walk with a particular gait and wince with their pain. The more as professionals we can develop and utilise synaesthetic awareness, the more we will be able to enter the patient's world and begin to understand what they are experiencing – whether or not it makes sense to our diacritic logical conclusions (4, p. 223).

Diacritic skills are those of thinking about the evidence, critically analysing, testing hypotheses and coming to conclusions that are logical and make sense. This is the scientific method and the basis of almost all medical training.

EXAMPLE 11.6: COMBINING WHAT IS OBSERVED WITH HOW THE PRACTITIONER FEELS

Patient and Practitioner Defences Combined

A patient tells the doctor that she has not slept for 2 weeks and is in tears all the time – yet during your time together does not cry and does not seem tired.

What do you conclude? First, it is a risky area questioning the account of a patient in distress and understandably the doctor will try to believe the account. To reduce the risk of conflict a common defence is to say that you believe every word, though knowing that in reality the account cannot be true. Your diacritic skills lead you to analyse what has been said and come to the conclusion that you must be cautious in believing this patient's account of their physical and mental state. But what if you were to utilise your synaesthetic awareness? Getting inside this patient's world leads you to feel that indeed she is so overwhelmed with grief that sleep seems alien. The logical fact that it is impossible not to sleep for 2 weeks is irrelevant when you need to know what the patient feels. Synaesthesia draws you to the feeling of constant painful alertness. You have a real link with the patient's reality. As a psychosexual practitioner your next task is to apply your diacritic skills and ask how, what you logically know can be used to assist. What you know is based on your clinical experience refined by your training. You know that the patient does not appear tired and is functioning. You know that sympathy can be evoked by exaggerating symptoms and you may have done the same in your life. So you look for an interpretation. You may offer 'I find it difficult to accept that you have not slept for 2 weeks but I know it can feel like that'. This is the exact summary of the atmosphere between the two of you. Her exaggerated distress and your cautious sympathy. This is the sort of response that may bear fruit enabling her to explain her grief. It is an interpretation because it involves your acknowledgement that in extreme circumstances anyone has a tendency to exaggerate, even you yourself.

EXAMPLE 11.7: SYNAESTHETIC AWARENESS ALLOWING A PATIENT TO VERBALISE DISTRESS

The Professional's Sensitivity as a Tool

A rather flambouyant divorced garage mechanic had trouble keeping his erection with a new girlfriend. He strode into the room with bravado almost pushing aside a receptionist who was clearly unhappy. He explained that he had no problems with doctors but wanted something different from sildenafil. He described his girlfriend as the 'ideal' partner. The (female) GP began to think what it must be like being his girlfriend and felt uneasy. His dress, manner, language and demeanour made her want to keep him at a distance. She didn't want the patient to invade any more of the consulting room. Another doctor had given him sildenafil but he wanted to ask his own GP if that was the best solution for him 'because my girlfriend says that she doesn't mind either way'. She queried what he meant. He explained that she did not mind him having to use tablets. The GP repeated 'She doesn't mind' and waited quietly. After a long pause the patient asked 'What do you think, doctor?' The doctor did not reply and there was another pause. Eventually the doctor repeated 'She doesn't mind?' After another pause she said 'I'm not sure you know exactly how she feels' and waited. The patient slumped in his chair and said firmly in a quiet voice 'She ought to mind. I do. I just wish she'd tell me how she really feels'. He said no more and left. His relationship was clearly not ideal and did not last.

Using silence is a skill that develops with practice. There may be times when it leaves a patient feeling too uncomfortable. It must be tailored to the circumstances.

Using the Physical Examination as a Psychosomatic Event

Doctors, nurses, physiotherapists and other professionals are required to examine in their everyday work. We are licenced to do so. It is often at these moments of close interaction when defences may be lowered that a special degree of understanding is gained. Frequently there is nothing found physically wrong but that does not matter. The examination is a special opportunity for the professional to understand how the patient feels about their private life. When clothes are removed and hands are laid on a patient may feel freed to talk intimately with someone they trust. Chaperones are always there to help provide a safe setting but it is usually most helpful if the chaperone can remain quiet not intruding in the professional-patient interaction.

> **EXAMPLE 11.8: AFTER SEVERAL ROUTINE EXAMINATIONS A PHYSIOTHERAPIST ENGAGES PSYCHOSOMATIC SKILLS**
>
> A man with long-standing bowel problems had been given various explanations about having an unusually large bowel and dietary intolerances. He did not believe that. He had occasionally enjoyed sex but they had stopped trying. He had become very lonely. The specialist physio had examined him several times to try to optimise his voluntary muscles in allowing evacuation. As he prepared to be examined again she noticed that he folded his clothes and placed them on top of the pillow on the couch. She commented on it. As she checked his pelvic floor he began to talk explaining that he had learnt to be very tidy and disciplined at his boarding school. He told a story of abuse by a master of other boys that he had been obliged to watch. She was the first person to whom he had ever disclosed this.
>
> She felt his emotional pain and tension in a new way saying how difficult it must have been for him to tell her. She reflected, 'Is this why you find it so difficult to relax?' In stages he began to 'let go' and his complaints of physical distress faded away.

It was during a physical examination by a professional engaging her synaesthetic skills that the patient felt safe to disclose the source of his intractable pain.

Making Interpretations

From the beginning of training it is important to acknowledge the value of reflective and interpretative interventions. The words *reflection* and *interpretation* are sometimes used interchangeably but in origin they are not the same. There is value in understanding the difference.

Reflections are the process of feeding back to the patient the emotions and feelings that they have understood in the developing interaction. A reflection may refer to something understood early, even before meeting the patient. Those who repeatedly cancel seeming to engineer difficulties may not understand that their behaviour may mimic what goes on in their sexual relationship. A comment such as, 'I note that it is not easy for someone to meet up with you' may bring a new understanding that is unavoidably obvious to the practitioner but that the patient has never before considered. Frequently one comments that 'This is difficult'. A defended patient may invite the observation 'there's some anger somewhere here'. All these comments are reflections, mirroring to the patient the feelings that the professional has felt in the room.

Interpretations are also comments made from observations of the atmosphere in the room but crucially require the practitioner to recognise his own response generated by the patient and use that unique understanding. This is appreciation of the countertransference. This sort of response requires a degree of self-understanding and surety coming from experience and training. The heritage of interpretative work extends from before Freud. He established the pattern of professionals undergoing one-to-one analysis addressing their personal difficulties. Once identified, the expectation is that the practitioner will tackle the matter in his own life and emerge stronger. If a patient is consumed with anger that someone in their life refuses to believe them and that they are untruthful, then the patient may also cast the professional as someone who will not believe them. If the professional can recognise the response in himself that he is being looked on as a poor judge he can, with skill, use his own response as an interpretation. An interpretation is more than an awareness of the feelings in the room. It is the practitioner using his life experience, tempered by seminar training, to give special understanding to a patient in distress (Figure 11.1). Neville Symington, psychoanalyst, stated that 'The analyst cannot make an interpretation

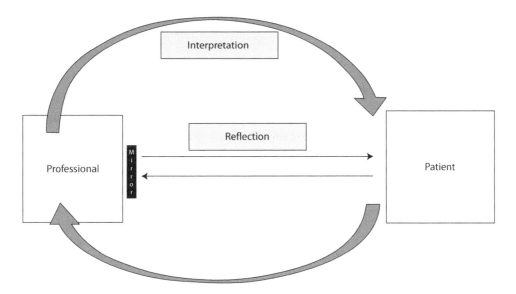

FIGURE 11.1   The interactions of reflection and interpretation (black arrows illustrate the practitioner holding a mirror to reflect back what the patient is projecting; grey arrows illustrate the effect of countertransference penetrating the practitioner's psyche and acknowledged in making interpretations).

when he is too anxious about the topic' (12), or in analytical language the therapist must appreciate the countertransference to be able to make an effective interpretation. Psychosexual training develops that degree of self-understanding. During training a practitioner acquires new skills of such a depth that one establishes a 'limited but definite personality change' (4, p. 230).

EXAMPLE 11.9: INTERPRETATION – A PROFESSIONAL DRAWING ON HIS OWN EXPERIENCE AND RECOGNISING HIS OWN DEFENCES

A quiet, caring, retired businessman active in his local church came in distress with his impotency. He wanted full investigations of his hormones and whether his penile vasculature was failing. He had searched long and hard and prayed for a solution. It began after family discord when his daughter broke away from home, in the process committing an offence. The police were involved though they did not press charges. He and his wife together decided that she must not be allowed to return. During a physical examination he tried to hide away his genitalia saying that 'perhaps their days are over'. The doctor paused, commenting how the man seemed to be rejecting that part of his body. But the doctor went further exploring his own reactions to hearing of the recalcitrant daughter and a wife with unshakeable boundaries. The doctor had in his life dealt with family issues. He knew that he was being influenced by the patient's emotional world and recognised his own defences in a reluctance to query the foundation of a seemingly contented marriage. He interpreted, 'I see it is impossible for you to feel angry with the people you love'. The man replied 'My daughter?' The doctor said, 'I was thinking more of you and your wife'. He left quietly, returning for follow-up saying that they had talked and that he had managed lovemaking again. He had also made contact with his daughter. He did not want to explain further. As a private man the shutters were drawn back across life at home.

Interpretation of his anger by a professional who could listen to his own response led to this man identifying what he wanted to do about it. This is the key to psychosexual medicine. Main described our work as 'applied psychoanalysis' (4, p. 242). Some prefer 'brief interpretative therapy'.

Summary

Working in general practice, physiotherapy, gynaecology, genitourinary medicine, prostate surgery, gender services or whatever field we occupy the principles are the same. We must approach with an open mind (in ignorance) regarding the patient as the expert. We recognise defences for what they are, honour them and move on. We must actively listen to understand the interaction. We examine our patients and ourselves with all our senses and must formulate interpretations that we know are soundly based. It is easily stated but takes years of experience to apply.

REFERENCES

1. Maslow A. *Motivation and Personality*. New York, NY: Harper and Brothers, 1954.
2. Winnicott D. *Human Nature*. London: Free Association Books, 1988.
3. Freud S. *Totem and Taboo*. http://www.gutenberg.org/ebooks/41214, 1918.
4. Main T. In J Johns (Ed.), *The Ailment and Other Essays*. London: Free Association Books, 1989.
5. Mathers N, Bramley M, Draper K, Snead S, Tobert A. Assessment of training in psychosexual medicine. *BMJ* 1994;308:969–972.
6. Stainer-Smith A. Dare we measure patient satisfaction? *IPMJ* 1996;12:11–14.
7. Bramley M, Brown J, Draper K, Kilvington J. Non-consummation of marriage treated by members of the Institute of Psychosexual Medicine. *BJOG* 1983;90:908–913.
8. Pollen R. Working with immigrant patients in a GP setting. *IPMJ* 2009;52:21–24.
9. Hobbs R, Muir W. Use of MYMOP to measure effectiveness in a psychosexual medicine service. *IPMJ* 2014;66:16–18.
10. Knowles M. *The Modern Practice of Adult Education: From Pedagogy to Andragogy*. Westchester, IL: Follett, 1980.
11. Harrison J. *Synaesthesia: The Strangest Thing*. Oxford: Oxford University Press, 2001.
12. Symington N. *The Analytic Experience*. London: Free Association Books, 1986.

12

The Psychosexual Genital Examination*

Jasmin Khan-Singh

Introduction

Embedded in the Institute of Psychosexual Medicine's (IPM's) logo are four words – 'unique training, enlightened approach'. These four words capture what is so different about the genital examinations carried out by members of the IPM, why such examinations are so pivotal, and why they then become known as the psychosexual genital examination.

The IPM prospectus (2014) (1) states:

> The doctor learns to conduct the examination in a safe setting that allows the patient to express their feelings about their difficulties. It also provides a less guarded situation in which to study the Doctor/Patient relationship. The attitude of the patient to the examination or prospect of examination and the feelings of the doctor when performing it may reveal something of what the patient feels about intimacy.

In this chapter, we explore what makes a genital examination psychotherapeutic and so unique, some of the factors to consider during such an examination, and finally address some of the concerns clinicians may have when carrying out an intimate examination.

You have read in the preceding chapters about the significance of the doctor-patient or clinician-patient relationship, working with the 'here and now' and the 'defences' of the patient and doctor. The understanding gained from this provides the foundation from which the psychosexual genital examination can bear fruit. During the genital examination, these same areas require attention, and may well illuminate further or – as can sometimes happen – throw a totally different light on the problem. The case studies presented in this chapter, assume this foundation work has been carried out in the consultation before getting to the genital examination, apart from Case 1. In Case 1 we look at the psychosexual genital examination *de nouveau*, when the only contact with the patient is for a genital examination.

For ease of reading, I refer to the relationship under study as that of the doctor-patient relationship (DPR), but it is meant to be interchangeable with the relationships of our allied colleagues such as nurse-patient and physiotherapist-patient. In addition, it is important to be clear about usage of the words *fantasy* and *phantasy*. Like Tunnadine (2) and Skrine (3) I hold that a distinction between the two words needs to be made, even though the *Concise Oxford English Dictionary* (4) gives the same meaning to both while medical dictionaries only define *phantasy*. The distinction is based on awareness. In 'fantasy' there is a *conscious control* of the imagination, for example when masturbating; but in 'phantasy' the imaginations are *unconscious* and may even be pathological or distorted, such as believing that the vagina will burst apart when penetrated, or that the penis will be damaged by the teeth of the vagina.

But first, a brief mention of Balint and Main. It was in the 1950s that Michael Balint and his associates started training groups of doctors, from family planning to use brief psychoanalytical skills in their everyday work. The proposal was not to import wholesale the psychotherapeutic techniques proper to another branch of medicine, but rather that each branch should aim to develop psychotherapeutic techniques appropriate to

---

* This chapter is dedicated to my mother, Halima.

its own particular setting (5). Tom Main, being one of those associates, soon started his own groups, and over the next 40 years was closely involved in the training and development of these pioneering doctors. He had the innovative thinking to train leaders from within the membership, recognising that you did not need to be a psychoanalyst to lead such groups. The goal was not to breed mini-psychoanalysts, but doctors with the unique skill of being able to use brief, focussed, penetrative psychodynamic psychotherapy in tandem with their physical doctoring. This was the original concept for what is now known as psychosexual medicine.

CASE 1

To dive straight in and illustrate the use of the psychosexual genital examination, let us consider a common everyday occurrence in our clinical work.

Your nurse colleague asks you to examine his patient, who has already had her smear done and swabs taken, and is lying on the couch. You are told that she has come in several times before with discharge and pain, and repeated test results keep coming back negative. You are of course busy with your own list.

You might come rushing into the room, apologise for keeping the patient waiting, introduce yourself, may even take a quick history and check if it is okay to examine them. You might then reassure that everything is normal, as you slip your gloves off and exit the room having been quite efficient. Job done.

The IPM-trained doctor is aware of their own irritation at being asked to examine a part of the body. The doctor introduces himself or herself, registers the grizzly baby in the buggy, and checks the history very quickly. (Something does not 'feel' right with this patient. 'What's going on here?' the doctor asks himself or herself. The doctor parks his or her irritation and is now fully present. The doctor notices an attractive woman, lying on the couch with her legs up in stirrups. The patient seems 'unusually' uncomfortable, and the doctor ponders why she keeps coming back.) The doctor checks consent to examine and carries on. (During the examination, the doctor notices the screwed-up face of the patient, and an overwhelming sense of disgust and horror, the genital examination is otherwise all normal.) The doctor then comments, 'You seem disgusted by all of this, I wonder why that is?' The patient immediately replies, 'I don't know how you can even look down there, it's such a horrible mess!' 'Why do you think that?' the doctor asks. The patient answers with some distress, 'It's all been split apart, my vagina is ripped apart'. 'Those are very strong thoughts and emotions; can you tell me more?'

Her narrative of a difficult delivery unfolded. The patient's partner had been in attendance and commented later to her that it was awful watching his wife being 'ripped apart'. This horrendous image had stayed with this woman. It prevented her having sex with her partner and caused her repeated attendances as she was not being 'heard'. The doctor was then able to address the phantasy and invited the patient to have a look for herself. The doctor slipped her gloves off and left the room. Job done.

What Is the Psychosexual Genital Examination?

Psychosexual medicine employs 'experiential learning' to foster an approach to the patient that simultaneously acknowledges the physical, psychological and social. Doctors are trained to 'listen' carefully, to use the imagination, to evaluate self-critically and to test the validity of professional intuition. The psychosexual genital examination is the core of this discipline. It is a skill that can only be acquired and maintained by practising regularly. We all know someone who is a great cook, a yoga master, a fixer of things that are in need of mending; they became that way by learning from both failures and successes and by the dogged application of regular practise.

When the IPM-trained doctor uses their skills during the genital examination, the examination then becomes a psychotherapeutic genital examination. IPM doctors occupy and work in the space where the body and mind are given equal importance. Intimate contact is used to get in 'touch' with the patient's innermost fears. It is not without significance that innermost thoughts and fears are often expressed when innermost parts are touched, both emotionally and physically (6).

Tunnadine (7) states the concept of the psychosexual genital examination is that the 'anticipation of' or 'reaction to' this intimate moment gives us insights into the individual's attitude to his or her personal sexuality, this is of course diagnostic.

Crowley (8) mentions 'the power to touch the body of the patient sits with the clinician, as the body is brought to us. This power given to us by the patient allows a closing of the literal gap between us, gratifies the infant need to be felt, and allows the body to speak to the body; this is enormously therapeutic'. Touch can take many forms in the consulting room, including emotional (moved to tears), physical (routine examination), psychosexual (genital examination), comforting (a hug) and so on (9). (See Digging Deeper 12.1.)

Our patients attend, more often than not, hoping there must be a physical cause to their sexual problem which the doctor will find. It is useful to remember all physical problems will have a psychological aspect to them, i.e. what the patient thinks and feels about it, sometimes impacting on the problem significantly. The reverse, however, does not apply.

The psychosexual genital examination is not a prying but an enabling moment for a patient, who may be able to get in touch with feelings they did not know they had. It reveals something about the whole patient and can allow a sharing of painful and personal emotions.

The psychosexual genital examination can be of great value, provided the timing is right. 'It can be used as "safe-ground" (to retreat to) by the anxious doctor at a stuck point in the consultation, looking for something to do. Equally, the avoidance of a genital examination may not allow exploration of feelings and phantasies' (10).

Skills Used in a Psychosexual Genital Examination

The skills employed during the consultation and examination can be remembered as the pneumonic LOFTI, thought up by my director of training colleague, Jane Botell.

Listening: 'When you have a talking mouth you have no listening ears. When you have listening ears, you have no talking mouth' (11). So when using our ears, not only does the doctor need to pay heed to what is being said and how it is being said, but also – and perhaps more importantly – what is not being said. Subtle clues like a laughing remark or a change in speech tone need to be picked up on during the examination.

Observing: This means observing all aspects of patients closely, including how they undress, in what manner they walk in and lie down, how they talk to you, and their general behaviour. Every detail needs to be absorbed, not forgetting to pay attention to the atmosphere in the room. In carrying out this scrutiny it can be easy to fall into the trap of making generalisations and assumptions.

EXAMPLE 12.1

Harry: The portly, elderly man in his dapper outfit and bow tie, always the gentleman, so pleasant, so disarming. I was taken in by his exterior marshmallow defence which hid an angry, vengeful sexual fantasy that allowed a potent erection only with the women he hated, totally at odds with how he presented himself to the world.

Here I had made assumptions about Harry based on his appearance and was resistant to seeing the true fantasy.

Feeling: Be aware of the feelings within the room. How does this particular patient make you feel? How easily do they show their feelings? Be prepared to stay with uncomfortable moments/silences and learn to tolerate any confusion and feeling ignorant. During the genital examination patients have wondered aloud why feelings of anger, sadness, fear or regret emerge at such a time. If they do not emerge, it is important to reflect on the patient's emotional aspect, i.e. how do they feel about their problem? Having picked up feelings, the doctor must have the ability to understand and interpret such emotions and *use* them in a therapeutic way.

EXAMPLE 12.2

Jenny: She came with an overwhelming list of complaints…dyspareunia, post-coital bleeding, infection and concerns around her delivery. Her story was about a partner who had been sleeping around the last year or so after she had given birth to their baby. The pregnancy was fine but the delivery was reported to have been 'awful' for her. The placenta was stuck and she had to go to theatre. It now hurt to have sex with him. The overriding feeling in the room however was of anger, particularly when talking about her partner. Examination confirmed her doors were shut with vaginismus. Anger bubbled up as she confirmed that this is what happened with sex. I suggested it must be difficult to have sex with someone you are so angry with. She was then able to link that her mind had some part to play.

Here one might have expected a number of feelings: horror, anxiety and helplessness. In reality only the anger was palpable.

Thinking: In terms of psychosexual medicine this is the ability to step out of one's mind during the examination, observing and reviewing what is happening. It is often referred to as using our 'internal supervisor' or 'the third eye'. Schon (12) clearly articulates the messy world of clinical practice and discusses the practitioner who is able to reflect *in* action, as well as *on* action. This reflective practitioner is the IPM member. It is necessary to give thought to what sort of a doctor you are being, what is going on between you and the patient (the DPR), and what are the defences of doctor and patient. What is the atmosphere, has there been a change in it, and what happened to bring about that change at that particular time? A moment of critical evaluation is needed.

Interpreting: This is the offer of the doctor's critical evaluation to the expert: the patient. The crux of the psychosexual genital examination is not only to hold in mind all that you have heard, observed, felt and thought about; but also to *act* on the information. This action needs to be made spontaneously in real time (can be a few seconds to a minute or two). This takes *courage* to expose the professional self. There is no room for procrastination or avoidance, as the 'moment' may be lost. If the latter does happen, then exploration of why, with reference to what was going on between the doctor and patient, needs to be considered.

I would like to further suggest the LOFTI skills are actually the component parts of what we know as *attention*, defined by the *Concise Oxford English Dictionary* as the 'act or faculty of applying one's mind'. We would all surely be quick to say that we pay attention to our patients, and of course we do, but only in the way that our medical model of working has trained us to do. The 'attention' that I am speaking of is something that becomes the very 'being' of the training doctor and is likely to change their professional life to the benefit of the many patients they will encounter. In the current world of National Health Service (NHS) targets, efficiency savings, and quantity over quality, I would argue that paying proper 'attention' to our patients is the greatest form of generosity and care. (See Digging Deeper 12.2.)

What Makes the Psychosexual Genital Examination so Unique?

The talking therapist's training, in sexual dysfunction, is not to touch the patient, as this is viewed as interference in the 'transference' analysis, even if the therapist comes from a medical background. Those who carry out genital examinations in the disciplines of sexual and reproductive health, obstetrics and gynaecology, urology, etc., are not trained to work with the psychology of their patients – this is alien to them. IPM doctors are trained not to separate the 'body and mind' and are fully aware that patients cannot split themselves for the convenience of practitioners or the service providers. The *uniqueness* lies in the training and the psychosexual genital examination being a truly holistic process.

I would posit that this uniqueness is the result of the doctor learning to access both the right and left sides of the brain simultaneously. This seems fitting as it parallels the doctor's effort to understand the whole patient: both their internal world of subjective truths and their external world that is on show. The creation of a *safe space* (13) that allows sharing of the internal world of the patient and doctor requires the doctor to accept that they are not the 'expert' and that they 'do not know' what is of significance to

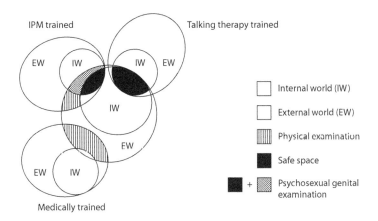

FIGURE 12.1 Areas of engagement by type of professional © Jasmin Khan-Singh, 2017.

this unique patient and their unique set of circumstances. This idea can be difficult for both doctor and patient to fully grasp and work with (see Figure 12.1).

Allen (14) reflects on the problem of knowledge being a favourite subject in Western philosophy. He states, 'grab hold of "don't know" and hang on tight. It's not easy; we are always tempted to consider our opinions as incontrovertible, but if you succeed in hanging on long enough you'll smile when you find that "don't know" is not mere ignorance but something fundamentally important and very exciting'.

The ability to sit with the 'not knowing' enables each DPR to be unique; one of equality, co-ignorance and co-endeavour (15).

Factors to Consider during the Psychosexual Genital Examination

There is a myriad of clues that can be picked up on just before, during and after the genital examination. Some are more obvious than others, e.g. as the doctor goes behind the curtain to examine and finds the patient is still fully clothed. The job of the IPM doctor is to understand why, and offer that understanding to the patient to accept or reject.

Offer and timing: Was examination suggested to get away from an uncomfortable moment in the consulting room, or because the doctor did not know what else to do, or as an avoidance to something unpalatable about the patient, or because the patient shares a physical worry? Or was it offered too early or too late, or – significantly – was an examination not even thought of, and so on? The considerations and possible defences of doctor and patient are many, but there is usually one unique understanding for that particular DPR that will throw light on the patient and the sexual problem presented.

CASE 2: TOM

Tom, a 30-year-old diabetic, presented with premature ejaculation. He is concerned that there must be 'something wrong' down there, eyes pointing to his genitals. During the examination, however, his eyes were held very tightly shut; when I pointed this out he admitted he was concentrating on making sure he did not get an erection. I wondered with him if during sex he was concentrating so hard on 'not coming' that he is not in the present moment and so ends up losing control. Tom then, as he had done throughout the consultation, made light of this with another joke around respecting me as a doc. I offered that his use of jokes, to deflect from critical emotional moments, perhaps meant there are some unacknowledged feelings behind them. He was then able to voice his 'fear of all the loss' that would be inevitable living with this 'silent killer', to my surprise he was referring to his diabetes.

Here I took up the request of 'examine me' that was clearly being voiced as a physical worry.

Refusal or acceptance: Did they freeze in terror, or show ambivalence, or appear to be very much at ease, or give the doctor excuses such as 'I can't be examined today – I haven't showered', and so on? Or did they just flatly refuse? Exploring and understanding why a patient is reluctant to have an examination, or the doctor is hesitant in offering one, can be just as therapeutic as carrying one out.

CASE 3: KYLIE

Kylie was a 22-year-old who complained of no libido, previously everything was good with sex. She had a 1950s style of dress sense, prim and proper with matching handbag. She flatly refused the genital examination; she does not allow anyone to see her body. She ensures her boyfriend never sees her body and sex takes place in the dark, under the covers. I was feeling it would be risky and dangerous to push it. This strong defence and where it might have come from was explored, I enquired has it ever felt risky or frightening to expose your body in the past. Then the painful tears flowed as memories were relived. She had been bullied over the mole on her face, for most of senior school, and had almost put it in the past but for the recent resurrection of the teasing by her boyfriend's sister. The doctor had barely noticed the neat and stylish mole on her face, but for the patient it represented rejection and pain by not only her peers but also her boyfriend, as he did not defend her against his sister. How could she enjoy sex with a man who had let her down?

Here even though the patient refused, it was possible to use that strong rejection to throw light on the underlying cause.

Preparation: How do they undress, which clothes are removed, how do they stow their clothes, how are they lying on the couch – all covered up or fully exposed? It is as if by peeling away the outer layers that the inner self is revealed, a metaphorical removal of their defences along with their clothing. This places the doctor in a very privileged position of experiencing an intimate connection with the patient, both emotionally and physically, giving the doctor an insight into the patient's sexuality (16).

CASE 4: RAVEN

The thin, truculent, demanding 15-year-old in her ripped designer jeans, tight crop top, oozing sexiness and availability; she had given all staff in the clinic a hard time as no method of contraception seemed to suit and was putting her off sex. This exterior prickly armour, once removed for the genital examination, exposed a child lying on the couch, clutching onto the barely adequate modesty tissue. I was taken aback by the personality change and wondered out loud how difficult it must be for her to be this sexy, in-control teenager on contraception, when really, she still felt like a child. Making this realisation a conscious event allowed the teenager to re-evaluate. She understood that she did not want to be sexually active and it was not too late to stop being that person.

Here the patient's journey of undressing and getting on the bed had exposed her real self, a child lying on the couch.

Reactions during: Do they stiffen or look embarrassed or chatter away incessantly, or are they totally detached from the examination? Do they engage fully or make remarks such as 'I couldn't do your job – how awful to have to look at private parts all day' or 'I'm too small for that speculum'? For some patients this feels like exposure, and they have used expressions such as feeling invaded or exposed. The trick is to balance 'containing' the patient and challenging them gently to think about the uncomfortable feelings. Sometimes connections are made there and then between body and mind, and these may or may not be shared.

CASE 5: STANLEY

Stanley was a traditional, gentle giant of a man, with a set of rosy cheeks and kind eyes. His 68 years were worn well. He had been unable to penetrate or have an orgasm since the death of his wife, 4 years ago. He accepted the offer of an examination with deference and once on the couch he was working hard not to show his feelings. Once I pointed this out to him, his eyes turned red, his face became flushed as he allowed himself a few tears. His sadness and grief filled the room. He admitted that he had not cried for his wife at all (because men do not), and felt guilt ridden that people may think he never loved her. His grief still felt raw, we wondered together whether having been unable to show his love for her by crying, the resulting guilt meant it would be disloyal to let her go, which is what he would have to do when penetrating another woman.

Here the picking up of a male generational pattern of behaviour allowed connection to his grief and guilt and the understanding of its impact on his ability to engage with sexual intercourse.

Feelings of the doctor: What the doctor feels is critical in helping to understand the problem. In the training groups I have led, trainees have often reported that they feel prying, abusive or all too powerful. They worried whether the patient really understood what the psychosexual genital examination was about. These strong emotions may be too uncomfortable to bear and the urge is to flee, but the skill is to pick them up and share them in a way that makes sense of that unique patient and their unique life. Ideally this should happen at the genital examination, but it can be delayed until they are dressed (recognising that as a defence) as long as the feelings and thoughts are studied. These feelings are clinical findings in their own right, and the trainee can learn to use them therapeutically. This can be difficult, as the tendency would be to ignore these feelings as they do not belong in the world of evidence-based medicine. This does the patient a great disservice.

Skrine (14) talks about the ability to allow mental images to flood the mind and then share them tentatively, enabling the patient to either accept or reject the interpretation. This I believe is *the definitive skill*, to be open and receptive so you do pick up these emotions and images.

CASE 6: MOLLY

This menopausal lady walked in, plain and greying, a sad troubled face, wearing comfy beige trousers and top, she was almost invisible. She could not have sex since her hysterectomy, a few months ago. It was a rushed decision as she was bleeding heavily, but she did not want to lose her womb. Her loss was palpable. She was told the offending fibroid was quite big but the surgeons had managed to 'cobble' things back together. I enquired what she thought had happened down below. Her phantasy was startling – she described it as 'shrivelled and dead, like a zipped off area with nothing in it'. I offered we take a look together. Her vulva was normal, and after some initial vaginismus, I put in two fingers. The patient seemed far away and I was stuck with her phantasy in my head; then an image of her vault, as a grave, flooded in, and I felt disrespectful going in. Once she was dressed and we were at the table, I related that it all feels dead, like a grave down there, not to be entered. Her tears trickled out. I offered there was a huge sense of loss here in the room, I wonder if you are mourning the loss of your womb. Somehow what is left after the operation has become a memorial to it. Now the tears flooded down her cheeks as she accepted the interpretation.

Here the vivid image of a graveyard, accompanied by the emotion of feeling disrespectful, was presented to and accepted by the patient. This helped the patient to understand what had become of her sexy parts and she claimed it back for herself, reporting in her review appointment that sex was now fine.

The 'Moment of Truth'

The case examples all show a moment in the examination when the truth emerges or a realisation occurs or an illuminating connection is made by the patient (Table 12.1).

Aptly named the 'moment of truth', this is the actual moment when doctor and patient know intuitively that they have reached the real feeling, thought or phantasy behind all the defences.

This moment trickles into the patient's consciousness and the patient recognises it for what it is, their subjective truth. Very often the moment announces itself in the room with a change of the atmosphere or as if someone has pressed the pause button, but it is always felt. It can be followed by silence or an intense emotion and the urge to fill this moment with chatter should be resisted. Other thoughts can then surface in the head of the patient and they may be shared with the doctor, or not, shared with the partner, or not, or never shared with anyone.

TABLE 12.1

Moment of Truth in Cases 2–6

Case 2	The fear of his diabetes
Case 3	The rejection and pain, signified by the mole
Case 4	Being conscious of the dichotomy of her personality
Case 5	Awareness of his guilt and sense of disloyalty
Case 6	Understanding her vault had become a memorial

Common Concerns over the Intimate Examination

The 2013 General Medical Council guidance on intimate examination state the following (17):

1. The guidance should not deter you from carrying out an intimate examination when necessary.
2. Explain to the patient why an examination is necessary and give the patient an opportunity to ask questions.
3. When you carry out an intimate examination, you should offer the patient the option of having an impartial observer (a chaperone) present wherever possible. This applies whether or not you are the same gender as the patient.
4. Keep discussion relevant and do not make unnecessary personal comments, during the examination.

The Royal College of Obstetricians and Gynaecologists (18) expects, as part of fundamental communication skills, trainees to demonstrate 'appropriate use of chaperones for intimate examinations, maintaining dignity at all times and being sensitive to cultural and religious issues'.

The IPM Chaperone Policy (2017) (19) states the following:

> Practitioners are required to follow the chaperone policy required of their professional legislative body.
>
> For doctors this will be 'Intimate examinations and chaperones. General Medical Council 2013' and any further standards advised by their specialist royal college.
>
> Nurses, physiotherapists and allied health professionals are similarly bound by policies issued by their registration and governing bodies in addition to what may be required by trusts and places of employment.

Consent: In my experience of leading seminar groups, trainees often show a resistance to offering a genital examination, particularly when there is no physical complaint or the patient has been recently examined. For example, if the patient is complaining of decreased libido or anorgasmia then it seems difficult to broach or justify the genital examination.

Point 4, previously mentioned, causes concern and confusion for the IPM trainee. It applies neatly to the 'black and white' medical model of working. However, it fails to take into account the unique scenario when the physical examination is integrated with brief psychotherapy. The whole ethos of IPM training is to comment on the subconscious, which is one of the most personal parts of our patients. Consequently, gaining informed consent is difficult when you are still grappling with understanding the need for it yourself. We do need to explain why an examination is necessary and how a psychosexual genital examination may throw some light on the problem presented. It may help to think of the psychotherapeutic examination as a clinical measurement in its own right, just like a blood pressure recording; it is *necessary* and lies firmly within the scope of work of IPM trainees as well as diplomates and members.

Chaperones: For the IPM-trained doctor, the presence of a chaperone is an added barrier to the way of working. This third person, an 'intruding other' (20), can have an effect in many ways; such as making it difficult for the patient to voice their fears and phantasies, hampering the clinician from using any recognised unconscious feelings of the patient and potentially changing the DPR from a two- to a three-way relationship.

Thankfully for those of us who routinely carry out intimate examinations, we know that in the real world of clinical practice it is only occasionally that the patient wants a chaperone present. More often than not, they are mortified at the thought of exposing their 'private parts' to more people than necessary. The offer and the declining or accepting of a chaperone is required to be recorded in the notes. A defensive local policy, whereupon it is decreed a chaperone has to be present regardless of the gender of doctor or patient, can result in delayed examinations. However, the General Medical Council requires any delays in examination should not adversely affect the patient's health. The tension thus created, may mean the choices made by practitioners are open to even more scrutiny.

It is more likely it will be the clinician who wants a chaperone present, e.g. in the case of a vulnerable adult, or sexualisation of the consultation, or male doctor with female patient and vice versa. Such situations require safeguarding of the doctor as well as the patient, and understanding in the context of the DPR. In the end both doctor and patient need to feel comfortable before a psychosexual genital examination can proceed. (See 'Practical Points' box.)

LEARNING POINTS

- The psychosexual genital examination is a unique enabling moment allowing connection to the patient's subconscious.
- During the psychosexual genital examination tolerating the 'not knowing' and the creation of a 'safe space', for both doctor and patient, are key skills.
- The 'moment of truth' often occurs during the psychosexual genital examination.
- A psychosexual genital examination is a necessary clinical finding and lies within the remit of those working and training in the field of psychosexual medicine.

DIGGING DEEPER 12.1

A comforting touch in clinical practice can have many meanings. Was it done to stop crying, or to show empathy, or considered inappropriate, did it feel wrong and right at the same time, or therapeutic? It is the understanding of that touch for both patient and doctor that is of importance.

Example: **Arthur:** A widower of 2 years with erectile dysfunction, he kept everyone at arm's length but also went up to complete strangers who seemed sad to make them laugh. We discussed his ambivalence over making 'connections' with people and that sex required a connection too. When it was time for discharge from the clinic, he stopped himself from shaking my hand and asked permission to give me a 'hug'; as I stumbled over my reply, he explained he should start making connections. The hug was heartfelt. We both understood this touch was the start of a new beginning for him.

DIGGING DEEPER 12.2

Tom Main clarified the skills that need nurturing as synaesthetic perceptiveness to gather empathy 'data' and diacritic perceptiveness to critically assess it (15). Doctors are usually comfortable with the scientific approach, i.e. the diacritic (questioning and telling method), but the 'feeling' approach (tuning in to subjective truths felt by a whole living person) can be quite a challenge. So perhaps it is of no surprise that a rare minority of trainees do not have or are unlikely to ever acquire the necessary perceptiveness, while others seem to have a talent for the work and quickly pick up the skills; the majority of us, however, have to wait for an inherent shift in understanding within ourselves.

PRACTICAL POINTS

As the genital examination in psychosexual medicine is pivotal in the work, proper consideration should be given to where and how an examination is carried out. You could bear in mind the following:

- Ensure your room is warm, privacy is maintained by either locking the door or drawing the curtains, there is sufficient modesty roll available and a chair for the patients' clothes.
- Try not to change rooms for genital examinations, as moments of connection can be easily lost or difficult to get back to and the ability to observe how the patient undresses and gets to the point of lying on the couch will be missed.
- Chaperones, if present, should be trained to be as discreet as possible, placed out of the direct sight of the patient, have a basic understanding of the psychosexual genital examination and not be too quick with offers of tissues or consoling at highly emotional moments.

REFERENCES

1. Institute of Psychosexual Medicine Prospectus. London, 2014. http://www.ipm.org.uk/17/our-therapy.
2. Tunnadine P. *Insights into Troubled Sexuality.* London: Chapman and Hall, 1992, 15.
3. Skrine R. Out of the woodwork – Body phantasies then and now. *Inst Psychosexual Med J* 2013;33:2–6.
4. *The Concise Oxford English Dictionary* (9th ed.). Oxford, UK: Oxford University Press, 1995.
5. Michael A, Balint E. *Psychotherapeutic Techniques in Medicine.* London: Tavistock Publications, 1961.
6. Rogers J. RL Skrine (Ed.), *Introduction to Psychosexual Medicine.* Carlisle, UK: Montana Press, 1989, 32.
7. Tunnadine P. That he who runs may read. *Inst Psychosexual Med J* 1993;6:11.
8. Crowley T. Touch or 'mind' the gap. *Inst Psychosexual Med J* 2007;45:8–14.
9. Roberts M. Touch and the doctor-patient relationship. *Inst Psychosexual Med J* 2003;33:8–10.
10. Gill M. In RL Skrine (Ed.), *Introduction to Psychosexual Medicine.* Carlisle, UK: Montana Press, 1989, 108.
11. Allen R. *365 Smiles from Buddha.* MQ Publications, 2003, p. 211.
12. Schon D. *Educating the Reflective Practitioner.* San Francisco, CA: Jossey-Bass, 1987.
13. Skrine R. *Blocks and Freedoms in Sexual Life.* London: Radcliffe Medical Press, 1997.
14. Allen R. *365 Smiles from Buddha.* MQ Publications, 2003, p. 272.
15. Main T. Training for the acquisition of knowledge or the development of skill? *Inst Psychosexual Med J* 2014;66:8–14.
16. Smith A. In RL Skrine (Ed.), *Introduction to Psychosexual Medicine.* Carlisle, UK: Montana Press, 1989, 64–71.
17. General Medical Council. Financial and commercial arrangements and conflicts of interest. London: GMC, 2013. http://www.gmc-uk.org/guidance/ethical_guidance/30200.asp
18. Royal College of Obstetricians and Gynaecologists. Part 3 MRCOG: Syllabus. London, 2018. https://www.rcog.org.uk/en/careers-training/mrcog-exams/part-3-mrcog-exam/part-3-mrcog-syllabus/
19. Institute of Psychosexual Medicine. London. https://www.ipm.org.uk/
20. Elliman A. Chaperones in the psychosexual medicine clinic. *Inst Psychosexual Med J* 2005;40:14–15.

13

Vaginismus and Non-Consummation

Claudine Domoney

Introduction

Sexual problems are frequently a source of shame to the woman/man/'patient'. None more so, perhaps, than the inability to have an intimate relationship, despite a present and willing partner. Non-consummation of a relationship often presents late with embedded behaviours that may take time to resolve. The couple or individual may not have been able to discuss the difficulty with anyone until there is a specific issue that needs to be addressed: for instance, fertility, calls for cervical screening, or other gynaecological problems. Vaginismus may have always been present and contribute to unsuccessful sexual relationships or develop after a traumatic experience, recognised or unrecognised.

Definitions

Non-consummation

Non-consummation is defined as the lack of penetration required for sexual intercourse and can be caused by female and male factors. Most often it is 'blamed' on the receptive partner although the dynamic between the couple may be independent but linked with features of the problem. Erectile dysfunction, also a cause of non-consummation, is discussed elsewhere in the book. In females the focus is often on a physical obstruction to a finger, penis, tampon or speculum. The physical demonstration of this may extend to the inability to expose the genitalia, either by covering up with clothing or blanket, adductor spasm of the thighs, intolerance to touch, or physical distraction with other interjections, such as talking or focussing on an accompanying child or partner during a consultation.

Vaginismus

Vaginismus can be a primary or a secondary symptom. It is useful not to think of vaginismus as a disorder in itself but a symptom that expresses psychological distress that may or may not be physical in origin. Involuntary pelvic floor spasm is the usual underlying disorder that is a protection from pain – pain being of the mind and/or body. Rationalising the physiological response may not enable the woman to control this. Understanding and interpreting the defences involved in this response is the aim of psychosexual treatment, using both the feelings of the woman and the doctor, during their interaction. Access to the denied or suppressed feelings of the patient by both the patient and doctor can enable access to the vagina (Figure 13.1).

Presentation

Overt

Referral from primary care to the psychosexual clinic or gynaecology clinic depends on the general practitioner (GP) or practice nurse's perception of the causes of the non-consummation or vaginismus.

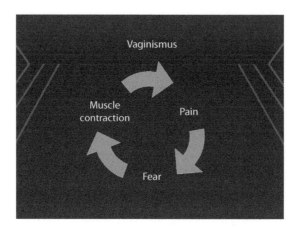

FIGURE 13.1   Mechanisms at play in vaginismus.

The patients themselves may have looked up their symptoms on the Internet and present with a diagnosis. The patient may wish to conceive but acknowledge that this will not happen without medical help. Often there are expectations of pregnancy after marriage that force the couple to progress (usually after some time) to seek medical help. Counsellors in fertility clinics frequently find that intercourse is not happening and may never have occurred. A call from the GP to have a cervical smear can expose the difficulties in penetration. Many in this situation believe they are placing themselves at risk because they have not had a smear, despite never having had penetrative intercourse and therefore have very little risk of human papillomavirus (HPV) infection. Those who have been able to succumb to a smear may have the unpleasantness of vaginal penetration reinforced, further compounding the problem. The doctor may be called upon to reinforce the perceived abnormality of the vagina – 'a vagina too small, a vagina with a blockage or the endless tunnel with access to the abdominal organs'.

Non-consummation is often explained by patients in terms of their cultural or religious beliefs and constraints. Yet the lack of evidence of widespread sexual problems as a result of these beliefs, suggests that acceptance of these factors is not sufficient. The experience of the individual and how she and her partner process the difficulties is more likely to be what needs to be tackled by the healthcare professional (HCP). Perceptions and stereotyping by the HCP are not likely to be helpful on their own.

Covert

It is often difficult for women to vocalise issues with penetration. There will often be another agenda presented to the HCP as there is much shame and isolation associated with an inability to have penetrative intercourse or have a cervical smear or examination. An expressed belief that something is wrong or the anatomy abnormal preventing entry is common. However, this is often combined with an understanding that the person or their partner is too fearful to allow entry or to enter. Inability to have a cervical smear or allow speculum examination, fear of prolapse, fantasies of a scarred (and scared), closed vagina, a vagina too small with or without surgical interventions, including episiotomy, deformed vulva, the sensitive bladder, the tunnel with no end where items can get 'lost' or the vagina that leaks discharge or urine, the vagina that passes flatus because it is too big – can all be 'calling cards' for the woman suffering with vaginismus, or on occasion, non-consummation. Non-consummation as a secondary problem is less common as women with issues around fear of penetration often will not feel able to commit to a relationship because of the risk of exposing their shameful secret. This is, despite the finding that a powerful defence to further harm, may be inability to have any form of penetration, whether it be with tampons, medical instruments or a penis or other penile representative, including fingers. It may be more acceptable to present with pain or sexual pain, even though this differentiation is not always on a conscious level. An understanding of the causes and reinforcing/maintaining factors may not be recognised. It is for the HCP to help guide the patient to that understanding through active use of the HCP-patient relationship dynamic.

Causes of Vaginismus and Non-Consummation

Physical

Direct physical causes must be excluded but are infrequent. The opportunity for examination is the advantage that practitioners of psychosexual medicine have over many other sex therapists. The examination itself is often a therapeutic event if used appropriately. It is common that treatment of the physical problem alone may not 'cure' the vaginismus. Learned behavioural responses to attempts at intimate exploration are deeply ingrained and may have been present for many years. Clumsy attempts by HCPs to reassure patients that they are now normal after various interventions, may leave the patient feeling even more isolated and abnormal as the psychological effects of the physical findings have not also been addressed as discussed below.

Rigid hymens are rare but do occasionally present to gynaecologists for surgical intervention – usually an examination under anaesthesia (EUA) will allow stretching or tearing with occasional recourse to excision. Yet more often an examination under general anaesthetic will reinforce the vagina as being a remote place that is abnormal and cannot be approached in a conscious state. The 'pain' may be transformed into another problem. Chronic pain after surgical intervention can be particularly difficult to manage when it has followed a procedure while unconscious.

EXAMPLE 13.1

A lesbian patient was accompanied by her partner diligently supporting her both physically and psychologically for weeks while she healed from a 'division of hymen' performed under anaesthetic. She did not feel she needed it, but it had been done while a hysteroscopy was performed.

Vaginal septums are sometimes detected in young women finding it difficult to use tampons or have penetrative sex but are not often linked to long-standing psychological issues. Managing female reproductive organ congenital anomalies needs care and sensitivity.

EXAMPLE 13.2

One young woman presented to a gynaecology clinic with vaginismus associated with a history of frequent examinations by gynaecologists as a child, when she was found to have an 'interesting' combination of uterine and vaginal anomalies, that required several operations. She was exposed to a number of humiliating consultations where she described large numbers of medical students looking and poking at her genitals such that she never wanted anyone to 'go there again' and described herself as a 'freak of nature'.

Shortened vaginas can be associated with congenital genital tract anomalies including Turner's syndrome and disorders of sexual differentiation, which are associated with other psychosexual difficulties. These children and women should be supported by behavioural and physical therapy, but this can cause difficulties through inappropriate exposure to multiple HCPs. They may develop feelings of abnormality, being a 'freak' and that their private parts are no longer their own.

More commonly in clinical practice are vaginal scarring, stenosis and shortening after childbirth and surgery.

EXAMPLE 13.3

A woman was seen in a clinic with an inability to have penetrative intercourse post-childbirth although her GP had referred her with pelvic floor prolapse. She had assumed that she had a psychological problem as her birth experience was described as traumatic. She was openly disappointed in her inability to resume her sex life which she felt was a very important component of her relationship and needed to 'put the birth behind' her. Her openness in discussion and willingness to embrace a psychological cause did not quite seem to follow the patterns of a psychosexual problem. So, it was with some surprise but delight that a complete introital stenosis of the lower vagina was found on examination. Surgical repair was completely successful and she did not require further psychosexual support.

Women with female genital mutilation are frequently referred to specialist clinics with non-consummation but occasionally women are seen in antenatal clinics having conceived with ejaculation at the introitus.

Skin and mucosal conditions are frequently associated with dyspareunia and therefore secondary (or primary) vaginismus. Lichen sclerosis can slowly reduce the introitus and fuse the labia and clitoral hood. Lichen planus can cause such significant stenosis that surgical separation is required although frequently steroid foam preparations can prevent recourse to surgery if the patient presents early enough.

EXAMPLE 13.4

A woman in her 40s only presented after her husband had had an affair. She described his fury with her inability to allow him to penetrate her. She had tried to allow him but the doctor could feel her anger was preventing her letting him in. He had sent her to be 'checked out'. Yet she had an almost complete occlusion of the vagina. Only after she mentioned frequent lesions in her mouth was a diagnosis of lichen planus made. Yet after surgical intervention she was still not able to allow him 'entrance' due to her anger with his attitude to her and his sexual needs.

EXAMPLE 13.5

A couple was seen in a psychosexual clinic with the woman having a diagnosis of vaginismus. She was in her late 60s and him in his mid-70s. She had had a series of vaginal operations, initially for prolapse then subsequent operations to try to repair the scarring and stricture in the vagina. There was a sense of defeat from the wife. He sat looking old and hunched in his raincoat during the appointment, saying nothing and seeming remote, resisting eye contact. It seemed she had suffered many operations to try to achieve a vagina 'fit for purpose' as she remarked, when he appeared to have little interest. 'We are too old for all this', he said but looking dejected. Yet, when the sadness was remarked upon, she was able to show her husband the disappointment that they had not been able to resume their sexual life, which she felt she had being doing for him. He looked up with a small glint in his eye. 'So, it's alright now then is it? We are not too old?' he asked the doctor. The doctor responded with a feeling of hope and enthusiasm as well.

There are many chronic pain conditions that will cause a secondary protective response which can result in vaginismus. Treatment of these conditions may need an understanding of the psychosexual impact in order to treat the vaginismus component. The mind may understand but the body not respond accordingly. Bladder pain syndrome, vulval pain syndrome, endometriosis, pelvic inflammatory disease, chronic discharge can all cause a pelvic floor response that may be direct or secondary to a learned response to the pain that will follow. Lack of diagnosis and lack of treatment further embeds the abnormal pelvic floor spasm, with its consequences for sexual intimacy.

Menopause

The physiological changes of menopause can cause significant problems for women not aware of the effects. The lack of information and care by healthcare professionals in the UK system who are not able to regularly advise women of the possible sequelae of lack of oestrogen, can create long-standing issues. Vaginal atrophy in particular, is poorly understood by both women and those responsible for their care. As many of the complaints are separated in time from the cessation of periods, they are not linked. They are thought of as the consequence of ageing. 'It is normal' not to want sexual intimacy any longer. Yet frequently it is the tissue changes that cause pain and discomfort, abnormal discharge, overactive bladder symptoms, urinary tract infections after intercourse, worsening prolapse symptoms.

The lack of information for women and their partners leads them to suppose it is in some way their 'fault'. The loss of libido that ensues is perceived as part of the ageing process, rather than the defensive behaviour of the mind and body to pain. The psychological difficulties are reinforced by the protective response of the partner, who unwilling to cause pain to their partner may develop erectile difficulties. Doctors reviewing these women may not acknowledge the physical changes and resort to their own prejudices.

Things that have been said to patients by unfeeling HCPs:

> If you hold out any longer your husband will lose interest.
> Masturbate more to lubricate your tissues then you will know what to do with your husband.

Women experiencing peri-menopause or post-menopausal women have a multitude of issues that are complex and, if left for some time in a cultural setting not expecting ongoing sexual activity, become a predetermined state of inactivity, with vaginismus being an inevitable consequence. The perspective of the menopausal woman addressing her changing life parameters can challenge her sexuality. How she deals with these challenges is in part determined by her partner and access to 'specialist' healthcare.

Psychological

The sexual transition from being a child to an adult woman (or man) is a process that can be dependent on many factors. Although there may be common themes regarding cultural restrictions on sexual expression, any individual's response to their upbringing is unique. Reactions to sexual awakening and awareness of genitals may be circumstantial and based on many influences. The child absorbs the feelings around them and responds in their psychologically protective own way. The family that does not verbalise conflicts around growing up, genitals or sexual behaviour or those that frame them as being 'dirty' or overwhelming or to be endured, can pass on these values to their children. The genitals that should not be touched even as a child, become shameful and mysterious. The woman who struggles with leaving childhood and/or their mother can find the move to adulthood and sexual relationships a challenge.

Fantasies

Fantasies that focus around the vagina are powerful and can be long lasting. It cannot be visualised, unlike the penis. 'A long thin tube, one that opens into the abdomen, a space that can swallow objects put inside, a long dark tunnel, a raw red tissue that bleeds, a tunnel with a bone blocking the way, a delicate flower that will be crushed'. All of these are fantasies of women striving to understand why their vagina does not 'work' like others. The vulvas that need to be always covered, shaven of hair, maintained 'clean', neat and tidy (with non-protuberant labia minora) are to be hidden from view. The mother has great influence over her daughter's emergence into a woman.

Taboos

Taboos around menstruation, its experience as dirty and shameful, can powerfully project a negative sexual experience. The girl told she cannot use tampons until she has been sexually active, that she will lose her virginity, perpetuates the ownership of her vagina by another, to be handed over from her mother to her husband. The 'good girl' does not explore herself or experiment. Growing up to accept an independent life, including sexual life may be challenging. The vulnerable or emotionally immature 'girl' can find it hard to feel big enough to allow a penis inside – that of an adult man – her vagina is 'too small' or will be damaged by his large organ. She is not 'big enough' to allow him in yet – emotionally and physically. Or if she does, she may be overwhelmed by sexual feelings she cannot control but should – as she has done for many years. This is often found with women and men who have not been allowed to have sexual relationships – usually before marriage – and have controlled their sexual urges for many years, only for the control to continue when they are allowed to express them.

Adults who have developed rigid thinking around the sexual act rather than its context, may experience the failure of 'appropriate' intimacy as the transition involves taking responsibility for sexual feelings and acting on them, rather than always denying them. Those that have reinforced those behaviours – mothers, fathers, elders in the community, may also be metaphorically present in the bedroom judging their behaviour and performance.

CASE 1

The primary school teacher with perfectly cut and blow-dried hair in a neat ponytail, wearing a tight pencil skirt with a high buttoned blouse, with high heels on sensible court shoes, explains she has not been able to have penetrative sex since her wedding 18 months ago. She was brought up in a strict Irish household as a good Catholic girl. She had managed to 'save' herself for marriage, despite having quite a few boyfriends and sexual experiences. Yet when it came to letting herself experience orgasm with penetrative sex, she found she was not able to feel anything but fear and disgust. She misses the days of foreplay and oral sex. She cannot even allow that now. She sits very primly, upright like a ballerina, hands held calmly in front of her. Her coat is folded carefully over her lap.

She makes the doctor feel intrusive for asking about sex. It feels like she might 'break'. It feels important not to push too much. 'It seems difficult to talk about your feelings about sex'. 'He doesn't want to hurt me so we don't get very far...' The doctor has the sense of a little girl dressed up like a woman but sitting on a very high stool, with her legs dangling, a woman on a pedestal. She is powerfully able to steer the conversation away from anything too sexual and directs it to the behaviours of her husband and her family that reinforces her own.

She is on the contraceptive pill and he uses condoms even though there has not been ejaculation anywhere near the vagina. 'What are you afraid will happen?' 'I don't think I am ready...' For sex, for pregnancy, for marriage, for penetration, for the sensation of loss of control with someone else perceived as being the powerful one? Although all of these thoughts are with the doctor, it is too much to challenge directly. 'Ready for what?' She then details her life plans for the next few years. She wants to be headmistress in 2 years then start a family of her own. 'Will that be when you have to have sex?' Planning ahead for then, having homework set and getting it in on time appears to be the agenda. 'I know it takes some time to treat vaginismus'. She has done some of her homework already. She declines examination on that day. Enough has been achieved. An appointment is organised and put in the diary for a later date.

At the next appointment, a very different woman presents. Her hair, although in a ponytail, is messy and her clothes are more youthful. She is in jeans and a fleece top. She is ready for her examination. Her pubic hair is perfectly 'manicured'. She has laid her clothes on the chair folded meticulously. She takes herself to the couch and places the blanket over her and lay waiting with her legs apart. The doctor started to tell her what she was going to do. It would be at her pace. She had prepared herself, seeming to be engaged, and said she was ready. Yet the moment she was touched, she recoiled and turned her head away. 'No, it's ok. Carry on. Just do it'. The doctor cannot continue without her agreement or engagement. The doctor feels she is perpetrating an abusive act. 'You seem to be forcing yourself to go through with this. We are both finding it difficult. Shall we leave it until another time?' 'No, I have to do it now. I promised myself I would grow up'. 'But it is not so easy to tell yourself to grow up. Perhaps you do not feel ready'. 'But I must'. They try together again but she is not able to allow any more than touching the external genitalia without closing her thighs. The consultation ends with an agreement that tampons and self-examination will be tried. The doctor reflects that it seems like a form of homework. The teacher laughs and comments she is good at that.

At the next consultation, a happy excited young woman bounces in. She is pleased to report that she has managed her homework well and has been able to insert two fingers and successfully used tampons with her last period. 'I read the instructions' she says. 'Can I try sex now? Do you think it will be OK?' The doctor is caught up in her enthusiasm and confirms that it is time to try again. She hopes that the less meticulous and more carefree woman can now allow herself to experience the freedom of sexual intimacy. She does not return, implying that she has reached her goal without further support or tuition.

Traumatising Situations

Any exposure to traumatising situations can be sensitising experiences. These may be minor issues, that at first mention may seem of minimal importance, but the expression of emotion implies the incident is of greater magnitude and the HCP needs to be alerted to its possible significance. The skill of psychosexual medicine is to note the change in mood at the details described: how the patient expresses themselves with verbal and nonverbal communication. The feelings evoked may be recognised as emanating from the patient. Why does the doctor feel protective now, how has the mood changed to anger, where has the sudden sadness originated from, the frustration directed towards the doctor who appears not to be listening or who cannot find out what is wrong or find a 'cure'?

Interactions with healthcare services are anxiety provoking for many individuals. When the most vulnerable parts of our private lives and bodies are exposed psychologically and physically to potentially damaging and unpredictable interventions, an adverse reaction is not unusual. The maintenance of a negative impact will depend on how the patients are managed and understood. Women who have been told their cervix is in the wrong place, have a retroverted uterus, a cervical erosion, have high-risk HPV and many other misinterpretations of pathologies, can be seen to develop defences against perceived damage. This may occur, just during gynaecological examination, but can also extend to any penetration. Exploration of when the problem started can evoke a re-creation of the trauma of the event. Even in an impatient or rushed consultation, with the patient feeling 'naughty' or 'uncooperative' or 'silly' or not being able to respond to a command to 'just relax', this, if recognised, could be used by the HCP to elicit better understanding of the development of a secondary problem. Also, the HCP can find themselves colluding with the patient's fantasy of the genital tract.

Loss of trust of the patient's own body can be caused by careless words or actions. This needs to be addressed by acknowledging the emotions engendered. Careful, cautious examination with the patient in control can reassure the traumatised individual that she can be 'normal' again.

The chaperone who holds the patient's hand during examination may further reinforce the expected trauma of the event, whereas the woman who can allow an examination at her own pace in a private, respectful fashion can find this a therapeutic undertaking. It is important to note that chaperones change the dynamic of a psychosexual examination such that it can be difficult to interpret the reactions coming from the patient and those projected from an inexperienced chaperone.

Many gynaecological interventions can be triggering factors for significant sexual issues. Most will be temporary or cause a change in libido that can be reframed as part of 'survivorship' in the case of those with gynaecological cancer or ageing in others. For some, a reduction in sexual activity is acceptable. Others may develop vaginismus with sexual pain or it may extend to an inability to have penetrative intercourse. It is important to establish what the patient herself has experienced and how she has reacted to the changes in her body. The psychological impact of any intervention will be unique and the tendency to stereotype expected responses, despite the HCPs experience, should be resisted. The difference between detection of HPV on a cervical smear and the treatment of a cervical cancer may seem enormous to an HCP, but in the mind of an ill-prepared, uninformed vulnerable patient, the impact may be equally as traumatic. Both have associations with the risks of sex.

Listening to the effect of a diagnosis and its subsequent management, supports the journey to recovery. Treatment of sexually transmitted diseases or the management of an excessive discharge are part of the spectrum demonstrating how the vagina can intrude into the psyche. The bleeding vagina can demonstrate damage or, be part of femininity. There are women who do not want periods and demand a hysterectomy compared to the women who do not feel feminine without regular bleeds. The changes caused by a cone biopsy, hysterectomy, labial reduction, vulvectomy, cervical cautery, the un-sutured perineum after childbirth, perceived scarring after prolapse repair – precipitate a feeling of loss. These losses can be transformed into lack of enjoyment or pleasure and a change in purpose of the vagina and vulva. Sex may be thought to cause damage or further recurrence both by the woman and sometimes her partner. Unscheduled bleeding may create anxiety. A psychological response may logically be protection from sexual activity by loss of libido and/or sexual pain due to vaginismus.

CASE 2

A woman in her 30s presented in a gynaecology clinic requesting labial surgery. She was immaculately dressed and very engaging, encouraging eye contact at all times. Every move of the doctor was observed, making the consultation feel restricted. The story of her life was told as if it had been told many times before. She had committed herself to the man she thought was the love of her life. She had 'his baby' then he started abusing her, commenting on her ugly genitalia and belittling her. A labial and 'designer vagina' operation was undertaken and then she had another baby because 'he wanted one'. The relationship again became intolerable. She had sought another operation. Her dialogue became quieter. 'The other doctor stood at the end of the bed. He didn't even need to touch me. I was so disgusting. He just said – I can sort that out'.

'Will you have a look?' she asks quietly. This doctor wants to tread carefully where so much abuse has been perpetuated, but a pause in her story necessitates a comment. 'You have been through a lot. I wonder how you feel now. Does this affect your sexual life?' 'I wised up. I'm not putting up with s… anymore. I got rid of him and was on my own with the kids for ages, but I have found a lovely man… but we can't have sex. When he used to try, there was a blockage. It felt like a bone in there. Now he doesn't try anymore'. 'Can you put anything inside – tampons, a finger – it seems important that you can control your genitals?'

She asks again whether she can be examined. Will the doctor reinforce the 'reaction' of the other doctor? On examination, the doctor is shocked at the tiny remnants of labia minora and struggles to control her reaction to this observation. The patient is closely watching her. But on touching the genitalia, the patient says, 'I can still feel them so that is good'. Yes, the doctor agrees. When a digital examination is performed, control of the pelvic floor is good. She can control the contraction by squeezing and releasing. 'You have a good, strong pelvic floor with excellent control'. This seems to be reassuring – an understanding of her ability to control her pelvic floor on command points to the suggestion of a situational vaginismus.

After dressing, she settles and remarks – 'So it's me and him not my body that's the problem. I thought so. I need to stop pushing him away. I'm so glad I don't need surgery – I think he will be happy too'.

Occasionally it may be helpful to use mirrors where women have been scared to look but want to explore their fantasies in a safe place with a patient and empathic HCP. Encouraging touching or parting the labia can be an important step to normalise, rather than reinforcing the expectation of penetration by a speculum or the HCPs fingers as has previously failed with a penis. Being able to control a pelvic floor spasm may be a further step to recognising the physiological reaction occurring but will generally not work in isolation. The training of physiotherapists in psychosexual medicine has created great support to women with non-consummation. Without any insight, the routine use of vaginal dilators and exercises only increases the sense of failure in those who cannot make progress.

The responsibility for the sensation and function of the vagina can be slowly handed back to a woman presenting with non-consummation and/or vaginismus. As she recognises the factors contributing to, and maintaining her perceived lack of control, she may understand the subconscious power her body is providing. Avoidance of the feelings of trauma, damage, danger, unsuitable or unwanted contact, the need to preserve childhood, etc. reinforces detachment and remoteness of the genital tract. Although often these women may be able to experience orgasm and satisfaction with other sexual activity, their inability to allow penetration is experienced as immature and not 'proper sex'. The isolation discourages exposure to potential new partners or HCPs, until its exploration is encouraged or necessary. Yet careful revelation of the underpinning beliefs that pertain to the unique woman – a sum of her past and present – may be helpful in allowing her to learn to take control and lead to release and experience of sexual pleasure.

Partner's Fantasies

Fantasies can often be shared with partners who collude and develop sexual problems themselves – erectile and ejaculatory difficulties. An example of these are the vagina with teeth, the vagina that has a blockage, a bone, a rigid hymen, a closed tunnel or the dirty vagina, dripping discharge that will infect her partner, the hairy vagina/vulva. Although psychosexual medicine techniques discussed here do not routinely involve couples seen together by invitation, they can often present. This then offers insight into the couple dynamic with their comments and nonverbal communication.

Psychosexual Medicine in Clinical Practice

In clinical practice, the consultation may start at the moment of reading the referral letter. This can distort the consultation into being defined by our own categories (those of the healthcare professional) rather than that of the patient. One of the most powerful techniques in psychosexual medicine is using the patient's own communication and understanding of her (or his) problem. This can involve their own use of resource tools, including peers or the Internet to find their 'diagnosis' or interventions to help resolve their problems, which can appear threatening to the HCP. Yet to allow the patient to be 'the expert', will ultimately be more revealing and therapeutic than the use of medical pathway driven algorithms of care. Insights gained from the general and intimate examination of the patient can facilitate therapeutic interactions.

Non-consummation is a problem often perceived as being within the remit of the gynaecologist. An examination under EUA can be suggested to be 'the solution'. However, this is generally a very unsuitable intervention as it reinforces the separation the woman feels from her genitalia, removing her from the responsibility to and responses from her pelvis. Both gynaecologists and patients seem surprised that the 'opening' of the hymen and vagina has failed to work, as if separating the physical from the psychological will be curative. This is often despite the disclosure in clinic of a multitude of factors that may have contributed to the discovery of difficulty in penetration. Even when there is a partner factor involved in the hesitation and fear of penetration, it is perceived as a receptive problem. Fantasies about the vagina and how it is to be treated can be reflected in comments by the patient about the doctor's *'dirty job' 'poor you having to do this', 'I'm sorry I haven't shaved…'*.

Dissociation from the genitals is a common defence. In its more primary form, non-consummation, most commonly in a first sexual relationship, protects the woman from her feelings, fears and/or fantasies. This can occur in a secondary relationship after other distressing events, whether psychological or physical: abusive relationships, difficult intimate examinations, surgical or oncological management, peri-menopausal changes as examples. Vaginismus or vaginal spasm/pelvic floor muscle spasm can be a physical reason for non-consummation but also causes sexual pain or inability to have speculum examinations without an impact on sexual function. Vaginismus can be a circumstantial problem only, commonly during gynaecological examination but not be a problem during sexual activity. Non-consummation is non-penetration, whereas vaginismus can be a cause of this. Vaginismus should not be thought of as an independent disease condition but a symptom that causes other issues, sexual and otherwise.

Women presenting to clinic have often searched for diagnoses and interventions for their 'vaginismus' and may have purchased vaginal 'dilators' to help ease or widen the vagina. Although there is an understanding of the abnormal contraction of the vaginal muscles, the degree of physical control is frequently misunderstood by both patient and HCP. The contraction of the pelvic floor muscles is not necessarily seen as a protective mechanism but as something to be overcome. There is perceived to be a state of contracture of the muscles, for example as seen in scarring, that needs to be actively stretched and eased, rather than engagement in the physical and psychological relaxation of the normally functioning but abnormally reacting muscles. This requires an ability to squeeze as well as relax. For this reason, the coercion of the chaperone in a consultation, or the partner during intercourse, to 'just relax' will be counterproductive. The use of alcohol or locally acting muscle relaxants will also generally be unsuccessful as any sensation of pressure or pain will cause an involuntary spasm that will reinforce the separation of the mind and body.

Non-consummation causes great feelings of failure which reinforce the shame of not being able to establish a 'normal' sexual relationship. Media perspectives and public discussions around sex isolate women and men who are not able to have penetrative sex. They may present after many years of unsuccessful attempts that have then been abandoned as repeated failure causes more suffering. The 'need' to conceive, often at the limits of the reproductive lifetime, under family and/or peer pressure, with fertility interventions that do not remove the need to 'succumb' can cause more despair. However, when tackling these factors, the experience with other 'non-consummators' must be put aside, even though themes of similar issues may be present. The women, or couple, bring their own unique set of circumstances, beliefs and experiences.

Treatment: Consultation and Examination

Non-consummation and vaginismus are managed from the initial assessment of the referral letter or the perceived reason for attendance in addition to any previous non-attendances or multiple attendances with other issues or 'medically unexplained symptoms'. Observing how the patient is in the waiting room, her reaction to being called and who and what she brings with her, are all clues to her dilemmas.

CASE 3

The young woman sat meekly in the waiting room with a childlike looking partner with his hair covering his face. An older woman sat upright next to them with many bags, keenly watching every time someone was called. She bustled into the consultation room ahead of her daughter and son-in-law when her daughter was called. 'Who is the patient here?' the doctor questioned. 'She is', said the mother pointing a finger in her direction while launching into a demand 'for something to be done'. She sat in the middle with the appearance of mother hen with her two little chicks, rounding them up. 'I see a lot has been done so far but perhaps we are not addressing the issues as your daughter sees them?' The daughter looks askance at the doctor. Is this doctor going to stand up to her mother? The doctor feels nervous and not sure if she is able to negotiate the dynamics in the room delicately, in a manner suitable for the childlike couple. Is it too much to ask the mother to leave? Will it leave the young woman feeling vulnerable? Will it be helpful for the mother to have a different perspective on how to address her daughter's problems?

'I see you were not able to be examined yet we have performed a laparoscopy to see what has been causing your pain?' The laparoscopy had not found any abnormalities in the pelvis, but an intact hymen had been noted. The indication for surgery had been dyspareunia. 'Are you comfortable with talking about sex with your mother present?' This seemed the most challenging question that could be levelled at the daughter (and acknowledged the possible role of her partner – husband as the mother corrected – as if this made it alright for them to be having sex – even though they both seemed infantilised by her approach to helping them). She says, 'yes', shyly, but looks at her husband, and tacitly agrees to discuss their problems with the doctor. 'What happens when you are intimate with each other?' More sexual, direct words seem inappropriate with this young, inexperienced couple. They look coyly at each other with the body and bags of the matriarch between them. 'They are trying to get pregnant. We really want a baby', interjects the mother, 'I would like to hear what your daughter wants from us, how she thinks we may help' retorts the doctor, wanting to protect the childlike woman in the room. However, the confrontation between mother and doctor brings out the rebellious teenager. 'I don't want a baby and I don't want to be here. We were getting on nicely until you decided we wanted a baby'. We were both being shut out of the issues. However, the silent until now partner then quietly brings it back to the relationship between him and his wife. 'But you know we can't do it. We are here now'. The mother and daughter look at him, as if 'how dare he say anything!' 'Well perhaps we can look at you now and see if your operation has made any difference to the examination'. It seemed like an opportunity to make some progress and hide from the mother behind the curtain. She agrees and even asks if her husband can 'come too'. The doctor feels like she is showing him where to go but they both seem excited by the ease with which a digital examination can be performed. They silently nod to each other.

They are seen once more and arrive without the mother, looking more like an adult couple. They confirm that penetrative intercourse has happened on several occasions and they request contraceptive advice, as they wanted to delay starting a family at present.

The consultation will provide a framework within which the patient's understanding of the problem will be revealed. A detailed sexual biography is not required but listening and observing how the issues are presented will give 'clues' to the causes and development of the defensive protection of nonconsummation or vaginismus. Reflecting the feelings this generates in the HCP can illuminate the construct of the symptoms and help resolution. Generalisations of stereotypical attitudes to sex before marriage or relationships with an 'unsuitable' partner are of limited value. Why these persist in relationships that are suitable may be more revealing. Those with cultural or religious reasons for restricting sexual experience will 'blame' this as being the reason for their limitations and fear, but the unique experiences of that individual and her reactions to her restrictions will be more revealing.

The pressure of family expectations for children may be the reason 'why now' they present, causing even more pressure to succeed. Yet resorting to *in vitro* fertilisation presents an acceptable alternative to natural conception. A woman may have little insight and wish to have a 'treatment' that will solve her penetrative problems. Gentle but challenging questions as to what they believe can help, may reveal how passive they feel sex may be – being a receptacle – within a sexual relationship as well as in a consultation. This can be reflected in the withdrawn woman looking away or at the wall during examination – a resigned, detached, 'just do it' type approach.

Looking at the beliefs and understanding as previously illustrated through use of the HCP-patient consultation is a therapeutic event that allows the problem to be evaluated and transformed into a different framework through which the individual can evolve into a fully functioning sexual adult.

LEARNING POINTS

Fears and Fantasies of the Non-Consummator

Pain from loss of virginity
Bleeding – reinforcing damage
Damage to the hymen/vagina
Endless tunnel

Dirty genitalia
Vagina too small
Vagina too delicate
Blockage – like bone/rock, etc.
Penis too big
Penis too hard
Ejaculate too messy
Menstrual blood as dirty
Fear of pregnancy
Damage to hymen that can be detected when woman 'should be a virgin'

Conclusion

Non-consummation and vaginismus commonly present after some delay. This can be due to the shame and isolation experienced by those who think everyone around them has an uncomplicated and satisfying sexual relationship. The embedded behaviours can be hard to address if approached on a purely physical basis, even though physical conditions may contribute to their development. The HCP-patient relationship is a useful therapeutic tool for intervention in understanding and changing the protective but disabling response of the body and mind to distress.

14

Female Sexual Desire

Annie Hawkins

Introduction

Human beings are complex. Desire for sexual activity with another or alone is an interplay between the mind and the body. It has been described as the ultimate bio-psycho-social event. Anatomy, hormones, medications, medical conditions and physical limitations are important, but no less so than past experiences and expectations along with cultural and social conditioning, relationships, plus the psychological and emotional landscape of that person and their self-perception.

Drive disorders include hormone deficiencies, affective and depressive disorders, physical severe or chronic illness. They can be drug induced. There will be a generalised lack of energy and interest in any sexual activity.

Desire disorders include psychological issues around sex, relationship problems and situational difficulties. They are often, but not always, partner specific.

Overview

I would like to take you through these different aspects that affect us all and influence our desire for sexual intimacy. What is normal? First, I would like to look at what we know about sexual behaviour and how it changes through life.

As far back as 1978, the World Health Organisation had recognised that health, including sexual health, was important.

> Health, which is a state of complete physical, mental and social well-being, and not merely the absence of disease or infirmity, is a fundamental human right. (1)

The *Diagnostic and Statistical Manual of Mental Disorders* of the American Psychiatric Association (*DSM-5*) classifies sexual dysfunctions by their end result. There is 'female sexual interest/arousal disorder' and 'male hypoactive sexual desire disorder' listed, along with other disorders such as 'female orgasmic disorder'.

I would suggest that sexual disorders overlap significantly and that there is more to be gained from understanding the root cause or causes of the problem than the way it exhibits itself. The presentation does however give clues and act as a starting point for discussion of the issues around this problem. A patient may present complaining of pain during sex. This may be due to lack of lubrication due to lack of oestrogen in the tissues of the genital tract – a hormonal cause. It may be due to decreased lubrication due to lack of arousal, which may be due to lack of desire, which may be due to relationship issues. It may be due to lack of lubrication due to anxiety due to pain during sex at the last encounter and anticipation of pain with this episode – a psychological cause.

It may also be perceived as more acceptable for an individual to present with pain during intercourse rather than lack of desire. It may be a more acceptable way to refuse a partner than the truth, or an easier

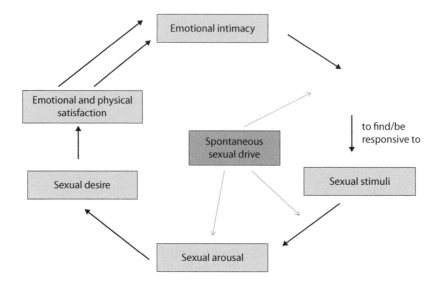

FIGURE 14.1   The intimacy-based sexual response cycle. (Based on Basson R. *J Sex Marital Ther* 2001;(27):33–43, with permission.)

thing to tell a healthcare professional. It may be that the referral letter has a different story entirely from what the patient brings to you. The patient may have not told the referring doctor the full truth or the doctor may have heard a different story.

It has been shown that 40% of those presenting with a desire disorder had a concurrent arousal or orgasm disorder (2).

This century started with a new international consensus on female sexual dysfunction. The definition states that sexual dysfunction is 'the persistent or recurrent deficiency or absence of sexual thoughts/ fantasies and/or desire for or receptivity to sexual activity which causes distress or interpersonal difficulty' (3).

The important part about this is that the issue 'causes distress' to the individual.

The same group came up with a new sexual response cycle for women, reflecting their concept that not all women have innate sexual drive or desire, but that desire can be awoken in the right context (Figure 14.1) (4). Emotional intimacy may motivate a woman who was feeling sexually neutral to be responsive to a sexual stimulus.

The global study of sexual attitudes and behaviours (5) was the largest study I could find. It covered 27,500 men and women aged 40–80 years, from 29 countries. The researchers asked about common sexual dysfunctions and noted those that were described as 'frequent or persistent'. The study showed that one or more dysfunctions were common, with lack of desire being a problem for 21% of those surveyed.

In 2009 a study from Massachusetts in the eastern United States (6) showed that of 10,429 women with self-reported low desire, only 27% were distressed by this. Having a lower level of sexual desire may not be a problem if the individual has no partner or the partner has an equal level of sexual interest.

The National Survey of Sexual Attitudes and Lifestyles (Natsal-3), a UK national survey of sexual attitudes and lifestyles, found that of women surveyed in 2010–2012, 34% had experienced low desire, but the context of their life was very influential on the amount of distress this caused (7).

The famous study (8) looking at age-related female hypoactive sexual desire disorder shows that while the probability of having low desire increases with age, the probability of being distressed by this decreases with age, leading to only a slight rise in the problem of low desire with age (Figure 14.2).

Thus, the problem of low sexual desire is only a problem if the patient comes to a healthcare professional raising it as an issue and asking for help.

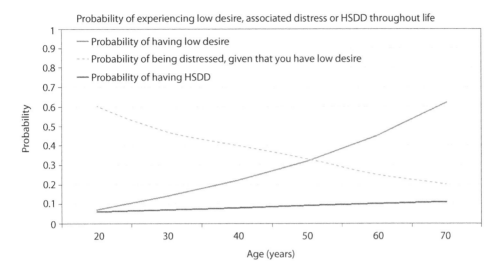

Probability of experiencing low desire, associated distress or HSDD throughout life

— Probability of having low desire
- - - Probability of being distressed, given that you have low desire
— Probability of having HSDD

FIGURE 14.2 Probability of experiencing low desire, associated distress or hypoactive sexual desire disorder throughout life. (From Hayes RD, Dennerstein L, Bennett CM, Koochaki PE, Leiblum SR, Grziottin A. *Fertil Steril* 2007;87(1):107–112, with permission.)

Causes of Low Sexual Desire

Medical Problems

It is clear that any severe illness or injury will reduce desire while the body directs its resources into healing itself. Chronic renal failure or other such debilitating illness can be associated with reduced desire for this reason. There are chronic illnesses such as diabetes mellitus where there is reduction in nerve conduction and arteriolar function which can have a direct effect on the ability to achieve erection and to feel sensation. Stroke and spinal cord injury can also directly affect nerve function. Chronic pain can limit desire and mobility. Mental illnesses such as depression are also often characterised by low desire (9). Such limitations can be temporary or permanent, depending on their nature and severity. It is also important to remember that it may be the partner who has the physical problem, and the change in the partner may be affecting their desirability to the presenting partner. This may be rejection but could also be from a need to nurture and care, changing the dynamic of the relationship. There may be fear of causing pain or damage in a partner who already seems to have suffered so much (10).

CASE 1: MRS MARRIAGE

Mrs Marriage was a 65-year-old breast cancer survivor who was referred to the sexual difficulties clinic with loss of sexual desire. On examination she was found to have severe vaginal atrophy, which, she admitted, bled significantly on any attempt at sexual penetration. She had been married for 43 years and, although her husband attended every appointment, he listened behind a broadsheet newspaper on the edge of the consultation room.

Despite my reassurance, she did not want to take any form of oestrogen, even local, as she was terrified it would cause a recurrence of the cancer. She worked hard with me using vaginal re-moisturiser, self-massage and dilators to regain her confidence and the use of her vagina. However, they still could not achieve penetration as he had developed erectile dysfunction as he did not want to hurt her. Subconsciously his penis preferred to stay outside. Similarly, during the consultation, he had exhibited no desire to be fully involved. He turned up but then hid behind his newspaper. His fear of hurting her was discussed and he was offered onward referral for further help.

Medications

There are many medications that can have an impact on sexuality and many do this by a direct effect on desire. It is well known that the selective serotonin reuptake inhibitors (SSRIs) reduce desire in 50%–85% of users (11–13), and there is no accommodation to this with time (14). It appears that most people who have this effect from one SSRI have the same problem with all of them, and although they are the most widely prescribed anti-depressants these days, this is rarely discussed. Other anti-depressants, anti-psychotics (especially if they increase prolactin) and anti-convulsants can also reduce desire (15). While no one would want to restrict access to potentially effective treatments for these serious conditions, it is important for the prescriber to discuss potential side effects and monitor and enquire after them.

Any enzyme inducers can affect desire, as they will increase metabolism of the sex hormones and so reduce their effect.

Anti-hypertensives, another widely prescribed group, can reduce desire in some cases, as can statins, digoxin and other cardiovascular medications. H2 receptor blockers can interact with hormones and of course any hormone or hormone antagonist or modulator will affect sexuality. Gabapentin also has effects. Most chemotherapy regimes are such an insult to the body that it will go into survival mode and shut down reproductive urges.

Anatomy

Human anatomy is very varied, within what is judged as 'normal'. People have always tried to change their bodies towards a concept of beauty, which changes in different centuries and different cultures. The current trend for low body mass index, depilation of pubic hair and cosmetic labial surgery are examples of women trying to conform to an ideal, perhaps disturbingly pre-pubescent norm. Some people do not see their anatomy as normal and can become very distressed by this perception. Some people react negatively towards what we would see as a neat and well-healed episiotomy or abdominal scar. Their thoughts and fantasies should be explored and shared as reassurance alone does not help change a fixed idea.

Then there are many issues that come as our bodies change and we age – for example there are changes in skin elasticity and texture, there are wrinkles and grey hair. Some anatomy has changed and become different, e.g. prolapse of the womb and vagina. Some surgery may be needed, e.g. vaginal repair or hysterectomy, and this will come with associated concerns and feelings in the patient that can impact on the patient's sexual life, especially with these parts of the body that are involved with sex and gender identity.

Occasionally there is a need for disfiguring surgery, e.g. vulvectomy for vulval cancer, limb removal or abdominal surgery with colostomy that can have a huge impact on the patient's self-perception and ability to feel desirable and to desire.

Cancer Treatments

Radiotherapy is exhausting and draining for the body. It not only depletes the body's resources and affects desire in some women, but can directly damage sexual function. Examples of this are prostate radiotherapy and brachytherapy – radiation directly in the vagina which causes scarring and stenosis. Radiotherapy and chemotherapy are also very likely to cause gonadal failure leading to testosterone deficiency in men and oestrogen and testosterone deficiency in women, both of which will have a marked effect on desire and sexual function. As healthcare professionals we can help with these issues if patients know they can come forward to ask for help.

During the time of acute cancer treatment, both clinician and patient are most interested in survival and cure rates, and too little thought can be given to quality of life after treatment is successful. It is very important in all these situations to talk about the patient's feelings towards that part of their body and how it has changed, to share the sadness and acknowledge the emotional pain. Sex does not have to be the price you pay for survival. It is also important to be practical and offer help where available, e.g. hormone replacement and lubricants.

Subfertility

If there was no psychological, psychosexual, hormonal or relationship problem before a couple starts down the road of infertility investigation and assisted conception treatment, there is likely to be by the end of it. Having your most private organs prodded and declared deficient in some way is not conducive to feeling sexy. It can feel as if they are on show for all to see this deficiency and labelled as 'empty' 'useless' or 'barren'.

There can be resentment and anger, blame and guilt between the couple, trying to work through how they came to be in this situation. Approximately 55% of subfertility is due to female factors, 30% male factors and in 25% there is no identified physical cause. In 40% there is an issue with both parties (16). Many relationships break down under the strain and only one-third go home with a baby. That means two-thirds try to work through the grief of being childless and reach some resolution.

CASE 2: MRS DISAPPOINTMENT

Mrs Disappointment was a 38-year-old French Christian woman who was referred to the sexual difficulties clinic because of loss of sexual desire. I mention that she was Christian only as her religion was very important to her. She had met her husband at the age of 35 and moved to the United Kingdom to marry. He was her first and only sexual partner. They both married wanting children. She had two first trimester miscarriages within 9 months. There was nothing unusual for the early pregnancy team looking after her, just her age. Only now she could not have sex, a problem on the way to creating that longed-for child.

There were no physical or hormonal issues, her periods had resumed normally. She had 'drive' but not desire. I reflected how sad she seemed and on discussion, it seems she was deeply disappointed with her partner's response to her prolonged grief. To her mind, she had lost two babies, to his, they just needed to move on and try again. She was very frustrated with him, she could no longer communicate with him. He would not listen. Despite her overwhelming desire to conceive again she could not bring herself to have sex. The doctor looked at ways in which they could re-establish communication.

Social Factors

It is very important to remember that although every patient will bring with them into the bedroom and into the consulting room their background, their cultural and religious upbringing, their previous experiences, education and social situation, they are not defined by them. It is important that the clinician should have an understanding of the patient's situation and ask about it if they are unfamiliar with the culture or unclear on the situation. However, feelings towards one's body and sexuality share a commonality across all types of people. The patient is the expert in their own life and will usually bring the answers of how to help them and what they need.

Similarly, there are often relationship issues that can be co-morbid with other physical, hormonal or psychological problems. It may be possible to make one partner feel differently about themselves and want to rekindle a sexual relationship, but the other may not agree. Long-term relationships may naturally go through periods of closeness and more sexual activity and then times where there are less of both. Often getting patients to talk about their relationship can bring insights into the interactions and problems within it, which may be appropriately reflected back to the patients, allowing them to use this information to decide how to move forward. Some people may then go home and talk to their partners, some may decide to work on their relationships and the sex will follow, some will decide to initiate sexual activity to try and rekindle the relationship, some will decide to end the relationship. Whatever they decide, the clinician is there only as a reflective mirror and support, not to direct in any way.

Hormonal Issues

In women both oestrogen and testosterone deficiency can cause sexual problems. Oestrogen has a secondary effect on desire and libido, while testosterone has a direct effect.

Treatments for Problems with Desire

Systemic Oestrogen Treatment

Think of the familiar symptoms of oestrogen deficiency – the hot flushes, central obesity, dowager's hump, tooth loss, dry skin, hair and nails plus wrinkles as the skin loses elasticity. None of that sounds very attractive and all these changes can affect self-perception and so desire. The night sweats, poor quality sleep and chronic associated tiredness of peri-menopause will reduce desire. The dryness of the mucus membranes and vulvo-vagina make sex more uncomfortable or frankly painful. The low mood, anxiety, memory loss and loss of confidence follow and all reduce the feeling of desirability.

Oestrogen replacement will relieve these symptoms (17). It will improve the dryness of mucus membranes, improve skin sensitivity, olfactory function and pheromone secretion. The maintenance of secondary sexual characteristics will have a secondary effect of improving higher psychological function, self-perception and so arousal and sexual desire (18).

Systemic oestrogen replacement is available as licenced preparations in Europe as tablets, gel and patches. Many patients can be successfully treated in primary care. Following the adverse publicity surrounding hormone replacement therapy in the early 2000s the use of peri-menopausal hormones to replace the natural decline in oestrogens has reduced significantly. However, the balance has been somewhat redressed since the re-analysis of the data from the Million Women Study and the Women's Health Initiative were first published (19).

In November 2015 the National Institute of Clinical Excellence (NICE) (20) released its first guideline on the use of hormone replacement therapy (HRT). While there is still a lot of research to be done it notes that in most women in their middle years, HRT is safe and appropriate, when symptoms indicate its need.

For most women in their early 50s who have no significant medical issues, obesity, smoking and excess alcohol consumption are increasing their risk of breast cancer more than a small amount of oestrogen replacement will do.

In Europe we generally prefer to give oestrogen in the form of 17β-Oestradiol, as is the physiologically natural molecule. We also, where possible, give it trans-dermally to avoid liver first-pass metabolism and the interaction with other drugs. This also reduces its metabolic impact and effect on the cholesterol pathways and means that it has no effect on the clotting system, so negating the increased venous thrombotic disease risk seen with oral oestrogens.

Local Treatments

Vulvo-vaginal atrophy is widespread and its effects are under-reported. Local oestrogen replacement is very safe and underused. Studies have found prevalence of 15% in pre-menopausal women, 10%–40% in post-menopausal women, 10%–25% in women on systemic HRT and 66% in women over age 75 (21,22).

The physiological changes include loss of elasticity and rugae of the vagina, thinning of the vaginal epithelium, reduced acidity in the vagina, reduced blood flow and reduced nerve transmission.

The clinical effects of this are decreased tissue elasticity causing discomfort and pain, shrinkage of the vaginal orifice, decreased discharge, decreased lubrication to stimulation, change in smell, increasing urinary infections and bladder irritation.

Practically it is therefore easy to see that this can lead to decreased desire, as penetrative intercourse can be less pleasurable and even painful.

Treatment can involve systemic oestrogen, but usually topical treatments are given.

Topical oestrogen is available in cream, pessaries and a vaginal ring.

There is virtually no systemic absorption and it can be used long term with an indefinite licence. Topical oestrogens can usually be given safely even in previous breast cancer sufferers, after discussion with their oncologist or surgeon.

Alternatively, there are non-hormonal vaginal moisturisers available in gels or pessaries. In the United Kingdom these are available over the counter, or on prescription. If used regularly they can make a significant difference to comfort.

Clinician should always recommend a topical lubricant for sexual activity. On the market there are water-based and pH-balanced forms such as 'Sylk' and 'Yes'. There is an oil-based form of 'Yes' (not compatible with condoms). There are many more on the market, but only pH-balanced osmotically appropriate forms should be recommended by healthcare professionals (23).

Progestogens

All women taking oestrogen preparations, who have their uterus, need a progestogen for opposition. Unopposed oestrogens can cause stimulation of the lining of the womb and thickening of the endometrium, which, if left untreated, can become atypical cell growth and, in time, malignancy. Progestogens licenced for opposition in Europe include oral synthetic progestogen tablets, micronized progesterone capsules, vaginal progesterone creams or pessaries and the levonorgestrel intra-uterine systems.

Progestogens can be given either continuously to prevent thickening of the endometrium or cyclically to produce withdrawal bleeds. Younger women (<52 and those still having menses) are usually given a cyclical (also known as sequential) progestogen and older women (>1 year since last bleed) a continuous regime.

There is now concern that the more androgenic progestogens such as medroxyprogesterone acetate 'Provera' may be implicated in the increase in breast cancer seen in women on combined HRT over those on oestrogens alone (24). In Europe the trend is to use less androgenic progestogens such as dydrogesterone and micronized progesterone itself to reduce this risk and the side effects.

There can be significant side effects from synthetic progestogens, where there is low mood, bowel changes, irritability and a full range of pre-menstrual type symptoms.

Any progestogen and progesterone itself in the natural cycle can have an effect on sexuality. Many women report a decrease in sexual encounters pre-menstrually (25), although in some drive is increased (26). 'He comes near me at his own risk' a patient with severe pre-menstrual symptoms once memorably said to me about that time of the month.

The gynaecologist specialising in female hormones will meet women suffering from pre-menstrual syndromes (PMSs) (27). More than 150 symptoms have been described as occurring cyclically in the luteal phase of the menstrual cycle and these can range from the mild and manageable to those that completely destroy careers and relationships.

While a hormonal sensitivity seen in PMSs can be very satisfying to treat, it is known that this population will also include women with psychological, psychiatric and psychosexual problems. In a specialist PMSs clinic studied, there was an over-representation of psychiatric disorder (67%, with 50% affective disorders) and 40% psychosexual problems (28). There is also an over-representation of sexual abuse survivors in this PMSs population, from 40%–95% in studies (29–31).

It is not surprising that if a woman is spending the two weeks a month where she feels well, trying to understand and apologise for her behaviours in the luteal phase, that this can have a significant effect on relationships, sexual behaviours and desire.

Testosterone

Testosterone is a normal female hormone produced from the ovary and the adrenal glands. Young women produce 300–400 mcg a day, which is three to four times the amount of oestradiol they produce. There is a gradual decline in the amount of testosterone produced in both men and women with age.

Testosterone is an anabolic hormone and has effects on bone density and muscle mass as well as energy levels and well-being. It has a direct relationship with sexual desire, arousal and orgasm (32).

There will be an abrupt drop in testosterone levels when the ovaries are removed. In the United Kingdom, 250,000 pre-menopausal women have had their ovaries removed. Other women who have ovarian failure induced by cancer treatment, autoimmune disease or idiopathic gonadal failure will all need hormone replacement to maintain quality of life and long-term health. The younger the woman is when her ovaries are removed, the more she will feel the lack of testosterone. Female androgen deficiency syndrome (FADS) is characterised by loss of energy, loss of libido, headache and low mood (33,34).

The younger the female is if the ovaries fail, the greater dose of oestrogen she will need and this should be continued at least until the age of natural menopause at around 50. This will protect the bones and cardiovascular system from long-term oestrogen deficiency problems. Consideration must be given as to whether women need testosterone replacement therapy along with their oestrogen replacement therapy at natural menopause and especially after a surgical menopause, as this can be vital for their well-being in the longer term in general, and the maintenance of a healthy sexual life.

Unfortunately, there are no licenced testosterone preparations for women in Europe. We have one 1% and one 2% testosterone gel preparations, licensed for men, that we can use off-licence through the National Health Service at a female physiological dose. At the time of writing we also have unlicenced products imported from the United States or Australia available, for those women who can pay to access them.

The amount of available oestrogen and testosterone in the bloodstream that can have a clinical effect is dependent on the amount of sex hormone-binding globulin (SHBG) made in the liver. This protein binds to the sex hormones rendering them inactive, so directly affects activity. Oestrogens increase the amount of SHBG that is made, and testosterone decreases it. Giving oestrogen alone will therefore decrease available testosterone even further. Decreased active testosterone will directly decrease sexual desire. This is especially seen with oral oestrogens that are metabolised in the liver. This is best assessed in practical terms by a blood test including oestradiol and free androgen index. In many women oestrogens and androgens need to be given together to achieve a physiological balance.

Other Treatments

Phosphodiesterase Inhibitors

The phosphodiesterase inhibitors (Viagra, Cialis) were trialed in women with sexual dysfunction in the early 2000s. Some small studies showed some benefit, but overall there was no clinically meaningful benefit in women (35).

Bupropion

Bupropion was originally used alone to increase libido (36). Its mode of action is unclear; it is thought to have an effect on noradrenaline and dopamine neurotransmission. In SSRI-induced decreased desire bupropion can be added to improve libido (37), and sildenafil has been shown to help in limited studies (38,39).

Flibanserin is a 5HT1 agonist and a 5HT2A antagonist that was shown to have some potential benefit to desire and is now licenced for use in women with low desire in the United States (40).

Flibanserin acts post-synaptically on the 5HT receptors in the brain. It increases 5T in the pre-frontal cortex and decreases 5HT levels in the hypothalamus. It acts as a monoamine modulator by targeting neurones that release dopamine and noradrenaline.

Dehydroepiandrosterone

Dehydroepiandrosterone (DHEA) is not available in the United Kingdom and trial data are limited as to its efficacy (40,41).

It is available over the counter as a dietary supplement in the United States and other countries, so is available over the Internet.

Institute of Psychosexual Medicine Approach

The understanding clinician dealing with any of these women described will realise that women are complicated and desire is multifactorial. The principles of psychosexual medicine (as taught by the Institute of Psychosexual Medicine [IPM]) are very useful when assessing and assisting these patients (41). Hormone levels do not tell the full story.

The IPM teaches a brief interpretative psychodynamic form of psychosexual medicine, where the clinician-patient relationship is studied in depth. The feelings in the consultation room are explored and where possible reflected back to the patient with interpretation and support.

It is often the patient who keeps re-presenting or where the symptoms do not fit the signs, who is asking for help with a psychological sexual problem rather than a hormonal or physical issue. The physical and psychological can coincide. The patient may be a 'good' or 'difficult' patient with unusual illness behaviour.

CASE 3: MRS EMPTY

Mrs Empty was a smart, sophisticated businesswoman who came for replacement of her hormone implants of oestrogen and testosterone. She made a point of showing me her new knee-high designer boots and telling me how much they had cost. She was overtly very sexy. We chatted about her job, she managed a team of men, she told me with a proud laugh.

As she agreed to complete the sexuality questionnaire that I was offering women on implants, and I sensed something was wrong and over time I learnt her story. She had a colposcopy for cervical intra-epithelial neoplasia at the age of 21. It was terrifying. She started having pelvic pain. She had three laparoscopies and endometriosis was seen. A transverse laparotomy, total abdominal hysterectomy and bilateral oophorectomy were performed when she was 26. The pain persisted, another laparotomy and the top vaginal cuff removed to treat her dyspareunia. The pain persisted, 12 years passed, multiple operations culminated in the removal of her sigmoid colon for 'functional problems'.

She was very medicalised in her descriptions, and very eager to please all the doctors, she would have done anything to get rid of the pain. It was hard to get to the sex. Her long-term partner seemed loving and long suffering. Sex was rare and involved careful positioning and lubricant. There was pain, but no feelings. The story was overwhelming.

During the examination we stopped to look together at the scars on her abdomen and there was a moment of intense sadness. She agreed that she had not owned her abdomen for the last 12 years. She described it as 'an empty void' echoing the difficulty in reaching the feelings. I reflected that all the fun with sex seemed to have gone and that her abdomen and vagina seemed to be associated only with medical procedures and pain. This was in contrast to her initial presentation with the sexy boots and I pointed this out to her. She laughed and said that maybe there was a bit of her that was still sexy and that she would need to work on it.

Simple, open-ended questions and statements are used to encourage the patient to reveal information and feelings and the psychotherapeutic examination is used to look at the distress. The clinician becomes more observant, picking up on non-verbal cues and feelings expressed in the room.

The consultation can be presented and discussed in an IPM seminar group, to look at the defences in the clinician and in the patient, the 'why now' and the patient's aims in more detail. This is to try and aid understanding of the root of the problem, enable the patient to air the distress, release it and move on.

Summary and Conclusion

In my practice when I am looking with a patient at her lack of interest in sex, I try and determine whether this loss of 'libido' is due to a problem with drive or desire. The first thing I was taught at medical school was to 'listen to the patient, the patient will tell you the diagnosis'. As a practising clinician, 25 years on, this is still the most important thing for us all to remember, when meeting any patient. She will tell her healthcare professional why she is there and what is troubling her and give clues as to what she needs and how you can help her as long as the healthcare practitioner sticks with the patient's agenda.

Patients bring to us their mind and their body and often in order to help them we must practise holistically and treat both as best we can.

REFERENCES

1. World Health Organisation. Declaration of Alma-Ata, September 1978.
2. Segraves KB, Segraves RT. Hypoactive sexual desire disorder: Prevalence and comorbidity in 906 subjects. *J Sex Marital Ther* 1991;17(1):55–58.
3. Basson R, Berman J, Burnett A et al. Report of the international consensus development conference on female sexual dysfunction: Definitions and classifications. *J Urol* 2000;163(3):888–893. Review.
4. Basson R. Human sex-response cycles. *J Sex Marital Ther* 2001;(27):33–43.
5. Nicolosi A, Laumann EO, Glasser DB et al. Sexual behavior and sexual dysfunctions after age 40: The global study of sexual attitudes and behaviors. *Urology* 2004;64(5):991–997.
6. Rosen RC, Shifren JL, Monz BU et al. Correlates of sexually related personal distress in women with low sexual desire. *J Sex Med* 2009;6(6):1549–1560.
7. Graham CA, Mercer CH, Tanton C et al. What factors are associated with reporting lacking interest in sex and how do these vary by gender? Findings from the third British National Survey of Sexual Attitudes and Lifestyles. *BMJ Open* 2017;7(9):e016942.
8. Hayes RD, Dennerstein L, Bennett CM et al. Relationship between hypoactive sexual desire disorder and aging. *Fertil Steril* 2007;87(1):107–112.
9. Appa AA, Creasman J, Brown JS et al. The impact of multimorbidity on sexual function in middle-aged and older women: Beyond the single disease perspective. *J Sex Med* 2014;11(11):2744–2755.
10. Corona G, Petrone L, Mannucci E et al. The impotent couple: Low desire. *Int J Androl* 2005;28(Suppl. 2): 46–52.
11. Zajecka J, Fawcett J, Schaff M et al. The role of serotonin in sexual dysfunction: Fluoxetine-associated orgasm dysfunction. *J Clin Psychiatry* 1991;52(2):66–68.
12. Zajecka J, Mitchell S, Fawcett J. Treatment-emergent changes in sexual function with selective serotonin reuptake inhibitors as measured with the Rush Sexual Inventory. *Psychopharmacol Bull* 1997;33(4):755–760.
13. Modell JG, Katholi CR, Modell JD et al. Comparative sexual side effects of bupropion, fluoxetine, paroxetine, and sertraline. *Clin Pharmacol Ther* 1997;61(4):476–487.
14. Sundblad C, Wikander I, Andersch B, Eriksson E. A naturalistic study of paroxetine in premenstrual syndrome: Efficacy and side-effects during ten cycles of treatment. *Eur Neuropsychopharmacol* 1997;7(3):201–206.
15. Clayton AH, Balon R. The impact of mental illness and psychotrophic medications on sexual functioning: The evidence and management. *J Sex Med* 2009;6(5):1200.
16. Fertility problems: Assessment and treatment. NICE Clinical Guideline 156; February 2013, Updated September 2017.
17. Cardozo L, Gibb DM, Tuck SM et al. The effect of subcutaneous hormone implants during climacteric. *Maturitas* 1984;5(3):177–184.
18. Bachmann GA. Prevention of menopausal sequelae. *N J Med* 1991;88(3):181–184. Review.
19. Roehm E. A reappraisal of women's health initiative estrogen-alone trial: Long-term outcomes in women 50–59 years of age. *O G Intnl* 2015;2015:713295.
20. Menopause: Diagnosis and management. NICE Clinical Guideline 23; November 2015.
21. Sarrel PM. Sexuality and menopause. *Obstet Gynecol* 1990;75(4 Suppl):26S–30S; discussion 31S–35S.
22. Bachmann GA, Leiblum SR. The impact of hormones on menopausal sexuality: A literature review. *Menopause* 2004;11(1):120–130.
23. Edwards D, Panay N. Treating vulvovaginal atrophy/genitourinary syndrome of menopause. How important is vaginal lubricant and moisturiser composition? *Climacteric* 2016;19(2):151–161.
24. Liu JH. Selecting progestogens: Breast, cardiovascular and cognitive outcomes. *Menopause* 2017;24(12):1419–1420.
25. Dennerstein L, Gotts G, Brown JB et al. The relationship between the menstrual cycle and female sexual interest in women with PMS complaints and volunteers. *Psychoneuroendocrinology* 1994;19(3):293–304.
26. Nichols S. Positive premenstrual experiences; Do they exist? *Fem Psychol* 1995;5(2):162–169.
27. Management of Premenstrual Syndrome: Green-top Guideline no. 48. *BJOG* 2017;124(3):e73–e105.
28. Chandraiah K, Kenswar DK, Prasad PLS et al. Sexual dysfunction, social maladjustment and psychiatric disorders in women seeking treatment in a premenstrual syndrome clinc. *Intl J Psych in Med* 1991;21(2):189.

29. Fonseca LC, Jones JE, Futterman LA. Sexual trauma and the premenstrual syndrome. *Miccio-J Sex Educ Th* 1990;16(4):270–278.

30. Golding JM, Taylor DL, Menard L et al. Prevalence of sexual abuse history in a sample of women seeking treatment for premenstrual syndrome. *J Psychosom Obstet Gynecol* 2000;21(2):81–91.

31. Paddison PL, Gise LH, Lebovits A et al. Sexual abuse and premenstrual syndrome: Comparison between a lower and a higher socioeconomic group. *Psychosom: J Consultation and Liaison Psychiatry* 1990;31(3):265–272.

32. Davison SL, Davis SR. Androgenic hormones and ageing – The link with female sexual function. *Horm Behav* 2011;59(5):745–753.

33. Sands R, Studd JWW. Exogenous androgens in postmenopausal women. *Am J Med* 1995;98(1, Suppl 1): 76–79.

34. Davis SR. When to suspect androgen deficiency other than at menopause. *Fertil Steril* 2002;S68.

35. Pomerantz JM. Viagra and medical necessity. *Drug Benefit Trends* 2002;14(10):33.

36. Coleman CC, King BR, Bolden-Watson C et al. A placebo-controlled comparison of the effects on sexual functioning of buproprion sustained release and fluoxetine. *Clin Ther* 2001;23(7):1040–1058.

37. Clayton AH, Warnock JK, Kornstein SG et al. A placebo-controlled trial of bupropion SR as an antidote for SSRI induced sexual dysfunction. *J Clin Psychiatry* 2004;65(1):62–67.

38. Clayton AH, Dennerstein L, Pyke R et al. Flibanserin: A potential treatment for HSDD in premenopausal women. *Women's Health* 2010;6(5):639–653.

39. Davis SR, Panjari M, Stanczyk FZ. Clinical review: DHEA replacement for menopausal women. *J Clin Endo Met* 2011;96(6):1642–1653.

40. Panjari M, Bell JR, Jane F et al. A randomized trial of oral DHEA treatment for sexual function, well-being, and menopausal symptoms in postmenopausal women with low libido. *J Sex Med* 2009;6(9): 2579–2590.

41. Skrine R. *Introduction to Psychosexual Medicine*. London: Hodder Arnold, 1989.

15

Erectile Dysfunction

Catherine Coulson

Introduction

Erectile dysfunction (ED) is defined as the difficulty in getting and maintaining an erection of sufficient power for intercourse. It was formally known as impotence for a good reason. A man with ED may feel weak, frustrated and powerless. He may come to see a doctor to get it sorted out, having not really considered that the penis is part of who he is. ED is often a symptom of physical or psychological disease. As doctors, we need to think about the mind and body together and help work out with the man in front of us, why he should have this problem. It is often more complicated than just a single factor.

It must be remembered that what appears to be ED may be a symptom of loss of sexual desire, often known as *libido*. This may also be due to a physical problem, such as testosterone deficiency, but is more often psychological or situational. ED itself can cause secondary loss of libido as the fear of failure limits desire.

Background

Prevalence of ED

Two major studies have looked at male aging in relation to sexuality: the Massachusetts Male Aging Study (1) (MMAS) and the European Male Ageing Study (2,3) (EMAS). Both studies show an increasing prevalence of ED throughout life. The MMAS shows the prevalence (Table 15.1).

As with many conditions the incidence is less in better-educated men and those with higher earnings. It is worse when there is concomitant cardiovascular disease and high blood pressure. ED predates the onset of cardiovascular disease by 10 years. The EMAS showed the overall incidence was 30% (community dwelling men aged 40–79 years), but only 38% were concerned about it on average. Peak concern was in the 50–59 years age group and declined after that (Table 15.2).

The frequency of sexual thoughts or any sexual activity gradually declined with increasing age. The common concomitant co-morbidities were hypertension (29%), obesity (24%) and heart disease (16%). All of these add to the possibility of ED.

TABLE 15.1

Massachusetts Male Aging Study

Age Range	Prevalence of ED (%)
40–49	12
50–59	29
60–69	46

TABLE 15.2

European Male Ageing Study

Age Range	Severe ED (%)	Moderate ED (%)	Concerns about ED (%)
40–49	1	5	42
50–59	5	14	57
60–69	13	23	42
70+	35	29	28

Psychosomatic Aspects of Erectile Dysfunction or Loss of Libido: Causes and Modifiers

- Prediction of negative outcome/anxiety
- Partner response
- Symptom of failing relationship
- Past experiences
- Abuse
- Upbringing
- Rape
- Torture
- Guilt
- Grief
- Cultural
- Family
- Societal
- Religious
- Infertility

Physical Causes of Erectile Dysfunction and Modifiers

- Cardiovascular
- Neurogenic/structural
- Prescribed drugs
- Hormonal
- Ageing

Cardiovascular Causes

The blood supply to the penis is via the artery of the penis, which is a terminal branch of the internal pudendal artery. It is unusual for there to be a specific block to this artery in the absence of other arterial disease. However, the small vessels are susceptible to arteriosclerosis and ED is said (MMAS [1]) to predate overt cardiovascular disease by 10 years. Hence the presentation of a man with ED should trigger appropriate investigation of blood pressure, weight, exercise tolerance, blood sugar and hypercholesterolemia. Although the aetiology is usually microvascular disease, large vessel pathology such as an aortic aneurysm should also be considered. Tumescence is maintained by nitric oxide pathway (NO).

CASE 1: PHYSICAL/POWERLESSNESS

Ed was 58. He had had no erections since his coronary artery bypass 2 years earlier. He was puzzled and bereft without his erections. He tried to masturbate on a semi-erect penis but it did not feel right. He had no sexual partner at the moment, living a comfortable life with his wife who had had no interest in a physical relationship for 20 years. He came from a job where he had gloried in his physical strength. He described the sense of disbelief he experienced as his heart attack progressed, his sense of helplessness as he realised he could not move and then the fear as he called 999. After the operation, he was upset by the painful scars on his chest and the unexpected scar on his leg from the venous graft. It had taken a long time to heal and despite the cardiac rehabilitation he had felt powerless. We talked about how his body had let him down in an unexpected way. The drugs that he had to take in order to stay well may have contributed but the ED mirrored this powerlessness. He was unresponsive to PD5 inhibitors and the work was to help him see, with sadness, his change in circumstances. We assume that the microvascular disease is the prime cause here but his sense of helplessness at the time of his cardiac crisis was also very powerful and seemed to have squashed his libido completely.

Diabetes Mellitus

Diabetes mellitus (DM) is part of a cluster of conditions which increase risk for cardiovascular disease including high blood pressure, increased low density lipoproteins and obesity. There is an increased risk for men with DM of developing ED. The MMAS (1) showed an age-adjusted risk of ED in men with DM to be twofold over those without DM and overall a threefold probability of having ED when compared to men without DM. The occurrence of ED predated the cardiovascular disease by 10–15 years (4) and the ED is worse and less amenable to drug treatment in men with DM. Moreover, ED is a marker of increased risk of cardiovascular disease, coronary heart disease, stroke and all-cause mortality (5–7). Type 1 and type 2 DM seem to be equal risk factors for ED and it is not known whether good glycaemic control will prevent the development of ED. There is, however, some evidence to show that lifestyle changes such as weight loss and increased exercise and good glycaemic control may improve ED (8,9).

Neuropathy, vasculopathy, central adiposity, insulin resistance and hypogonadism are factors in the aetiology of ED.

Briefly the mechanism of erection is as follows: Parasympathetic stimulation via nitric oxide pathway causes relaxation of the smooth muscle of the arterioles and increased blood flow into the corpora cavernosae. Pressure builds but is restricted by the tunica albuginea and tumescence follows.

Men with DM have:

- Endothelial dysfunction, a pro-inflammatory response which interferes with this process
- Increased insulin resistance and central adiposity and hence
  - Hypogonadism with decreased testosterone levels
- Increased chance of being hypertensive and having cardiovascular disease
- Increased chance of being on
  - Hypertension drugs
  - Anti-depressants

Diabetes causes endothelial dysfunction which is associated with microvascular disease. This can cause autonomic neuropathy with reduced genital sensation and decreased parasympathetic activity leading to decreased nitric oxide mediated smooth muscle relaxation.

Diabetic men are likely to be taking drugs for cardiovascular disease and anti-depressants which may also add to the burden on the erectile process.

Treatment

PD5 inhibitors have been shown to help men with ED and long-term use (as opposed to required use) may have a better effect.

Interestingly there are some papers to show that treatment with PD5 inhibitors may be enhanced when combined with statins (11).

CASE 2: PHYSICAL/ABUSE

Peter was 63 and referred because of ED. He had a new partner who was very kind and understanding but although they were able to enjoy their sexual intimacy together he was unable to penetrate her. He was a large cuddly man with lovely blue eyes and a mop of greying curly hair that had once been blond. He had type 2 diabetes that was well controlled and was taking metformin. He was hypertensive and on medication for that. The erectile dysfunction had been present for much of his life however. He had been sexually abused at school and had been upset by the erections he had got when he had been touched by one of the teachers. He had felt ashamed and dirty. He married young to a woman he met at church. They had waited until they were married to be sexual and at that point he discovered that she was only interested in sex until she became pregnant. After that he felt excluded and ultimately had a depressive breakdown and moved out of the marital home. He felt relations with his children had been poisoned by his vindictive ex-wife. It would have been easy to dismiss the ED as a function of the high blood pressure, diabetes, his central adiposity and the β-blockers he took for his blood pressure. However, discussion about his past, his coming to terms with his sense of being powerless in the face of sexual abuse and a powerful first wife, and with gentle encouragement from a new and loving partner allowed him to become fully potent again. His physical problems may have predisposed him to ED but his sense of impotence derived from his past experiences.

Neurogenic Causes

Various conditions such as multiple sclerosis can present with ED.

Spinal cord injury will impact on erections. If the injury is lower than L3 the man may be able to obtain either a psychogenic or reflex erection, although the disruption of the sensation also impacts on his sexual pleasure. PD5 inhibitors may be expected to help (10). Lesions around S2–S4 affect the parasympathetic nervous supply to the penis and so erection is adversely affected.

Pelvic Surgery and/or Radiotherapy

Specific nerve damage as a result of radical prostatectomy is another culprit even when nerve-sparing surgery has been used. Once again PD5 inhibitors may help (12). Other pelvic surgery to the rectum or bladder may cause nerve damage.

Peyronie's Disease

Approximately 80% of men with Peyronie's have ED. The condition produces fibrous inelastic scars in the tunica albuginea. This causes plaques that cause a curvature of the penis making penetration difficult or painful. The mechanism of ED appears to be related to anxiety and pain as well as corporeal veno-occlusive dysfunction secondary to the structural changes. Research indicates that daily use of PD5 inhibitors may produce amelioration of the plaque and symptoms, at least in the short term (13).

Tight Foreskin

A tight foreskin is rarely the cause of ED and if tight, a foreskin can usually be coaxed to retract comfortably. However if this is not enough, it is possible that a circumcision may help although an anxious man may find that the operation adds to his trauma.

CASE 3: INFERTILITY/TIGHT FORESKIN/NAÏVITY

Tracy and Tom were referred by the infertility clinic. Both were in their late 30s and neither had been in a sexual relationship before. They seemed naïve. It was difficult to find out what was the problem they were experiencing. Eventually we were able to discover that Tom had a very tight foreskin that would not retract on penetration, or if it did so, he would experience pain and then a failure of his erection. He was anxious about his penis, anxious about damage and pain. Tracy had had no other lovers and so neither of them knew what to expect. Unusually the role of the doctor for this couple was education. Tom tried to massage the foreskin back using a mild steroid ointment but eventually had a circumcision. He was quite anxious after the operation but eventually was able to have intercourse that was easier and not painful for him.

Prescribed Drugs

The 'medicated well person' is a feature of life in developed countries. Sometimes it is the condition itself that causes the ED and sometimes the medicine used to treat the condition. Response to drugs may be idiosyncratic. For example, a man may get ED with one β-blocker prescribed for his high blood pressure and less side effects with another. Many drugs also affect sexual desire. The current British National Formulary can be consulted and also, many hospital trusts have pharmacists who can look into side effect profiles.

Prescribed Drugs that Can Cause ED

- Testosterone lowering drugs
- Alpha-blockers for urinary symptoms
- Beta-blockers for hypertension
- Thiazide diuretics
- Anti-psychotics
- Anti-depressants

The intended mode of action of some drugs will have an adverse effect on erections. Treatment for prostatic cancer aims to reduce the testosterone levels and ED is almost inevitable, partly due to loss of desire. Gonadorelin analogues will certainly reduce testosterone and anti-androgens such as cyproterone acetate, dutasteride or finasteride may cause ED.

α-Adrenoceptor blockers may cause a problem.

β-Adrenoceptor blockers to reduce blood pressure may have no effect at all but if the blood pressure does drop then ED may be a consequence of that.

Thiazide anti-diuretics are often to blame for ED.

Sexual dysfunction is a common reason for poor adherence to the use of anti-psychotics. Loss of interest and ED are common. Anti-psychotics reduce dopamine which in turn raises prolactin and this may reduce testosterone via the pituitary gland. The anti-muscarinic effects will adversely affect arousal and the α-adrenoceptor antagonist effect will reduce erection. Some anti-depressants cause delayed ejaculation, especially selective serotonin re-uptake inhibitors.

Depending on the condition being treated, it may be possible to change the medication to see if that helps. The onset of ED in relation to the medication under suspicion is obviously relevant.

Hormones

Hypogonadal younger men are liable to sexual dysfunction including ED. The cause of the deficiency needs investigating and treating by an endocrinologist. Causes may derive from the hypothalamo/pituitary axis, a raised prolactin due to drugs or pituitary tumour or gonadal failure, among others. Usually testosterone replacement is effective. Although these men may present with ED, on questioning, it may be that they also have loss of desire.

TABLE 15.3

Age and Testosterone Levels

Age	Testosterone Level nmol/L
40–49	8.7
50–59	7.5
60–69	6.8
70+	5.4

In older men, the situation is not so clear. The drive to find the 'andropause', the male equivalent of the female menopause, and the lure of fixing a problem with some hormones is seductive.

The MMAS (14) demonstrated that there is a normal decline in testosterone levels in men as they age. Table 15.3 gives their suggested normal levels.

The EMAS (15) looked for a causal link between low testosterone levels and ED. The testosterone level is associated with sexual drive, interest and spontaneous erections and is associated with overall sexual function but not ED. Men continue to be active sexually and higher sexual activity is associated with higher testosterone levels. Lower testosterone and decreased sexual activity were not associated with distress. There seems to be a threshold level of serum testosterone of 8 nmol/L in older men and below this level there was an increased risk of ED.

The estradiol levels however were associated with sexual distress in that a higher level was associated with more distress. Higher estradiol levels are associated with central adiposity and increased distress regarding sexual dysfunction.

Therefore, there is no indication to replace testosterone unless abnormally low levels are found.

The MMAS (16) found that obesity predicted a decline in testosterone and sex hormone-binding globulin with age but were not able to identify whether the central obesity causes the low testosterone or the low testosterone causes the obesity.

Ageing

In addition to the normal changes associated with ageing such as the increased risk of cardiovascular disease and other chronic conditions, there are social changes that may be equally relevant. Loss of status at work, loss of financial freedom, illness of partner or partner's loss of interest, family upsets or grief and loss all contribute to both loss of desire and ED.

Psychosomatic

Given the complexity of the process of erection, involving the mind and imagination and tactile, auditory, visual and olfactory stimuli, translated into outflow into the sympathetic and parasympathetic nervous supply and the ensuing vascular response, it is not surprising that it goes wrong from time to time. The willingness to be sexual, conscious or unconscious is modified by past experiences both good and bad. It is further altered by mood, partner's emotional and physical input to the encounter and emotional tensions in the relationship and in the man's life generally. For a man, there is huge pressure to perform. There are myths of male sexuality that are prevalent in society. These myths present a phallocentric view that magnifies and scrutinises a man's performance. For intercourse, there is requirement for controlled aggression in order to penetrate his partner and he may be frightened of aggression.

Common Myths about Male Sexuality

- We're liberated folk who are very comfortable with sex.
- Real men aren't into feelings and communication.

- All touching is sexual and should lead to sex.
- A man is always interested in and ready for sex.
- A real man performs in sex.
- Sex is centred on a hard penis and what is done with it.
- If your penis isn't up to it, there is a pill that will take care of everything.
- Sex equals intercourse.
- A man should make the earth move for his partner.
- Good sex is spontaneous with no planning or talking.

Source: Zilbergeld B. *The New Male Sexuality.* New York, NY: Bantam Doubleday Dell, 1999.

Brene Brown (18) describes some societal perceptions of 'maleness':

- Emotional stoicism
- Primacy of work
- Control of women
- Outward disdain for homosexuality
- Violence

Given these stereotypes it is not surprising that many men find it difficult to suffer from ED and to talk about it with their partners or their health attendants.

CASE 4: ANXIETY

Barry was 55. He bounced into the room, dressed in a stylish casual manner. He looked healthy. He had been married previously but for the last 10 years had been in a relationship with Sue. It was a wonderful relationship and sex had been excellent for the first few years. His erections had been progressively less dependable for the last 5 years. He had no trouble by himself but when he was with Sue, the erections often faded soon after penetration and he would become sweaty and distressed. PD5 inhibitors worked for some of the time but he disliked having to take them. Tests for cardiovascular disease were normal.

He was at a loss. He was a successful car salesman and he told me proudly how he had built up the business from nothing. He was proud of the way he could overcome obstacles. I sympathised that sex was one part of his life that he could not overcome with hard work. What happened 5 years ago I wondered? The business had grown so much that he had to take on extra staff and it was difficult to control them. Life had been easier when he was in control. He had become anxious but did not want to burden Sue with his worries, as he was a good coper. I pointed out that he was taking it all on himself and was it like that with sex?

He knew that he would lose his erection and as soon as he had that thought he would indeed lose it. His first wife had had an affair and in a moment of spite, had compared him unfavourably to her new lover. Since that time, he had harboured doubts about himself sexually and these had been reactivated when he became overstretched and anxious with his business. He was able to discuss it with Sue, he had some mindfulness training to help with the anxiety and realised that he did not have to take control of everything. He and Sue were to be less focussed on his performance and take more pleasure in intimacy.

CASE 5: GRIEF/PARTNER REACTION

John was 40. His first wife had died in childbirth, leaving him a young widower with a baby to care for. He had been well supported by his family. His daughter was now 8 and he had remarried a younger woman, Eve. Externally they were a happy little family. He was finding it increasingly difficult to get an erection and had little interest in sex. They attended together and sat holding hands. Eve stroked his arm and prompted him as he described his failures. They wanted a baby together to make them into a real family. I wondered aloud about whether he was afraid of losing her. He denied that, explaining that his first wife had had an underlying congenital heart problem that had contributed to her death. Eve was so supportive and she was always so kind to him when his erection failed. She was such a good mother to his daughter.

I really wanted to separate them. Responding to this I took him into the examination room to examine him. He lay there on the couch and looked down at his genitals. He said, 'It feels dead down there' and his eyes filled with tears.

'Dead?' I repeated. He told me about his first wife and the grief was palpable. At the time, he had just had to get on with life and now the prospect of a wanted, but frightening pregnancy, had brought his grief to the fore. Eve was reacting to his loss of desire in a motherly and caring manner reactivating the sense of care he had experienced from his own mother in the aftermath of his loss.

As he worked through these feelings and as Eve began to understand, they were able to become sexual once more.

The reaction of a partner of a man with ED can be critical. If he or she reacts as overly caring or maternal, that can be experienced as emasculating (not sexy). If he or she is critical, frustrated or angry then that can be upsetting and if he or she becomes overly sexy that can be experienced as too much pressure.

CASE 6: PAUL

Paul was a shy young man in his early 20s who had such severe ED that he had only managed intercourse a few times in his life. He could do so with PD5 inhibitors although he said he could 'sabotage' them. When masturbating by himself he had no difficulty but as soon as he was with a partner, he worried his erection would fail and as soon as he had that thought, he would lose the erection. He seemed to deliberately choose a long-distance relationship and keep himself aloof. He avoided any sexual encounter if he could. He was difficult to get to know and was withdrawn in the consulting room. I observed that he found intimacy difficult.

Some men need to be intimate to feel sexual but many men need to be sexual in order to feel intimate. Paul would benefit from some long-term psychotherapy to help him look at these reasons for avoiding intimacy.

CASE 7: AN ASPECT OF HIS PERSONALITY

Simon dipped in and out of coming to the psychosexual clinic. Perhaps he was ambivalent. He and his wife wanted a baby but he was unable to keep his erection, especially over the fertile time of her cycle. They were both frustrated. He wanted a baby so much and yet he could not do the most basic thing in the world. He described himself as someone who tends to think too much and to obsess about problems. He seemed shy and quiet, rather self-deprecating and not at all pushy in all aspects of his life. His sexual difficulties had been present on and off for most of his life and usually he was not too bothered as they were happy together.

Finally, his wife got pregnant through infertility treatment and then they did not wish to be sexual during pregnancy in case they damaged the baby. After the pregnancy they were busy being parents and the time was never right to address the sexual problems.

For Simon, the focus on his sexual difficulties was not helpful. They were happy as they were.

CASE 8: SHAME

Jay was quite a presence in the consulting room He was a powerfully built attractive man of 40. He was in a relationship with a man who wanted him to come to the clinic to find out why he lost his erections at times. He told me how he had come from a culture where homosexuality was considered unnatural. He had always known he was attracted to men but had not made any long-lasting friendships until he was 35. He had always felt ashamed of his arousal and although he got physical relief from a sexual encounter, he had always felt bad afterwards. His partner had provided him with a sense of peace but the reaction of his family had been very destructive to him. His eyes watered as he told me about it. As he had begun to settle into his new loving relationship, he had confided in a friend of the family, a much-trusted friend. She had told his secret to his uncle and soon the entire family had known about it. They had ostracised him and refused to talk to him and he had not been allowed to go to the funeral of his beloved grandfather earlier in the year. He had always known that his sexual orientation would be a problem in his culture but was unprepared for the venom of his family. For him, the work was to find the confidence to move away from his family and follow his heart. As he mourned the loss of his family of origin, he was able to be more sexual with his partner although he had to work hard not to feel shameful.

Conclusion

Men are often problem solvers and try hard to fix the problem in a very mechanical way. The treatments open to them are varied and outlined elsewhere in the book. These vary from mechanical drugs to talking treatments and behavioural therapy to self-help material (17,19).

As healthcare providers, we need to listen attentively and respectfully, listening to the story itself, the emotions that go with that story and what is said and found during the examination.

A man who is confident sexually may experience a loss of erection during lovemaking. If he is confident he will wait for it to return and when it does so, will remain confident. If he is naturally an insecure person, or at least insecure sexually, he will be anxious, obsessing about his perceived failure and running a negative loop in his mind.

When finding out the story, we need to know when and how the problems started and what was happening in the man's life at the time. Does it happen every time or is it just in some situations? Can he masturbate without difficulty or is he without any desire at all? What reactions from his partner(s) has he had? Does he get morning erections?

But rather than asking all these questions we could just wait and see what he tells us and then fill in the gaps later.

In a scientific model, it is satisfying to find cause and effect. If we can understand why, then we can fix the problem. All sexual problems are complex and especially with ED, there is a huge interplay between physical and emotional, between not wanting sex at all and losing the erection once sexual intimacy starts.

As we can see from the case material, when problems arise there are often echoes from the past which resonate with the current experience and so mind and body become intertwined in a web rather than a single thread of cause and effect.

REFERENCES

1. Johannes CB, Araujo AB, Feldman HA et al. Incidence of erectile dysfunction in men 40–69 years old: Longitudinal results from the Massachusetts male aging study. *J Urol* 2000;163:460–463.
2. Corona G, Lee DM, Forti G et al. EMAS Study Group. Age-related changes in general and sexual health in middle-aged and older men: Results from the European Male Ageing Study (EMAS). *J Sex Med* 2010;7(4 Pt 1):1362–1380.

3. Lee DM, Pye SR, Tahar A et al. EMAS Study Group. Cohort profile: The European male ageing study. *Int J Epidemiol* 2013;42(2):391–401.
4. Feldman HA, Goldstein I, Hazichust DG et al. Impotence and its medical and psycho social correlates: Results of MMAS. *J Urol* 1994;151(1):54–61.
5. Dong JY, Zhang YH, Qin LQ. Erectile dysfunction and risks of cardiovascular disease: Meta-analysis of prospective cohort studies. *J Am Coll Cardiol* 2011;58(13):1378–1385.
6. Ponholzer A, Temmi C, Obermayr R et al. Is erectile dysfunction an indicator for increased risk of coronary heart disease and stroke? *Eur Urol* 2005;48(3):512–518.
7. Arauyo AB, Travison TG, Ganz PA et al. Erectile dysfunction and mortality. *J Sex Med* 2009;6(9):2445–2454.
8. Maiorino MI, Bellastella G, Esposito K. Diabetes and sexual dysfunction: Current perspectives. *Diab Metab Syndr Obes: Targets Ther* 2014;7:95–105.
9. Camacho EM, Huhtaniemi IT, O'Neill TW et al. EMAS Group. Age-associated changes in hypothalamic-pituitary-testicular function in middle-aged and older men are modified by weight change and lifestyle factors: Longitudinal results from the European male ageing study. *Eur J Endocrinol* 2013;168(3):445–455.
10. Rizio N, Tran C, Sorenson M. Efficacy and satisfaction rates of oral PDE5is in the treatment of erectile dysfunction secondary to spinal cord injury: A review of literature. *J Spinal Cord Med* 2012;35(4):219–228.
11. Cui Y, Zong H, Yan H et al. The effect of statins on ED: A systematic review and meta-analysis. *J Sex Med* 2014;11(6):1367–1375.
12. Wang X, Wang X, Liu T et al. Systematic review and meta-analysis of the use of phosphodiesterase type 5 inhibitors for treatment of erectile dysfunction following bilateral nerve-sparing radical prostatectomy. *PLOS ONE* 2014;9(3):e91327.
13. Ozturk U, Yesil S, Goktug HNG et al. Effects of sildenafil treatment on patients with Peyronie's disease and erectile dysfunction. *Ir J Med Sci* 2014;183(3):449–453.
14. Mohr BA, Guay AT, O'Donnell AB et al. Normal, bound and nonbound testosterone levels in normally ageing men: Results from the Massachusetts male ageing study. *Clin Endocrinol* 2005;62(1):64–73.
15. O'Connor DB, Lee DM, Corona G et al. European Male Ageing Study Group. The relationships between sex hormones and sexual function in middle-aged and older European men. *J Clin Endocrinol Metab* 2011;96(10):E1577–E1587.
16. Derby CA, Zilber S, Brambilla D et al. Body mass index, waist circumference and waist to hip ratio and change in sex steroid hormones: The Massachusetts male ageing study. *Clin Endocrinol* 2006;65(1):125–131.
17. Zilbergeld B. *The New Male Sexuality*. New York, NY: Bantam Doubleday Dell, 1999.
18. Brene B. *Daring Greatly: How the Courage to be Vulnerable Transforms the Way We Live, Love, Parent, and Lead*. London: Penguin Life, 2015.
19. McCarthy BW, Metz ME. *Coping with Erectile Dysfunction*. Oakland, CA: New Harbinger Publications, 2004.

16

Ejaculation Disorders

Gareth Hughes

Introduction

In this chapter we look at how we combine the skills that we have learned from our Institute of Psychosexual Medicine (IPM) training to help those men who present with ejaculation disorders. The most common problem seen in men is premature ejaculation. Less common problems are retarded or non-ejaculation, retrograde ejaculation and painful ejaculation.

Problems of Ejaculation

- Premature ejaculation (PE)
- Retarded or non-ejaculation
- Retrograde ejaculation
- Painful ejaculation

As with all sexual problems the possibility of a pathological or drug-induced cause should automatically occur to us. The main pathological causes of ejaculation as in the following list are covered in more detail elsewhere:

- Metabolic problems including diabetes and thyroid disease
- Neurological conditions including multiple sclerosis and degenerative disorders
- Spinal or pelvic surgery
- Radiotherapy
- Diseases or treatment of prostate problems including prostate cancer
- Urological problems such as urinary tract infections or prostatitis
- Chronic mental illness such as obsessive-compulsive disorder (OCD), chronic depression, schizophrenia, severe generalised anxiety and borderline personality disorders

Commonly Used Drugs That May Affect Sexual Function

Anti-Hypertensive Drugs

The most common side effect of anti-hypertensive drugs is erectile dysfunction (ED). ED can, in turn, have an effect on ejaculation, especially when the man is aware that his erectile function is diminished or unreliable; he is more likely to 'let go', while he can, and so ejaculates rapidly.

β-*Blockers*, e.g. atenolol, bisoprolol, metoprolol and propranolol are probably the most recognised anti-hypertensive drugs that cause ED.

α-*Blockers*, e.g. alfuzosin, doxazocin, tamsulosin and prazosin, can block some of the effect of the α-receptors that control the bladder neck muscles and this can lead to retrograde ejaculation.

Ace inhibitors, e.g. enalapril, lisinopril and ramipril; *angiotensin II receptor blockers*, e.g. irbesartan and candesartan; and *calcium channel blockers*, e.g. nifedipine, are more likely to affect erectile function.

It must be remembered that hypertension, diabetes and sexual dysfunction can be more common as age advances and so it is often difficult to be sure if the sexual dysfunction is a direct effect of the drug therapy or the disease.

Anti-Depressant Drugs

The following groups of anti-depressant drugs can cause delayed or absent ejaculation:

- *Tricyclics*, e.g. amitryptiline
- *Selective serotonin re-uptake inhibitors (SSRIs)*, e.g. paroxetine, fluoxetine, citalopram and sertraline
- *Serotonin-norepinephrine re-uptake inhibitors (SNRIs)*, e.g. venlafaxine, sibutramine and duloxetine
- As discussed later, dapoxetine, an SSRI gained a license in 2014 for use in PE.
- *Psychotropic drugs* may all have an effect on ejaculation but great care is needed with this group of drugs and discussion with the original prescriber would be wise.

Recreational and Performance-Enhancing Drugs

As most readers will know, one of the most commonly used drugs, alcohol, can have an inhibitory effect on ejaculation but this is probably a secondary effect to a general numbing of both the erectile response (Brewer's droop) and the other phases of sexual reactivity. However, this is dose related as small amounts of alcohol can initially release inhibitions and cause a heightened awareness and responsiveness, especially of the libido. Other recreational drugs can have similar effects; some, such as amphetamines, initially enhance energy, social confidence and libido but then cause the opposite as alertness wanes and side effects kick in. γ-Hydroxybutrate (GHB) has a stimulating effect on sexual desire in small doses but is a strong sedative and anaesthetic in a higher dose. Anabolic steroids are taken for various reasons: to build muscle, to look good and to enhance performance in sport or bodybuilding. These are man-made versions of testosterone but they suppress testicular function with resultant negative effects on sexual function.

Most importantly, it is always advisable to ask about the use of prescription and non-prescription drugs when taking the history. It is important to see if there is a clear association between the introduction of a drug and the onset of symptoms. If so, assuming the benefit of stopping the drug outweighs the risk, a trial without the drug may be worth trying. Finasteride is an example of such a drug as it is now commonly used for prostatic hyperplasia and, in a small dose, to prevent hair loss. This can reduce libido and the ability to attain and sustain an erection. It can also reduce ejaculatory volume.

Management may be more complicated if certain associated medical or surgical conditions co-exist but the psychosexual doctor may still be able to offer help that others cannot by helping the patient look at the problem from a wider perspective. Patients have thoughts and feelings about the physical conditions they have and a diagnosis alone can provoke a psychosexual problem.

Before we look at the individual problems outlined above, I review the normal sexual response to see where ejaculation fits in. Later in the chapter I briefly refer to the behavioural approach to treating ejaculation problems where it is especially important to understand the normal sexual responses.

The Normal Sexual Response

In their 1966 work entitled *Human Sexual Response* (1) William Masters and Virginia Johnson described the normal sexual response as having four phases but in 1979 Helen Kaplan added another phase that preceded the others, desire (2).

As this is covered elsewhere in this book I focus on the plateau and orgasmic stages as it is mainly here where understanding the mechanism of ejaculation is helpful. We can then start to understand the mysteries and myths in this area.

The five phases of the normal sexual response according to Kaplan 1979 are as follows:

- Desire
- Excitation
- Plateau
- Orgasm
- Resolution

Following the desire and excitation stages, the body enters the plateau stage. This is traditionally depicted as a straight line before orgasm occurs. However, perhaps we should think of it as a wavy or undulating line, fluctuating within the plateau, as sexual excitement can increase or decrease in this phase. Ejaculation will usually occur but it is not necessarily inevitable.

Imagine that above this wavy line lies a second but straight line that I call the line of inevitability. If any single wave of excitement is high enough to reach the second line, this triggers the ejaculation process. The anticipation and buildup is over, the cork pops and the champagne flows.

Another way I like to think of this is to compare this wavy plateau to the height of waves in a bath. If the waves (of excitement) become too high then the bath water spills over. At this point, sensors announce that the water is starting to overflow but it is too late to stop the spillage.

Understanding this process gives us insight into the management of orgasmic and ejaculation disorders. See further Figure 16.1.

It is here where unconscious psychosexual factors seem to play a part. Working with our patients in this area, recognising possible conflicts and increasing awareness can give back a level of control in some way, as if adjusting the amplitude of a sine wave on an oscilloscope.

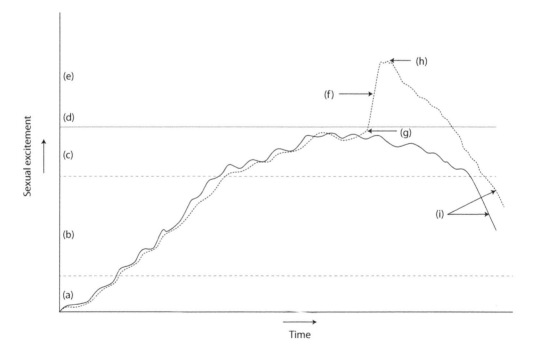

FIGURE 16.1 Patterns and phases of male sexual response: non-orgasmic response (solid line); ejaculation or orgasm (dotted line); (a) desire phase; (b) excitement phase; (c) plateau phase; (d) line of inevitability; (e) orgasm/ejaculation phase; (f) emission; (g) ejaculation/orgasm; (h) end orgasmic stage (height and length may vary); (i) towards resolution.

Those men who have PE have a very short or no time between the excitement stage and the orgasmic stage. It seems that they have a very small or no gap between the plateau and the line of inevitability.

In those with retarded ejaculation the waves build up but either take a long time to reach the trigger or never reach it at all. Normal variation should be taken into consideration as men are all different and any individual's response will vary at different times, depending on factors such as partner, environment and age.

Male Orgasm: A Two-Phase Process within the Plateau Phase

Orgasm in the male consists of two phases, emission and ejaculation.

Emission occurs, and can be felt, when semen is squeezed out of the seminal vesicles, where it has been stored, into the urethral bulb. This occurs as the waves of excitement build but does not necessarily trigger ejaculation if the wave is not high enough to reach the line of inevitability. Awareness of this sensation can provide a key to developing ejaculatory control. If a wave of excitement from the plateau stage does touch the line of inevitability, the male then senses that it is too late to stop, the countdown is over, the launch button has been pressed and rhythmic contractions of the muscles at the base of the urethra produce ejaculation.

For most men, ejaculation is the climax of sexual excitement and they should feel a sense of relaxation, relief and fulfilment. This is the case with or without a partner and, as with the female orgasm, is associated with 'letting go' of control and abandonment to the sensation. In the ideal world, there would be a degree of being able to choose when to let the control go so that both partners get to enjoy the experience and can relax, feel enriched and satisfied by it. However, in some cases, something gets in the way and interferes with the process. The key question seems to be: what is happening that affects the plateau stage?

The Mind-Body Link

What goes on consciously or unconsciously in the mind can interfere with any phase of the sexual response. This is just as important for the orgasmic phase, incorporating ejaculation, as any other phase. As we have looked at the normal sexual response as a physical process, let us now consider some of the emotions involved. What about our patient's developmental factors?

Boys are aware of pleasure in the genital area from an early age so shame, guilt and secrecy could ensue if parental attitudes to developing sexuality are negative. Once puberty is reached and 'wet dreams' occur, erections and seminal emissions are difficult to hide.

Growing into adulthood, they should be free to experience these feelings and develop a healthy awareness of sexual excitement including orgasm and ejaculation with or without a partner. Messy bed sheets caused by pubertal nocturnal emissions could lead to embarrassment and guilt and then produce powerful inhibitions to ejaculation in later life, as can exposure to any form of sexual abuse. Can we sense a fear or block in 'letting go' and 'feeling safe enough to let go', 'allowing abandonment with a partner present'? Ejaculation is often described as an explosive event. In some circumstances could this 'explosion' reflect subconscious feelings towards partners, past partners or other significant women? On a positive note this may reflect great emotional connexion and pleasure or, on a more negative note, a release of pent-up suppressed resentment or anger; the individual's history may provide a clue.

At the other end of the spectrum with increasing age, levels of arousal, the strength and duration of erections and forcefulness of ejaculation can decline. It may take longer to achieve orgasm and this can be compounded by loss of erections as both partners try too hard. This can be seen as loss of manhood and cause further negative emotions. Fear of losing an erection can produce a hurried ejaculation response or worse still, avoidance of sexual activity with a partner, leading to avoidance of intimacy and strain on a previously close relationship.

Factors That May Interfere with the Mind-Body Link

- Ignorance and inexperience, youthful or otherwise
- Guilt
- Embarrassment or lack of social privacy
- New relationships, problems with intimacy, peer expectations or body image
- Anxiety or depression
- Stress and distress, perhaps relating to a history of abuse or previous traumatic sexual experience
- Strict or repressed upbringing
- Problems with relationships
- Significant life events such as bereavements, unemployment and divorce

The history should give us a good picture of how and when the problem presented, if it has been permanent or intermittent. It is fairly common for most men to ejaculate quickly when finding their way through their first sexual experience, especially if this is associated with ignorance, inexperience, anxiety or embarrassment. Cultural and social backgrounds are likely to be factors if associated with a strict or repressed upbringing, as they may provoke conscious and unconscious feelings of conflict and guilt.

Early sexual relationships may occur as one night stands, often under the influence of alcohol and little thought may be given to the feelings of the partner. Why 'hold on' if you have nothing to hold on for? Equally, being too preoccupied with your partner's feelings may block your own feelings and not allow them to build up to a level where they reach the point of inevitability. To achieve orgasm and ejaculation through masturbation may not be a problem as it may involve fantasy and therefore detachment from personal involvement.

A revelation of abuse or previous traumatic experience may come to light. This may not be immediately apparent in the history as, understandably, many patients are reluctant to open up about such things with feelings that include embarrassment and guilt, loss of confidentiality and possible recriminations. Recollection of the event interferes with natural responses and, due to deep defences such as repression, it may take time to surface even in what we may feel is a safe therapeutic environment. Using a similar bath water analogy to that used earlier describing orgasm, with skilled therapy, memories from the past may surface and spill over into the conscious, depending on the depth of emotion and the height of the waves.

Although events in childhood or adolescence may be linked or responsible, negative experiences such as a traumatic sexual relationship can happen to any man at any stage, even those with no previous difficulties. Experiencing a traumatic emotional or sexual event can produce any number of different feelings such as loss of confidence and self-esteem, embarrassment, questions about manhood and masculinity or anxiety and fear with regard to intimacy. In some circumstances, the patient may fear some internal physical damage.

Premature Ejaculation

Definitions and Expectations

Some definitions are based on whether the woman reaches orgasm; some quote different lengths of time after penetration before the woman reaches orgasm and some even quote the number of vaginal thrusts required.

We no longer use these definitions. For one thing, they do not take into consideration that, although figures vary, up to 75% of women will never reach orgasm through vaginal penetration alone. Additional clitoral stimulation, either before, during or after vaginal penetration is necessary for this group to achieve orgasm.

Various people and bodies have defined PE going back to Greek mythology (3).

In 1974 Helen Kaplan proposed a definition of PE that was adopted by the World Health Organisation (WHO), who use the *International Classification of Diseases* (ICD) and the American Psychiatric Association (APA) who use the *Diagnostic and Statistical Manual of Mental Disorders* (DSM) to classify diseases.

The WHO classifies PE as ICD-10 F52.4: The emission of semen or seminal fluid during the act of preparation for sexual intercourse before there is penetration or shortly after penetration occurs.

The APA classifies PE as DSM V 302.75: A disorder characterised by persistent or recurrent ejaculation before or after penetration and before the person wishes it.

It is interesting to note that PE is defined as a 'Disease' and a 'Mental Disorder' in these classifications.

The British Association for Sexual Health and HIV (BASHH) describes PE as a dysfunction rather than a disease, using the following main definition: *The male sexual dysfunction characterised by ejaculation which always or nearly always occurs prior to or within about one minute of vaginal penetration, and the inability to delay ejaculation on all or nearly all vaginal penetrations, and negative personal consequences, such as distress, bother, frustration and/or the avoidance of sexual intimacy.*

BASHH also name subtypes that include the intravaginal ejaculation latency time (IELT). The idea of an IELT was first introduced by Marcel Waldinger in 2005 (4).

CASE 1

John was a 30-year-old bachelor. He arrived a few minutes late. He was smartly dressed but looked a little harassed, or perhaps just anxious, blurting out that he was sorry for being late. He explained that he had to finish an important email at work and he did not want to keep me. He thought, from his Internet research that he had PE. He was due to see his girlfriend at the weekend and wanted to sort it out before then.

I told him that he was my last patient and that I had not worried that he was a few minutes late, hoping it would help him relax a little. I asked him to explain what was happening but could he first clarify what he meant by PE as I wanted to be clear what the exact problem was. He seemed to relax a little.

He had just started a new relationship, describing 'this incredible woman he'd met through work' and, following one of their after-work 'dates' they'd ended up in bed. He said he could not really believe it as she was one of the bosses but they got on really well and that she seemed to really like him. He had been so excited that it all happened rather quickly 'I came as soon as I entered her and then, to make it worse, I lost my erection'. The second time he felt 'really anxious' and even started worrying that he would not get an erection. The more I tried to hold back, the worse it got and 'I came as soon as we undressed and she started touching me, I could see that she was unhappy'.

Reflecting how difficult this must have been as she was his boss, he admitted to feeling awful about it and very embarrassed. He had never had difficulty before. We talked about the normal male sexual response and the fine line that men sometimes tread between excitement and orgasm, how this could be affected by his anxiety and how pressurised he must feel to perform well. He smiled when we talked about how he had put her on a pedestal, and in doing so had perhaps put pressure on his penis.

He had read about the 'squeeze' and 'stop-start' techniques on the Internet but worried that there would not be an instant fix, adding that the following weekend they planned a trip away; what could he do?

There was nothing in the history to suggest anything other than what I would describe as situational anxiety. Examination was normal (he declined a chaperone). I discussed the phases of the normal sexual response and would normally have suggested that he experiment and try and gain more awareness of his arousal and try to talk to his girlfriend.

Under the circumstances however, in the light of their plans and the weekend looming, I suggested that he try a rescue remedy in the form of 30 mg of dapoxetine. I suggested that he try it on his own, before the weekend, to make sure it did not cause him any undue side effects and we went through the various pros and cons. We agreed that, if it helped, it could give him some confidence and control and he may then be in a better place to look at the underlying factors later.

The following week we met again and I was pleased to hear that the drug had no ill effects and that the idea had been a great success. He had initially tried it on his own, his erection had been fine and he took much longer to achieve orgasm. His weekend date had been transformed. After making love successfully, he had been brave enough to share what had happened since the first date. He was pleased to get a supportive, helpful response from his girlfriend and he felt much more positive about the future. He asked if he could stay on the drug for a little longer but after a few more appointments announced that he no longer needed it.

He said how helpful he had found our discussion about 'the normal sexual response' and that he had become more aware of where he was in the plateau phase. He also felt less anxious about his new girlfriend being his boss, especially as it did not seem to worry her. Being more aware of the peaks and troughs of excitement had helped, especially learning that a trough in his excitement could be accompanied by a waning erection but that this could quickly recover.

Incidence of Premature Ejaculation

Studies vary but at least a third of all men can suffer from PE at some stage in their life. Once a physical cause has been excluded, we can concentrate on the psychological aspects that are reflected in our approach.

Pre-Conceived Ideas

Before we meet our patient, we may have read a letter outlining the problem and we may, consciously or otherwise, have formed some pre-conceived ideas based on the age or, in general practice, previous knowledge of the patient.

Once the patient has had the courage to seek help, we often find that the desperation and urgency felt by him projects onto all those involved, however long the problem has existed. I expect that many of us have had messages from secretaries or colleagues explaining the urgency and importance of a particular referral. During the consultation we understand that, for some patients, everything in their life seems to be urgent and important. They cannot hold back. Perhaps here, I am also being guilty of making assumptions.

Once the patient arrives, as with all problems, we listen to the story and obtain a history. As we listen we also watch, assess what we see and perhaps most importantly try and recognise how or what we feel.

In this case this initial impression is important as we decide how to respond. With psychosexual problems I often consider the patient to be the expert, my role being to help them find a solution by us working together.

I try to be more reflective than directive but if I sense a lack of understanding and general awareness of the normal sexual response I am more likely to make an exception and alter my management slightly.

So perhaps it is especially important here that we do not get too excited and 'ejaculate' our thoughts prematurely.

Retarded Ejaculation

Retarded ejaculation (RE) is said to occur when ejaculation occurs after a delay or, less frequently, not at all. In the latter case, it is also sometimes known as an-ejaculation.

It is more unusual to see men who have retarded or absent ejaculation. These patients are more likely to present to a psychosexual consultation after prior attendance at a urology clinic. The clinic may reassure the patient that they have no physical cause. Sometimes patients would prefer a physical cause that can be treated. Knowing that they have no physical cause can add to their distress when the symptom remains with no offer of definitive treatment.

Once again, the assessment may start even before the patient arrives. There may be clues from the letter or we may have to wait until we meet and listen to the history. If the problem is new and a physical cause has been excluded then, once again, it may help to try to focus on the 'why now'.

We should enquire if he has ever been able to ejaculate or are there some circumstances when he can and others when he cannot. If ejaculation occurs with masturbation but not with vaginal thrusting, does it feel different? Is ejaculation pleasurable or painful? Does he feel as if he has an orgasm but no semen is ejaculated?

Listen for possible covert anxieties and fears about emotionally letting go. Could this relate to physically letting the semen go? We see patients in the consulting room who find it immensely difficult to 'release' their emotions about past events that would appear very traumatic, and in some this ability to stay controlled encompasses all their feelings including during sex. Exploring the mind and body connexion can illuminate how the subconscious can affect their ability to orgasm and ejaculate for some men.

Anxiety and fear can both have a negative effect on the arousal mechanisms. Could a fertile male have a covert fear of fatherhood or fear of producing further offspring? This may become apparent from his social circumstances, relationship, job and financial security.

In the same way that PE may be caused by lack of conscious control, could RE be caused in some men by over-control and shutting off? Perhaps they are too focussed on trying to please their partner and deny their own pleasure. Could they be angry with their partner and want to deny them an opportunity to become pregnant? Could they resent having undergone a vasectomy and fear that by letting go and being orgasmic they could cause internal damage now that they have tubes that are tied off?

Retrograde Ejaculation

This describes where the man ejaculates but the semen is ejaculated internally into the bladder rather than ejaculating externally through the urethra. It is sometimes called dry ejaculation. This may not necessarily worry the man if he experiences normal orgasmic feelings but does become a problem if the couple is trying to conceive.

There is usually a pathological or developmental anatomical reason for this and involvement with this group is likely to follow investigation by the urologist. Prostatic surgery is the most common cause and it can also occur as part of diabetic neuropathy, spinal cord lesions and multiple sclerosis. α-Blockers are another possible cause.

Those people who practice tantric sex can, in some case, cause self-induced retrograde ejaculation. Tantric sex has evolved from the Hindu culture where men hold Shakti, the female goddess, in high esteem. Men are encouraged to stop ejaculation by holding and tensing their pubococcygeal muscle thus forcing semen into the bladder.

If the physical cause is untreatable then we may still be able to provide psychosexual insight and support.

Painful Ejaculation

This describes those men who experience pain when they ejaculate. If the urologist cannot find a reason, could this tie in with emotional pain resulting from previous ejaculations, such as fathering a child unintentionally, especially if it produced significant painful repercussions?

Ejaculation and the Consultation

When we meet our patient we may learn that finding a solution to their problem has defied the usual route. This can immediately make the consultation more interesting but also more challenging. What is going on? Failure to give the patient a credible answer changes the doctor's position from being the 'knowing expert' to one of 'ignorance'.

Let us review those skills gained from our IPM training. Past medical experience and training have incorporated many skills into our autopilot but in a psychosexual consultation we need to readjust and focus in a different way.

What is the patient really saying and how are they saying it? What is their body language telling us? Is the patient having an effect on us? Are we aware of the effect we are having on the patient? Is anything about them changing? Concentrate on listening and observing while registering our feelings and then observe the patient again. Let us hold back from ejaculating our thoughts too quickly.

We are looking for underlying causes of the sexual dysfunction, including those in the unconscious. Remember the 'here and now' of the consultation, the feelings we have and the feelings the patient may express. Where have those feelings come from? Are these feelings our own feelings or have they come from the patient? Can we interpret this in relation to the patient's symptoms? Is the sexual dysfunction a symptom of something rather than just a problem to be solved? Why are they here now? Have they been sent?

As in any medical history, we need to ask some questions but we try not to bombard with too many. Also, it is often helpful to know what the patient thinks as we cannot read their mind.

What Does the Patient Think?

- I wonder what was happening when it started.
- I wonder why you have asked for help now.
- I wonder what you were hoping would happen today.
- I wonder what it is like for you to talk about this.
- I wonder what you think is the cause of the problem.

If there is an awkward pause, the patient may be finding it difficult. Most of us also find this difficult, as it is almost the opposite of our basic training and previous experience. If we feel we have to break a silence, rather than another question, a reflective comment may be more helpful.

Reflective Comments

- It sounds as if this is difficult to talk about.
- You sound quite angry about this.
- That must have been difficult for you.
- That may have felt very embarrassing.
- No wonder you do not feel like having sex if this is happening.

With practice and perseverance, we often find that this builds up confidence in both the patient and ourselves and will produce helpful information.

Who Is the Patient?

There are many reasons why men (and women) want to have sexual relationships and these change with age and circumstances. Psychosexual therapists will be well aware of these factors but, on the whole, we are helping people who will not have our insight and experience.

When a man presents to us with an ejaculation disorder, as with other sexual difficulties, it is usually interfering with his sexual relationship and causing a problem for himself and/or his partner. Perhaps he has been sent to 'sort out his problem'. The underlying dynamic could range from sexual enjoyment and satisfaction to interference with conception.

In most of the scenarios where ejaculation is the problem the concept of internal emotional turmoil is never far away. There is often no single cause and this is one area of psychosexual medicine where there is a good argument to use a combination of approaches, rather than be too dogmatic that we should just stay with the traditional IPM model. With the changes in approach that have taken place over the last century and are well recorded, why not be prepared to mix and match and take advantage of what is available. I wish I knew what Tom Main, the founder of the IPM, would say.

CASE 2

Many years ago, when confronted with a young, fearless, athletic giant of a rugby player I sensed an inner fear of him failing to live up to his macho image. He was the youngest of three very competitive brothers and it appeared that most of his sex education had come from them. His parents were both keen sports fans and the house revolved around sport. He went to an all-boys' school and there was no one that he would not take on. He came in looking very embarrassed and explained that he had just started having a sexual relationship but he could not last ... was there something wrong with him?

I did not find anything initially in the history to suggest that he would have a physical problem. He seemed unduly anxious so I suggested a physical examination and he seemed pleased. He declined a chaperone. I asked if he was worried about anything being physically wrong and he just said he wanted to know if he looked normal. He thought, that being so fit, he would be able to perform better. Examination was completely normal and he seemed to relax a little.

I complimented him on being brave enough to ask for some advice and asked if he might know what was going on. He replied that he had no idea but that he became very excited and could not control what happened, despite thinking of anything that he could to distract himself. He also asked why, when he had seen some porn films at the rugby club, the men in the films could keep going for ages?

We chatted about his background and especially his prior knowledge and experience of sex, reflecting that there was no reason why he should be an expert in this area. I commented that porn films probably caused more harm than good and were responsible for all sorts of myths, misconceptions and false beliefs. I added that they could separate fantasy from reality and that the editing was highly selective.

I briefly adopted a 'teacher's role' and spent a few minutes talking about what I understood was normal. I explained how the normal sexual response varies from man to man, from partner to partner and from situation to situation. We looked at how and why anxiety and lack of awareness in the excitement phase can have adverse effects. I encouraged him to ask his girlfriend how she felt and what she wanted or expected. He agreed about the anxiety so I encouraged him to think of sex and sexual intimacy with his girlfriend as something that should be enjoyable, relaxing and fun, not a game to be won or a performance to prove. He admitted that he had never really talked to anyone about sex before and never thought about it in that way. He did not make another appointment but the next time he saw me was in the club bar after a match; he looked over at me, gave me a big smile and a 'thumbs up' sign. Hardly an auditable event but I think he inferred a positive outcome.

Other Approaches to Treatment for Premature Ejaculation

The Behavioural Approach–Squeeze Technique and Stop-Start

The first reported use of the stop-start technique was by urologist James Semans in 1956 (5). It was made popular by William Masters and Virginia Johnson in their work published in 1970, *Human Sexual*

Inadequacy (6). They blamed PE on a false learning or behavioural process and were more widely recognised, recommending a behavioural approach adding a squeeze technique to the stop-start approach.

To understand the behavioural approach, as already stated, it is important the patient understands the basic sexual response. The man can then work, with permission and with a better understanding, of what he is trying to achieve and why it may work. Depending on his circumstances and current relationship status he may or may not feel that he wants to involve his partner. Whatever he decides, this may change with time.

The theory behind this stop-start and squeeze method is to heighten sensory awareness within the undulating plateau of pleasurable excitation. As the man is stimulated, either alone or by his partner, he should concentrate on the sensation that he is feeling. He, or his partner, can then stop, slow down or squeeze the penis just below the glans. This allows the wave of excitement to diminish and he learns to recognise the level of excitement. He can then resume and recognise when he is likely to climax. This is the same theory used by the ancient Eastern tantric massages where the endeavour is prolonged sexual arousal and pleasure without the goal necessarily being orgasm and ejaculation.

The Chemical Approach

The first use of a chemical to help PE was reported by Bernard Shapiro in 1943 when he successfully treated 33 patients with a topical local anaesthetic, 3% dibucaine cream (7).

The use of local anaesthetic creams to numb the penis has reported limited success and there is a danger of spreading the local anaesthetic to the partner, resulting in genital numbness and skin sensitivity. Neither these creams nor wearing condoms really address the underlying problem and most patients find them unhelpful.

In other situations, drugs are produced to target certain conditions and side effects are recorded that are, occasionally, beneficial. Two such groups are the SSRI and SNRI anti-depressant drugs and are mentioned in the section 'Commonly used drugs that may affect sexual function'.

I became aware of these effects first hand as a general practitioner in the late 1980s when changing the treatment of my patients with depression from the tricyclic anti-depressants to the newer SSRI anti-depressants fluoxetine (Prozac) and paroxetine (Seroxat). Very quickly both men and women started to come in complaining to me that their mood had improved and that they felt very much better. They volunteered, on a positive note, that as a result of feeling better, they had re-engaged in the sexual side of their relationships but found that they were having difficulty achieving a climax. Looking back, this was the first time that I remember talking so often, in such frank terms, to a group of patients about their sex lives and certainly the first time that I remember women complaining that they were having difficulty being orgasmic. I learned much more from my patients than I did from the drug company information. The only references to these symptoms that were easy to find in the middle of a consultation were that they could cause 'sexual side effects'. A woman who found that the drug delayed her orgasm confessed that her husband was taking it as it helped him last longer.

Dapoxetine

In May 2014, the NICE (National Institute for Health and Care Excellence) approved the use of dapoxetine for certain patients with premature ejaculation. The NICE website shows the key points:

> Dapoxetine is a short-acting selective serotonin-reuptake inhibitor (SSRI). It is the first pharmacological treatment for premature ejaculation to be licensed in the UK. In a pooled analysis of 4 randomised controlled trials (RCTs) in men with premature ejaculation there was a statistically significant increase in intra-vaginal ejaculatory latency time (IELT) with Dapoxetine 'on demand' compared with placebo 'on demand', although an increase in IELT was also seen with placebo.

I have found dapoxetine most useful as an adjuvant when working with patients who have PE, especially those who are more anxious.

Conclusion

So much has changed since the last edition of this textbook was published in 2001. The Internet has changed the way we access and share information, Facebook was launched in 2004, YouTube in 2005 and Twitter in 2006. Everyone can find more information about sex and sexual problems. Easy access to pornography can influence the perception of what is normal and what is expected. Ejaculation, male and female orgasms are no longer subjects that few talk about; it has changed the map of sexual expectation. We, in turn, face increasing challenges as more people, including those from different religious and cultural backgrounds, gain confidence and feel empowered to talk about their sex lives, each bringing different problems and expectations as they look to us for help. Many will for the first time feel able to voice and share their personal situations, women expect more than just a few thrusts from their partners and many men are also becoming more aware, noticing their disappointment and feeling inadequate if they underperform. As therapists, together we grapple with those intertwining difficulties.

As with other psychosexual problems, no two patients who experience difficulty with ejaculatory control are the same. We can now supplement our counselling skills with some specific treatments outlined in this chapter but we must remember that previous knowledge or experience may blind the health professional to what is going on in the case in front of him or her. If we feel stuck then we must have the confidence to use the core skills that our training has given us.

REFERENCES

1. Masters WH, Johnson VE. *Human Sexual Response*. Boston, MA: Little, Brown, 1966.
2. Kaplan HS. *Disorders of Sexual Desire and Other New Concepts and Techniques in Sex Therapy*. New York, NY: Brunner/Hazel Publications, 1979.
3. Ehrentheil OF. A case of premature ejaculation in Greek Mythology. *J Sex Res* 1974;10:128–131.
4. Waldinger MD, Quinn P, Dilleen M, Mundayat R, Schweitzer DH, Boolell M. Ejaculation disorders: A multinational population survey of intravaginal ejaculation latency time. *J Sex Med* 2005;2:492–497.
5. Semans JH. Premature ejaculation: A new approach. *South Med J* 1956;49:353–358.
6. Masters WH, Johnson VE. *Human Sexual Inadequacy*. Boston, MA: Little, Brown, 1970.
7. Schapiro B. Premature ejaculation, a review of 1130 cases. *J Urol* 1943;50:374–379.

17

Problems with Female Orgasm

Fiona Cowan

KEY POINTS

- An orgasm is a natural reflex leading to a pleasurable alteration in conscious and physical state.
- Causes of anorgasmia predominantly have a psychosocial or psychosexual cause.
- Organic causes of anorgasmia are rare.
- Secondary anorgasmia can occur at any stage of a woman's life.
- Interpretation of the professional-patient relationship and the psychosomatic examination are useful skills in understanding and treating psychosexual causes.

Problems with Female Orgasm

The female orgasm is a sensation of heightened pleasure, a natural reflex which leads to a pleasurable alteration in conscious and physical state (1). These sensations are accompanied by involuntary contractions of the uterus, anus and striated muscles surrounding the vagina, in particular pubococcygeus. Achieving a successful orgasm requires the correct erotic stimulus of genital and non-genital areas for that individual. In addition, it is essential the woman has the psychological ability to lose her inhibitions.

For some, the ability to experience an orgasm may be perceived as impossible. The female orgasm has been a focus of medical and psychological research for decades (2). Initial research was by Masters and Johnson in the 1950s with some of the first recorded data on the anatomy and physiology of human sexual response. While the precise aetiology of female orgasmic disorder remains uncertain, studies indicate a multitude of risk factors including co-morbid medical conditions, psychological, physiological and socio-demographic factors (1). Insufficient stimulation and organic causes should be ruled out including endocrine, neurological, malignant and dermatological conditions. Medications including selective serotonin re-uptake inhibitors (SSRIs) and anti-psychotics can negatively impact on orgasm potential (1).

Psychological factors can arise from and include anxiety and depression, relationship problems, anger towards the partner for reasons such as dishonesty, financial difficulties, the patient's or the partner's infidelity, poor communication in the relationship, mistrust, lack of libido, bereavement, past history of sexual abuse, rape, termination of pregnancy, hospital treatments, body dysmorphia and negative religious views on sex.

In most cases when a patient presents with the inability to orgasm, there is a combination of problems with an interplay of other sexual disorders. A prime example may be a woman with genuine urinary stress incontinence causing vaginal soreness who has also become incontinent during orgasm. This combination of physical discomfort and the psychological fear and embarrassment of incontinence when pleasured can lead to anorgasmia and perhaps even avoidance of sex altogether. Each patient therefore needs a comprehensive assessment including psychosexual history and examination.

Anorgasmia

Orgasms can occur from an early age with recognition of pleasurable feelings when the genital area is stimulated, for instance while riding a horse or bicycle. Later in adolescence there is the desire for self-exploration of the genitalia with experimentation of rubbing and different levels of pressure over the clitoris to provide pleasure. Masturbation may become a normal behaviour. The stimulus to orgasm differs between individuals and so in order to have satisfying foreplay and sex, communication is essential between the couple. A number of relationship and psychological factors can however contribute to a difficulty in reaching orgasm. The media and pornography often portray an unrealistic view on what men and women should perceive as 'normal'. The patient and her partner may have very differing, unexpressed views on this. Women may feel under pressure to achieve a purely 'vaginal' orgasm without clitoral stimulation or to reach orgasm successfully to avoid her partner feeling a 'failure'. *Anorgasmia* is the medical term for regular difficulty reaching orgasm after ample sexual stimulation, causing personal distress. Primary anorgasmia where the woman has never experienced an orgasm is not uncommon. Secondary anorgasmia occurs in an individual who has previously been orgasmic but now has significant difficulties and an inability to orgasm. Patients can present with primary and secondary anorgasmia when the actual problem is that there is no libido and sex is unwanted or not enjoyable. Although it is useful to differentiate, this is less important than exploring and interpreting the patient's feelings.

Physical Causes of Anorgasmia

Neurological

The ability to orgasm relies on an intact sacral reflex arc and for psychogenic arousal, the integrity of sensation at T11–L2 (3). Our knowledge of the neurology of arousal and orgasm has been enhanced by human studies of individuals with spinal cord injuries. In patients with multiple sclerosis, studies have shown lesions in the right occipital area of the brain to be associated with impaired arousal and left insular lesions associated with decreased lubrication (4). The chronic neurological disorder, epilepsy, has been associated with anorgasmia, however this is not entirely understood. The condition can cause a number of downstream pathological alterations (5). Reproductive endocrine disorders have been associated with epilepsy including hyperandrogenemia, polycystic ovarian syndrome, hypothalamic amenorrhoea, menstrual abnormalities and infertility. Enzyme-stimulating anti-epileptic drugs (AEDs) such as phenytoin, topiramate, phenobarbital, oxcarbazepine and carbamazepine, increase the hepatic synthesis of sex hormone-binding globulin (SHBG). This results in a decrease in the accessibility of testosterone. Sexual dysfunction occurs with greater prevalence in patients taking phenytoin and carbamazepine than in patients taking valproate or lamotrigine (6,7). Case reports have been published of gabapentin-associated anorgasmia in epileptic women (8). Those taking valproate for bipolar disorder have been reported to have significantly decreased libido and anorgasmia. It may be challenging to establish whether difficulties with orgasm are due to the disease, medication or a combination of the two. It would be important to discuss this with the patient including a review of whether changing the timing or reducing the dose is at all possible.

Endocrine

An endocrine disorder may present itself as anorgasmia. This is often due to hypopituitarism, resulting in hypogonadism. Endocrine conditions leading to sexual dysfunction may include diabetes mellitus, hypothyroidism, Addison's or Cushing's disease. Secondary hypopituitarism is rare but may be the result of Sheehan's syndrome where there is ischaemic necrosis of the pituitary gland following a major obstetric haemorrhage. A hormonal profile including luteinizing hormone, follicle-stimulating hormone, oestradiol, testosterone (total and free), prolactin and thyroid function testing in addition to a thorough history and examination are useful in ruling out an endocrine cause. There has been little research conducted on the effect of diabetes on arousal and orgasm in women.

Malignant Disease

Sexual dysfunction, in particular anorgasmia, is common following radical pelvic surgery (9). This may in part be due to disruption of the neuronal pathways essential for orgasm. It can be difficult to differentiate between anorgasmia caused by neuronal damage and that of psychological distress due to loss of fertility, feelings of guilt, shame, disfigurement or feeling less desirable. The patient may feel her past enjoyment and freedom she experienced during sex has contributed to her condition and so can lose the ability to relax and enjoy sexual activity. After hysterectomy, a woman may feel 'less of a woman' or have concerns about 'what is at the end of the vagina' (10). This can affect partners who can be similarly impeded during intercourse with anxieties of causing further harm.

> What is in there now, doctor? Is it a hole? Will her guts eat my penis? (Male partner who developed erectile dysfunction after his wife's vaginal hysterectomy)

Such phantasies can be largely eradicated by examining the woman with a supportive discussion regarding anatomy and reassuring the patient of normality. Women with reduced libido and anorgasmia can appear fearful and defensive during the examination but may well disclose during this process when they feel most vulnerable. It is sometimes helpful to suggest that the woman examines herself. This can be done at home if she feels uncomfortable doing it in the healthcare setting.

> Since I had cervical cancer my vagina belongs to the doctors and not my husband. I can't think about sex anymore because it's so frightening to think that I almost lost my life from an area that had given my husband and me such pleasure. (Survivor of cervical cancer with low libido and subsequent anorgasmia)

Dermatological

Sexual activity and the ability to orgasm can be detrimentally affected by dermatological conditions of the vulva. These can include vulvovaginitis caused by candidiasis, herpes, trichomonas, atrophic vaginitis, vulvar dermatosis such as lichen sclerosus, lichen planus or eczema that can sometimes be a chemical irritation due to soap, washing powder or perfumes. There can also be provoked vulvodynia, hymenal abnormalities, pelvic radiotherapy causing vaginal stenosis or trauma and scarring such as from previous vaginal surgery or episiotomy (11). Lichen sclerosus gives a classic 'figure-of-eight' pattern of white patches surrounding the vulva and anus which can be itchy and sore. Often there is a loss of normal architecture and the clitoris may become buried by affected skin leading to a loss of sensation. Both lichen sclerosus and planus can lead to vulval and vaginal adhesions also affecting function. A detailed history and genital examination must be taken to rule out an organic cause, however there is often a combination of physical and psychological factors for failure to orgasm.

> I just can't get aroused, every time he comes near me my labia and vagina burn like he has set fire to them. I can't even remember what an orgasm feels like anymore.

Medication

The female sexual response can be impeded by the use of medication for other conditions. As well as anti-convulsants, these can include anti-depressants, psychotropic drugs or narcotics. β-Blockers and α-adrenergic drugs commonly used in hypertension have been found to reduce sexual desire, arousal and sexual pleasure (12). SSRIs and serotonin noradrenaline re-uptake inhibitors can reduce vaginal lubrication and impair orgasm in 5%–71% of patients (12). Tricyclic anti-depressants and monoamine oxidase inhibitors are associated with reduced sexual desire and orgasm. Anti-psychotic use has been linked with diminished desire, changes in orgasm quality or anorgasmia.

It is believed the reduction in free testosterone when taking oral contraceptives can contribute to reduced desire however, it is always worth considering other confounding factors such as fear of sexually transmitted diseases and pregnancy. An alternative contraceptive, depot medroxyprogesterone acetate, can lead to weight gain, depression, vaginal atrophy and dyspareunia with decreased libido in up to 15% of women (12). It is important to talk to the patient about all the factors before attributing the loss of orgasm to a specific drug.

Psychosocial and Psychosexual Causes of Anorgasmia

Psychosocial

Social and relationship difficulties can play a major part in developing anorgasmia. This may be due to situational difficulties such as living as a couple in a busy home with little privacy in close proximity to other family members. The fear of being heard by a relative, while having pleasurable sex, can cause many women to become anorgasmic. During the consultation, the woman may divulge that she is able to orgasm and find sex more enjoyable when on holiday or at home when the family is away.

> We used to have such a pleasurable sex life before we got married. We were made to move in with his parents after marriage. How could I climax and enjoy myself with them in the next room? We rarely bother having sex anymore.

Relationship difficulties can often be responsible for inhibition of the orgasm reflex. These can include poor communication and misunderstanding, mistrust, infidelity or another form of betrayal. This can dramatically impact psychologically on an individual. Other causes of anorgasmia can be deep rooted in the woman's psyche and need to be explored in a psychosexual consultation. Psychosexual therapy with an Institute of Psychosexual Medicine (IPM) trained therapist may be sought but marital or relationship difficulties may benefit by input from a College of Sexual and Relationship Therapists (COSRT) trained professional.

Psychosexual

We cannot assume there are specific psychological causes but need to work with the patient to unlock and understand any current or past factors. However, the following have been encountered in psychosexual consultations as contributing causes in these patients to difficulties with orgasm.

Childhood Sexual Abuse

Childhood abuse may lead to a variety of psychosexual problems. The IPM conducted research into adults who had been abused as children and found that almost a quarter of the subjects complained of an inability to achieve orgasm (13). Often this had originated from being confused and upset by any feelings of sexual excitement as a result of the inappropriate actions of the abuser. In later life, the previously abused teenager or adult may subconsciously suppress such feelings resulting in anorgasmia.

> When I was a child our house was a brothel. My mother a prostitute, my father her pimp. Everything seems tainted including sex. When I see milk I just think of semen. I cannot orgasm as I'm too ashamed.

In addition to the shame felt by the graphic sexual acts she was exposed to as a child, the patient also expressed the need to 'hold back' and an extreme fear of 'letting go'. If she 'lost control' she would be concerned of where this would lead and whether she would become promiscuous or what she described as a 'bad woman' like her mother, the prostitute. Psychosexual counselling helps the patient to bring subconscious thoughts, feelings and anxieties to the surface, enabling her to acknowledge and begin to cope with reawakened disturbing memories from childhood. By discussing and working through such feelings, she can then establish sexual feelings on her own terms in order to use her sexuality for her pleasure and therefore allow her to become orgasmic.

CASE 1

Valentina was a 45-year-old Spanish patient who presented to the gynaecology clinic with vaginal soreness, dyspareunia, loss of libido and the inability to orgasm. She was petite and strutted into the consulting room with skinny jeans and an oversized red bomber jacket. As she walked in I could sense her dissatisfaction in seeing me. I detected intense anger and she gave me a look as if to suggest I would be far too young to understand her issues. I started the consultation despite her failing to make eye contact with me. Her general practitioner (GP) had provided the results of a number of investigations which were all normal. 'Sex is just non-existent now and I do not find it pleasurable and I just shut down. I get so sore', she said. I could see the frustration in her face. The problem had been ongoing since the first two years into her 15-year relationship. Prior to this sex was enjoyable with her partner. She did not seem to think the pain on sex was due to any particular sexual position. Relationships in the past had been short-lived and she took pride in telling me she used to be 'hot blooded' and had previously had 'a number of flings'. She pronounced, 'sex was always fun and carefree but now my partner and I just hold hands like old people'. I asked her if she and her partner had been under any stress recently or if there were any problems in the relationship. She said no but at this moment I felt her close down and become even more distant.

I found this an appropriate time to examine her. To my surprise she was incredibly relaxed during the genital examination and in fact opened her legs readily before I even asked her to. Her genitalia were entirely normal. When back in her seat I openly reflected on how she seemed 'so relaxed' and asked her why she cannot be as relaxed with her partner during sex. I could tell she was becoming more agitated. I reflected this back to her, 'Am I right in sensing some anger and agitation?' She paused and then the tears ran down her face. For the first time in the consultation she made eye contact with me. 'Intimacy' she said, 'the fear of getting too close'. Considering she had been in a 15-year relationship I found this an interesting statement. I asked her why she fears intimacy and what the potential trigger had been considering sex had been so 'fun' at the start of the relationship. The atmosphere in the consulting room changed entirely and I felt I began to build a good rapport with her. The doctor-patient relationship dramatically changed from intense projected feelings of mistrust and anger to that of being a close friend. Valentina explained that at the age of 12 when she lived in Spain her mother sadly passed away. One night her father crept into her bedroom and started to touch her inappropriately. Shocked, scared and still raw from her mother's passing she promptly ran away to live with an aunt. She had told her family members that her and her father were no longer seeing eye to eye and up until this consultation she had not disclosed the actions of her father to anyone. A constant stream of tears was now running down her face. I sensed her sadness but also immense relief in disclosing this information. I asked her how she felt towards her father and she replied, 'Resentment. He took my childhood from me when I needed him the most'. I asked her if she had considered talking to her partner or at least close friends and she was unable to in fear of 'opening a can of worms'. I explored with her what in particular it was about this relationship that had triggered such strong feelings. She explained sex was always carefree until the relationship became serious. Valentina said, 'Things get bad when I start to depend and put my trust in someone. I put my trust in my father and look what happened to me'. She saw this as the ultimate betrayal. I asked her why she had come now after all this time. She thought perhaps it was because after years of lost contact her father recently wanted to make amends. Valentina also commented that at times she finds her relationship hard as ironically her partner on occasions drinks the same whisky and smokes the same cigarettes her father did when she was a child. This seemed to be a trigger for her. At the end of the consultation I reflected back how she seemed to be much more relaxed and I started to see her vivacious character come through. I offered to see her again but she felt she understood her issues so much more now and could see a way forward. I left open access to the clinic but she never returned. I would hope she was able to regain pleasure in sex and once again become orgasmic.

Rape

A sexual assault can result in secondary anorgasmia. A happy, satisfying and orgasmic sexual relationship can be destroyed by rape. Often the victim will be attacked by a close acquaintance. The woman may have lost her ability to trust and to 'let go' sexually following such a destructive and traumatic event. She may initially present to your consultation covertly with anorgasmia, loss of libido, or a physical symptom such as pelvic pain, dyspareunia or a persistent, irritating vaginal itch. During the consultation it is important to reflect back to the patient any transferred feelings onto you and in the room. She may appear angry, reflecting her subconscious anger at the attacker and frustration at the difficulties she finds herself in. Often during the genital examination, you may observe the patient to be 'frozen' or disengaged.

As highlighted later in this chapter as clinicians we need to be mindful of 'medical rape'. What is seen to us as a routine procedure can result in significant psychosexual consequences. An example of this would be a difficult catheterisation with an audience of doctor, nurse and medical student. The patient may see this procedure as a violation and her small, obscure urethra confused with her vagina resulting in a fear of painful intercourse and being anatomically 'abnormal'.

CASE 2

Jemma was a 29-year-old who worked in public relations. She presented with persistent vaginal itching. She came into the consulting room fidgety and agitated. She could not sit still. Jemma was dressed conservatively head to toe in dark grey baggy clothing. Her issues had been ongoing since the beginning of her pregnancy 2 years previously. She had pressure of speech, 'The itching is all the time, it's relentless, I've tried Canesten, I've been to the GUM clinic, changed my washing powder and nothing. Nothing helps but I know there's something wrong with me'. I was aware of a feeling of intense anger in the consulting room. On enquiring she was not currently having sex and had no desire to. She no longer had a partner. The father of her child she said, 'was not nice'. She even said she had no urge to masturbate and the times she did she had been unable to orgasm.

When I asked Jemma why she thought the problems started at the beginning of her pregnancy and what she thought may have triggered this she became very aggressive and more agitated. I reflected back to her that I sensed a lot of anger in the room and thought out loud, 'I wonder why this might be'. 'This is pointless', she shouted back, becoming a brighter shade of scarlet as she did so. I explained to her, 'I hope you appreciate I am trying to help you. Did you not have a good pregnancy?'. 'Why do you ask?' she snapped back. I went on to say 'because by raising this, it has caused you to become very agitated. What was it about the pregnancy that has caused you to feel this way?'

There was a long pause and a very deep sigh. Her head dropped to look at her hands clasped tightly on her lap. Her eyes were quickly filling with tears, but I could tell she put every effort into not crying. I allowed a period of silence and told her to take her time. 'My previous partner was abusive. My child is the result of him raping me. I had had a busy period at work and, when I told him I was too tired to have sex he forced himself on me asking me, "Why are you always so tight when I want to get in?"'

I asked her how this made her feel. She responded by saying 'violated, used, filthy and worthless'. There was a pause between each word which seemed put emphasis on each of the powerful words she used. She wept as she said, 'and now I have this awful itch that plagues me and even when I want to pleasure myself there's no point, I cannot reach climax, it's just all dead down there'. She spoke in a resentful way, looking down to her lap every time. I had a deep sense of her feelings of being 'unclean' which I reflected back to her. She agreed and said she felt 'damaged', like her 'privates' were not her 'own'. The pressure of speech returned, 'I've tried Dettol to clean but it doesn't help. Why? Why am I still so dirty?' I asked her why she chose to use a product which is so harsh on an area so delicate; 'to try to scrub away the harshness of what he did to me. I'm desperate to feel normal again and get my body back'.

I asked her how her bond with her son was. She explained she sometimes finds it hard and some days sees his father but exclaimed, 'my son is my life now and I want to get better for him'. I asked her if sex, the ability to orgasm and a future relationship would be important to her. 'Yes, I just want to be loved'. When I asked her if she believes she could be loved, she responded, 'I hope so'. The atmosphere in the room changed from a pressure cooker to one of calm. The doctor-patient relationship changed from me feeling her resentment towards me as though I were her enemy to that of a friend or sister. I commented on how Jemma seemed much less agitated and that the anger had subsided. She responded, 'Yes, I do feel it has helped to lighten my load somewhat'. Jemma declined an examination as she did not feel it necessary. I noticed as we had been talking she gradually became less fidgety and the itch did not appear to be bothering her as before.

Sexuality

Some female patients with anorgasmia are in heterosexual relationships with hidden homosexual feelings. This can place incredible stress on the partnership with the woman consumed by her homosexual thoughts and urges with feelings of guilt and dishonesty towards her partner. The woman may not become orgasmic until she breaks away and forms a homosexual relationship. Perhaps the woman had tried to live the type of life expected of her due to religious or family views. She may have struggled with her feelings due to children or other dependents involved. A psychosexual consultation enables a safe environment to release her conscious and subconscious feelings, empowering her to make the correct choices for her and ultimately allow her to gain pleasure in sex again.

Women who are transitioning or battling with feelings surrounding gender identity disorder may also present either covertly or overtly to a consultation with anorgasmia.

Termination of Pregnancy

The decision to terminate a pregnancy can be incredibly difficult. Ideally, the patient would have the emotional support from a partner, friends or family but in reality, many women feel isolated and unable to discuss their feelings. Many still see termination as a 'taboo' subject. Following the termination, feelings of guilt, regret or even post-traumatic stress can be expressed. These feelings can manifest as symptoms such as persistent vaginal discharge, loss of libido, anorgasmia or loss of sexual pleasure where no organic cause is found.

> I have had persistent vaginal discharge and unable to have pleasure with sex after I had a termination 6 years ago. I'm worried doctor. Do you think the scissors are still in there that they cut my baby out with?

To some patients, sex which was previously a fulfilling and enjoyable experience can be tainted by the subconscious thoughts surrounding termination. In a psychosexual consultation, the feelings projected by the patient, e.g. anxiety, fear or anger, can be reflected back and thus used. This, often in combination with a psychosexual genital examination, can help the patient to unlock their deep-rooted fantasies. In unlocking such thoughts and feelings during the doctor-patient relationship you can start to work with the patients' fears.

Childbirth, Motherhood and Medical Interventions

Pregnancy, childbirth and motherhood are significant events in a woman's life. The changes occurring to her body and her new role as a mother can have a major impact on her sexual activity and relationship with her partner. Postnatally a woman may present to the GP or gynaecology clinic with superficial dyspareunia, loss of libido and anorgasmia since the birth of her child. She may present feelings that her vagina is 'too tight' following repair of perineal injuries or 'too loose to be a lover'. To your surprise on examination, the genitalia are often entirely normal with no scar tissue and there is inability to recreate the discomfort she experiences. The woman may however transfer feelings of violation, disengagement, anxiety or frustration. It is often useful to interpret this back to her. Often during a psychosexual consultation, the woman will recall throwaway comments from medical staff which have made her feel less normal.

> I've got no sex drive anymore. Sex is no longer fun, and I can't seem to orgasm…I remember the midwife telling her student to 'cut' me as I was 'far too tight'. I just think of the words 'tight' and 'cut' when my husband comes near me. Why aren't I normal?

Similarly, anorgasmia can be a result of childhood memories of medical interventions associated with being exposed during sex with cold, stark flashbacks to clinical interventions.

CASE 3

Agata was a 27-year-old patient who had been referred by the colposcopy nurse. It had never been possible for her practice nurse, GP or the colposcopy nurse to perform a cervical smear. She gracefully walked into the room tall and slim with fair hair, a pale doll-like face and large piercing blue eyes. She was dressed in a tight black polo neck jumper which completely covered her arms and tucked under her chin with long black trousers and black boots. There was a childlike innocence to her, she seemed timid and I instantly felt I developed a parental role. She explained that she always had an issue with smears. She commented that she 'cannot let them in' and that her 'genitals cannot accept the device'. I asked if she was in a relationship and had problems with sex. She explained that initially sex is difficult, as she relaxes she finds it more comfortable but then has difficulties in letting herself go enough to climax. I wondered why this was and she said she was unsure. As I asked her, she seemed to become more nervous, becoming distracted by the large buckle on her oversized handbag which was placed like a large pillow for comfort on her lap.

I paused for a moment. I gently asked her why she thought her vagina could accept a penis but not a speculum. 'I…well…I'm not sure' she replied as she swept her hair behind her ears, pursed her lips and then looked at my computer screen. I told her she seemed distracted when I talk of the speculum and I asked her what it is about the device that she fears the most. There was a long pause. She looked me directly in the eyes and said, 'I had a happy childhood until I got sick. My memories are hazy, but I remember having lots of tummy pains and constipation when I was nine or ten'. She recalls her parents mollycoddling her and the resentment she felt from her siblings. Her eyes filled with tears which emphasised her striking blue eyes and she explained, 'I remember lying on a cold table, the harsh hospital lights were focussed on me and all these people I didn't know staring at me. The doctor put something into my bottom…now I am scared of hospitals and scared to let myself relax intimately with my partner. I just see sex as something clinical. Maybe that's why I can't let go and have an orgasm either'.

I asked her how she feels when she is about to have a smear or when her partner wants to have sex with her. She explained she feels she 'goes back there to that cold, stark room'. I asked her if she masturbates and interestingly she is able to have an orgasm when she relaxes and is on her own. I highlighted the fact that she seems to be particularly anxious when someone else is involved whether it be a nurse or doctor attempting to perform a smear or her partner wanting to have sex with her. She said she feels a 'loss of control' and I explained she could gain the control back by starting off by taking a small speculum home to insert herself and to see it as an extension of her own fingers. Perhaps then, after open discussion with her partner, she could allow him to gently insert this. She nodded with enthusiasm and I felt the mood lighten in the room. I offered examination however she did not feel ready to do this at this stage. I imagined her genitalia would be entirely normal however I wondered if she would be frozen, detached and project feelings of violation during the examination. Following a period of reflection I had a strong feeling urging me not to examine her and my concern was that perhaps an examination at this stage would exacerbate her problem. She left the consultation happier and more confident.

I saw Agata back in clinic a few months later. She wore brighter, more colourful and less constricting clothes. She appeared to have more confidence and was enthusiastic when she told me her and her partner had managed to insert the speculum. I felt she was more ready to be examined this time and she accepted. Behind the curtain however she sat like a child, semi-naked with her knees drawn to her chest. I reflected that she seemed apprehensive and asked if she was okay to proceed. Although she still felt anxious and she explained that the examination couch reminded her of her childhood experience, she seemed to have a new-found determination to overcome her fears and phantasies. I cautiously proceeded noting her normal external genitalia. She appeared at times to be frozen with her eyes fixed on the ceiling and I felt compelled to keep checking if she was okay. To both our surprise I managed to insert a small speculum with ease and was successful in taking the smear test. She immediately jumped from the couch very animated with tears of joy streaming down her face. 'I feel I have more control now, thank you so much, I am so relieved' she said as she jumped around behind the curtain. I felt an overwhelming sense of relief and on concluding the consultation, Agata left elated.

Conclusion

The ability to achieve an orgasm is an important factor for men, women and their relationships. Achieving a pleasurable sexual experience and ultimately the ability to orgasm require the correct stimulus for that individual and their ability to 'let go'. Women who suffer with either primary or secondary anorgasmia can become incredibly frustrated and depressed, convincing themselves they are 'abnormal'. The media and pornography industries have painted unrealistic ideas of what is 'normal' sexual functioning and within the relationship, there can be huge, unspoken discrepancies in what each consider acceptable. Women may present either overtly or covertly but initially many will expect you to find an organic cause. These are however rare compared to the psychosexual reasons which can be as varied as the patients themselves, occurring at any time of life.

Patients with anorgasmia can commence therapy in a psychosexual consultation. The woman may have certain beliefs or 'phantasies', a less conscious form of 'fantasy' regarding their bodily functions which can impact negatively on their sex lives. During the consultation and examination, deep-seated feelings and emotions of the patient can become apparent. These may include anger, guilt, fear or shame. As clinicians, we interpret the emotions transferred to us from the patient unlocking the puzzle with the patient. Often the psychosomatic examination can reveal the most insight, when the patient is at her most vulnerable, yet feeling that she is in a safe environment. This will often allow the woman to reveal her phantasies about her genitals. In the ensuing consultations, the psychosexual clinician can help the woman to work through her difficulties and lose her anxieties and inhibitions in order to become orgasmic.

REFERENCES

1. Cohen SD, Goldstein I. Diagnosis and management of female orgasmic disorder. In LI Lipshultz, AW Pastuszak, AT Goldstein, A Giraldi, MA Perelman (Eds.), *Management of Sexual Dysfunction in Men and Women*. New York, NY: Springer, 2016, 261–271.
2. Stephenson K, Kerth J, Truong L et al. Female orgasmic disorder in couple and family therapy. In J Lebow, A Chambers, DC Breunlin (Eds.), *Encyclopedia of Couple and Family Therapy*. New York, NY: Springer, 2017, 1–5.
3. Alexander M, Marson L. The neurologic control of arousal and orgasm with specific attention to spinal cord lesions: Integrating preclinical and clinical sciences. *Auton Neurosci* 2018;209:90–99.

4. Winder K, Linker R, Seifert F et al. Neuroanatomic correlates of female sexual dysfunction in multiple sclerosis. *Ann Neurol* 2016;80:490–498.

5. Atif M, Sarwar M, Scahill S. The relationship between epilepsy and sexual dysfunction: A review of the literature. *Springer Plus* 2016;5:2070.

6. Herzog A, Drislane F, Schomer D et al. Differential effects of antiepileptic drugs on sexual function and hormones in men with epilepsy. *Neurology* 2005;65(7):1016–1020.

7. Gutierrez MA, Mushtaq R, Stimmel G. Sexual dysfunction in women with epilepsy: Role of antiepileptic drugs and psychotropic medications. *Int Rev Neurobiol* 2008;83:157–167.

8. Harden CL. Sexuality in women with epilepsy. *Epilepsy Behav* 2005;7.2–6.

9. Corney R, Crowther M, Everett H et al. Psychosexual dysfunction in women with gynaecological cancer following radical pelvic surgery. *BJOG* 1993;100(1):73–78.

10. Cowan F, Frodsham L. Common disorders in psychosexual medicine. *TOG* 2015;17(1):47–53.

11. Connolly A, Britton A. *Womens Health in Primary Care*. Chapter 8: Management of patients with psychosexual problems in primary care. Cambridge: Cambridge University Press, 2017.

12. Conaglen H, Conaglen J. Drug-induced sexual dysfunction in men and women. *Aust Prescr* 2013;36:42–52.

13. Vanhegan G, Tunnadine P, Kwantes P. Treatment of psychosexual disorders in previously abused patients. *Br J Family Planning* 1996;2:191–193.

18

Sexual Pain Disorders

Nikki M.W. Lee and Leila C.G. Frodsham

> Vulvodynia and the associated sexual dysfunction destroys the lives of women who suffer from it. Loneliness, isolation, feeling like a freak, taking disappointment after disappointment, but looking normal on the outside.
>
> **Patient with vulvodynia**

Introduction

Sexual pain disorders are common and can be so debilitating that they can break relationships or affect a woman's ability to function at work and home. Prevalence in the general population is estimated to be 7.5% (1), but they account for approximately one in five gynaecological outpatient visits. Even if their primary presentation is physical (e.g. endometriosis), in most cases there is a concomitant psychosexual element. The healthcare professionals involved in their care should ideally be able to examine the 'whole patient', and address both the physical and psychological issues.

Presentation

Overt

Some women may choose to present with a direct appeal to a healthcare professional for help with a sexual difficulty (2). Painful sex is a common complaint in gynaecology, sexual health and family planning clinics. A patient's interpretation and feelings about the problem will mean she will appeal for help from the person whom she feels comfortable or trusting. This could be a nurse doing a cervical smear or a family doctor who already has an established relationship with the patient. It is important that these professionals feel comfortable talking about sex, as women expect healthcare professionals to be able to talk to them about these issues in a confident manner. Women are more likely to disclose to someone who uses both open communication and open body language.

Covert

If a woman feels too embarrassed, frightened or uncomfortable to tell someone directly that they have a sexual problem, presentation can take the form of repeated non-attendance at smear clinics, persistent dissatisfaction with contraception methods, pelvic pain, disassociation during physical examination, distaste or disgust with the genital region, or recurrent chronic vaginal discharge. Pain with sex may be a secondary presentation, only disclosed when patients have found a person that they trust.

Physical or Psychological?

Pain during sex is a physical symptom and so there may be pressure on healthcare professionals to find a physical cause. A patient may have expectation or hope for a robust explanation for her pain and wish her doctor to offer some course of treatment. However, the most important principle that a clinician must embrace is that sexual pain disorders are a complex interplay between physical and psychological factors. Consequently, in order to help these women, the interaction between clinician and patient requires a lateral rather than a traditional vertical 'doctor makes diagnosis and administers treatment' model. This can be a novel concept to many doctors, and some may struggle to make the leap to consider psychosexual pathology.

> Our first attempts at sexual intercourse were excruciatingly painful for me, but it was my embarrassment that hurt me more. Each time we tried, I would be clenching my muscles before he was even near me – subconsciously setting myself up for a failure each time. My legs would be locked in a rigid position and the pain would start in the vagina and spread through to my abdominal muscles and upper thighs. Inside it felt as though my partner was hitting a wall that was unbreakable.

Patient with non-consummation

Physical Causes

It is useful to consider the anatomical locations of pain – 'superficial' (external genital) or 'deep' (internal, pelvic structures). Box 18.1 lists the causes of superficial and deep dyspareunia; however, it is worth noting that there is considerable overlap.

BOX 18.1 CAUSES OF SUPERFICIAL AND DEEP DYSPAREUNIA

SUPERFICIAL
- Recurrent candida
- Herpes simplex virus
- Vulval dermatitis (exclude common allergens, urinary incontinence)
- Postnatal (often vulvovaginal atrophy)
- Vulvovaginal atrophy (postmenopausal)
- Genital dermatoses (e.g. lichen sclerosus, lichen planus)
- Vulvodynia
- Psychosexual

LESS COMMON CAUSES
- Iatrogenic (post-operative delivery, perineal trauma, radiotherapy)
- Neurologic (neuropathic pain, neurological disease)

DEEP
- Endometriosis
- Adnexal/pelvic pathology (cysts, fibroids)
- Pelvic inflammatory disease
- Iatrogenic (vaginal shortening, narrowing)
- Chronic pelvic pain
- Pelvic floor dysfunction (mechanical, anatomical factors, prolapse)
- Pelvic congestion (post-coital ache)
- Psychosexual

CASE 1

Mrs J was a 62-year-old woman who was referred to the general outpatient gynaecology clinic by her general practitioner (GP) for pain during sex. She was a Caucasian British woman, thin and petite in build. Her hair was tied tightly in a high ponytail and she wore jeans and a short denim jacket. She moved quickly and confidently into the consultation room when the doctor called her name, smiled on rising and started chatting immediately while following the doctor through. She gave off a slightly anxious energy, and her constant flow of conversation made it difficult to interpret her feelings. However, she was keen to answer the doctor's questions and to engage with the consultation on a physical level. Sex was painful with her partner of more than 30 years. She had tried lubricants, topical oestrogen and different positions for a couple of weeks to no effect, but now she was unable to have intercourse because 'he can't get in'. Her description of her difficulties was conveyed in a jovial way, and she chuckled (with slight effort) when she said, 'There's no point anymore; he has a go but he just can't get in there because it's so sore. He gets halfway in and then has to stop because it's impossible. Now we just can't be bothered'.

The doctor commented that it seemed difficult to talk about how this felt. She paused and suddenly looked deflated. She explained that it was difficult to discuss with her husband and sexual contact had declined.

Mrs J looked anxious at the suggestion of examination and folded her clothes carefully. She looked at the ceiling and refused to make eye contact. When the doctor commented that this seemed difficult for her, she just nodded and looked away. The nurse commented, 'it's always difficult for us women – you just have to think it will be over in a minute'.

Examination revealed an atrophic vulva; the skin was slightly shiny, thin and pale in appearance. Speculum examination with a well-lubricated medium speculum demonstrated a normal cervix and vagina. There was no evidence of dermatitis or fissures. Digital examination did not demonstrate any pelvic masses and was well tolerated. There was no spasm of pelvic musculature.

Diagnosis of post-menopausal atrophic vaginitis was made; a regime of oestrogen pessaries and cream was prescribed and advice given to use vaginal moisturizers and lubrication during intercourse. She did not return. The doctor was left with an overwhelming feeling of sadness despite the patient's apparent joviality and wondered what had not been said.

Comment

Post-menopausal vaginal atrophy can be undiagnosed for many years because women can complain of symptoms long after the 'menopause' has been complete. If systemic hormone replacement therapy (HRT) is not an option, then local oestrogen creams, vaginal moisturizers and lubrication can help restore the skin's integrity and elasticity (3). In this case, the doctor tried to explore the feelings but the patient seemed reluctant to engage. Perhaps the nurse's 'helpful' comments had inhibited disclosure.

Diagnosis

Careful history taking, followed by an examination (not necessarily physical – it may be listening) is needed to make the diagnosis of dyspareunia. A mixture of open-ended and direct questions asked in a sensitive and non-judgemental manner is extremely important. It is helpful to clarify exactly what the patient means by painful sex; even if a woman has a clear physical cause for her symptoms she will have feelings about her pain that must be understood. The listening during history taking and the questioning can be simultaneously an information-gathering and treatment process when carried out skillfully. In Case 1, the doctor may have enabled the patient to see the issues more clearly if it had been possible to reflect back to the patient that their problem felt 'very sad'. Another opportunity could have been used during the vaginal examination but was inhibited by the nurse's comments.

The Exploration of Psychosexual Problems

Table 18.1 summarises the Institute of Psychosexual Medicine's approach with the LOFTI acronym (listening, observing, feelings, thinking, interpreting), which is useful when assessing patients.

Physical Examination

The physical examination is part of the psychotherapeutic consultation in psychosexual medicine. It is important to note and reflect back the patient's feelings about this being attempted. Women fear loss of control and so may appreciate a comment that this can be taken to a level that they feel comfortable with, so that they are 'in control' of the examination process. If they are unwilling to be examined, it is important to explore this. Often women will decline examination because of menstruation so following up when they are not bleeding is important to remove a common defence; if it still feels difficult, it can be explored further.

Start with abdominal palpation – an abdominal or pelvic mass is unusual but should be excluded. The vaginal examination can only be considered when the patient trusts the clinician. It is always limited to what the patient finds comfortable. Examine the vulva and perineum for tears, fissures, erythema, candidiasis, skin bridges or dermatosis. If the posterior fourchette has microfissuring, this may indicate dermatitis. Note if there is evidence of lichen sclerosus or lichen planus (including typical figure-of-eight depigmentation). If post-menopausal, signs of vulvovaginal atrophy, such as hypopigmentation, non-elastic smooth tissue or shiny epithelium, may be present.

If the patient is comfortable with a speculum, make sure to use plenty of lubrication. If a patient requests a small speculum, be wary of colluding and ask why they feel that this is necessary. It might help the patient with pain or vaginismus to insert the speculum themselves. Use the opportunity to take swabs for microscopy, culture and sensitivity (including chlamydia and gonorrhoea) if there is abnormal discharge, but beware of positively reinforcing a 'dirt fear' if these have already been done.

Vaginal examination of the vaginal walls and pelvic floor may reveal tender areas or nodules. Anatomical variation in the vagina or uterus may be identified rarely, such as a vaginal septum. A thickened uterosacral ligament or an immobile uterus may indicate endometriosis.

More often than not, the examination is normal and reassurance in this case should be resisted. It can be helpful to ask what the patient feels is 'going on' or what they think you might find as this may lead to disclosure of a physical fantasy – 'phantasy'. While you may feel that everything looks completely normal, this may be far from the patient's feelings.

> I feel so sorry for you – doing this job – it must be horrible.
> Sorry, I haven't had a chance to wax.
> Can you see it doctor? [Wide, wild eyes] The wound? Is there still infection?
>
> **Patient 2 years after delivery when multiple doctors and midwives had expressed horror at her awful wound**

> The worst [speculum exams] have been the hesitant Doctor who lacks assertion and says nothing throughout, which can feel more uncomfortable and embarrassing.
>
> **Patient with dyspareunia**

Psychological

For women who have had no physical cause identified, or have exhausted their physical treatment options, the pain will remain real and distressing. In contrast to the physical causes of dyspareunia, the psychological or psychosomatic causes are not so easily categorised and so may be a frightening area for

TABLE 18.1

The Institute of Psychosexual Medicine LOFTI Acronym

Listening	Open questions and periods of silence allow the patient to divulge and elaborate on essential information.
	The doctor asked her if she'd ever been able to have sex. A long period of silence followed. Finally, a tense nod was the only indication that she'd heard the question. The doctor waited further. He asked if she ever thought about those experiences. More silence met his inquiry. After what seemed like ages, the patient slowly started to recount the first time she'd had sex, and her story began to unfold…
	What is the patient's tone/style of language?
	Note what is/is not said? How and when?
	Tolerate silence.
Observing	Patterns of behaviour, i.e. frequent cancellations/avoidance of appointments.
	The doctor suggested an examination. Mrs A stiffly removed her underwear and gathered the folds of her skirt into tense, white knuckled fists, held at groin level, seeming to block the doctor as she nervously lay on the examination couch, jaw tense, staring anxiously at the ceiling.
	Urgency, demeanour, style of dress and mannerisms.
	She had several layers of poorly applied makeup. She wore an old leather jacket, which was tightly zipped up. Her face was tense, her chin angled downwards as she stared aggressively at the doctor whilst sitting in the consultation chair. When asked whether she'd ever been pregnant, she turned away angrily, then suddenly started to cry. Streams of tears left mascara stains on her cheeks, and she confessed to a second trimester termination 20 years ago.
	Referral letters from the GP may be detailed and pressurised, emphasising the urgency of the referral (an example of transference, the unconscious redirection of feelings from the patient to the GP).
Feelings	Be aware of feelings in the room. How does the patient make you feel?
	She'd never been able to have a smear; no one had managed to put a speculum inside her. Sobbing, she desperately pleaded to the doctor to try. It was no good; it was as though her knees were a vice and nothing could persuade her to relax. The doctor was suddenly overwhelmed by a sense of grief and sadness; she felt she had failed her patient. Quietly crying now, the patient revealed her twin sister had died of cervical cancer 10 years ago.
	Feelings aroused in any doctor by the patient's language, behaviour and the attitude of the doctor to the patient are seen as possible evidence of the patient's own less than conscious feelings.
Thinking	Note what sort of doctor you are being in the consultation – a parent or a teacher?
	Why is the patient presenting now? How did the patient come to have the consultation/what is her motivation?
	Reflect upon how you feel before and after the consultation.
Interpreting	Interpreting is more complex and goes beyond simply understanding underlying issues. It involves *relaying* your interpretation of a patient's feelings or behaviour back to the patient with a therapeutic effect.
	Assess the overall picture – is the patient displaying certain types of behaviour or attitude as a defence mechanism or a means of hiding anxiety or fear such as tears or anger?
	Defence mechanisms include regression, dissociation, introjection, sublimation or denial. Disassociation can suggest a history of sexual abuse.
	The doctor imagined the examination was going to be very limited; the patient, a 27-year-old, was unable to consummate in her marriage. She had been a victim of sexual abuse between the ages of 12 and 17. However, she jumped onto the couch and flopped her legs open without bothering to cover herself with the sheet. The speculum examination was not met with resistance, and it was unremarkable.
	The doctor interpreted this lack of inhibition back to the patient; she looked quizzically back and then started to cry, admitting she 'blocked' off her body in order to numb herself to the painful memories of abuse.
	What do you notice from genital examination? Is there avoidance, i.e. patients menstruating at every appointment or always having difficulties with smears?

Source: Lee N et al. *BMJ* 2018; 361.

'conventional healthcare professionals' to explore. Healthcare professionals often describe this as opening 'Pandora's Box' and worry about time constraints in clinics. However, in reality, discussing the main issues with patients will save time and costs as this avoids unnecessary investigations and procedures. In psychosexual medicine, every patient is unique and the approach to identifying and elucidating the nuances of each patient's story will vary from case to case. The patient is the expert and so communication skills are key.

Pain can be a physical or psychological response to a multiplicity of problems, ranging from causes that are psychological, emotional, social or relationship based. A doctor may find a patient is in a dysfunctional, troubled or abusive relationship. A patient who has many surgical or invasive procedures (without benefit) may be angry, frustrated and lack trust in healthcare professionals. This can inhibit people from feeling able to help them and label them as 'heart sinks', which is further compounded by not feeling they have the skills to manage their pain.

CASE 2

Mrs J was a 30-year-old solicitor who had been married for 4 years with one child, aged 2. She was referred because she was complaining of pain during sex with her husband, that had started about 3 years into their relationship. They had been together for 6 years. She arrived at the clinic alone, dressed simply in a beige pair of trousers, cream cotton shirt and wore a pair of small pearl stud earrings. Her hair was swept neatly and loosely into a low ponytail. She appeared confident and poised and met the doctor's gaze easily.

Tests such as swabs and scans were normal. She complained that sex was painful and unpleasant. She said she loved him and was physically attracted to him; he was fit and good looking and they had a loving relationship. When they were first together they had sex three to five times a week; it was exciting and she had no problems orgasming. She did not experience pain then.

She now finds excuses to avoid intercourse, and for the last 3 years they had sex once every 3 months. Her husband still wanted sex regularly; her refusal was making him frustrated and sad. She resented his attempts to initiate intercourse and found herself withdrawing further from him. The doctor examined her; it was unremarkable.

The doctor noted that Mrs J made her feel a little tense and it was difficult to ask her intimate questions; she reflected that she felt Mrs J might try to avoid divulging more by diverting or dismissing her enquiries. The doctor confessed this to Mrs J, and queried it. They explored the possibility that Mrs J felt a little anxious in the doctor's presence (despite her confident poise). 'Had medical consultations always been that way?' She considered the question then shook her head. 'Had something triggered the change?' Three years ago, after a routine smear following the birth of her child, she was referred to colposcopy and had been found to be human papillomavirus positive. She had been terrified she had cervical cancer, and extrapolating, rationalised that intercourse had caused the infection which caused her 'cancer'. This was having a direct impact on her ability to become aroused. The lack of arousal meant she was not well lubricated and the pain was caused by dryness.

Comment

The doctor noted correctly that despite Mrs J's confident appearance and poise, the tension she noted in herself was a direct reflection of the patient's anxiety related to medical consultations. This was caused by her negative experience associated with colposcopy. Mrs J's belief that sex led her to have a pre-cancerous condition had directly impacted her ability to become aroused. She improved after discussion around these issues and an explanation that her vagina was now normal and healthy and that the pain was caused by lack of lubrication and muscle tension.

It seems relatively easy to get help to address the physical aspect of dyspareunia, but it is much harder to find a doctor who is forthcoming or even willing to address the psychological element of it. Whether symptoms start as physical, soon enough a psychological impact will be felt. There was never time for further exploration for a wider context, which, for me, meant two operations under general anaesthetic and a week off work each time, for tweaks that I put great hope on; with hindsight, this addressed only a small element of my overall problem.

Patient with dyspareunia

Management

Approaches will depend on the aetiology of the pain in combination with factors related to the individual patient. Diagnosis may take a number of consultations with the right professionals to fully understand the problem. Specific physical causes of pain (e.g. endometriosis) should be managed by appropriately trained healthcare professionals, but there are general principles that may be useful and can be applied to all women with sexual pain disorders:

- Reduce all allergens: supplement inert oils (such as olive oil) for all other washing practices (no soaps/shower gels/wipes), change to unbleached, undyed sanitary protection and use non-biological, unperfumed laundry goods.
- Use an inert oil twice daily for perineal massage – coconut oil is easier as it is solid until application. Thumb is easier for self-massage. This reassociates women with their genitalia, acts as a barrier, reduces vaginismus and can be helpful in vulvodynia (5).
- Consider a desensitising lubricant such as one that is a menthol-based or water-based lidocaine preparation.
- Perform a ferritin level test as 5% of patients will have pruritus and soreness secondary to iron deficiency (6).
- Swab for candida and treat with an additional anti-fungal in case of resistance. Consider referral to sexual health.

Specific physical conditions:

- In post-reproductive or postnatal women, vaginal atrophy can be the cause of pain, and exacerbate the situation even when using systemic HRT. Consider local vaginal oestrogens (which are safe in breastfeeding) (3).
- Under the care of an appropriately trained professional, vulvar dermatosis should be treated with a pea-sized amount of a potent topical steroid cream daily for 1 month, and then alternate days for 1 month and then twice a week for 1 month (5).
- If condition does not improve or if there is a raised lesion, refer to gynaecology or dermatology urgently.

Doctor M has taken me on a journey. With patience, kindness, listening, advising and suggesting to me she has earned my trust. Trust at first was so fragile that I managed the tiniest things. These baby steps led to a little more and a little more. After 18 months of seeing Doctor M every few months, my life is transformed. I have a lovely boyfriend and with the support and guidance of Doctor M, I have managed to have a physical relationship with him. It has been like growing up all over again. Am I cured? No. But I am slowly learning techniques that are possible and satisfying and every so often that includes full sex. Who would have thought it? Most definitely not me.

Patient who has received psychosexual therapy for dyspareunia

SUMMARY

- Doctors may be pressured to find a physical cause for sexual pain – for themselves and/or by the patient. Despite many doctors trying to 'put things right', the pain may persist because no one stopped to ask a different question – why are they wrong?
- Treatment should always be holistic; even in women with a clear physical cause for their pain, there will be concomitant psychological factors that perpetuate or aggravate the pain cycle.
- Note any feelings the patient arouses in yourself. Is this evidence of a subconscious feeling a patient may have? Perhaps this can be used to help the patient make connexions with their pain.
- Remember that the patient is the expert in her pain and chooses the person she wants to speak to about it. This may happen at a time that is not ideal, i.e. a busy outpatient clinic, but exploring the real cause for her pain will save time and resources in the long run.

REFERENCES

1. Mitchell KR, Geary R, Graham CA et al. Painful sex (dyspareunia) in women: Prevalence and associated factors in a British population probability survey. *BJOG* 2017;124(11):1689–1697.
2. Coulson C, Crowley T. Current thoughts on psychosexual disorders in women. *Obstet Gynaecol* 2007;9(4):217–222.
3. Kingsberg S, Kellogg S, Krychman M. Treating dyspareunia caused by vaginal atrophy: A review of treatment options using vaginal estrogen therapy. *Int J Women Health* 2010;9(1):105–111.
4. Lee N, Jakes A, Lloyd J et al. Dyspareunia. *BMJ* 2018; 361.
5. Nunns D, Mandal D, Byrne M et al. Guidelines for the management of vulvodynia. *Br J Dermatol* 2010;162(6):1180–1185.
6. Edwards SK, Bates CM, Lewis F et al. 2014 UK national guideline on the management of vulval conditions. *Int J STD AIDS* 2015;26(9):611–624.

19

Tocophobia

Leila C.G. Frodsham

KEY POINTS

- Defined as primary/secondary
- Increases requests for caesarean section
- Increases length of labour
- Increases medical intervention
- Associated with psychosexual dysfunction
- Associated with previous traumatic birth
- Associated with anxiety/depression
- Associated with low birth weight
- Associated with postnatal depression and bonding issues with baby
- Associated with post-traumatic stress disorder
- Increased requests for sterilisation

Definition of Tocophobia

A morbid fear of pregnancy/childbirth

CASE 1

Mrs X attends the gynaecology outpatients clinic and sees the training doctor. She is very tense and had questioned when she would be seen, to both reception and nursing staff. There is much eye rolling from staff when the registrar comes in to ask if she could be seen by the consultant. The doctor looks very flustered and unhappy and says that she struggled to get the patient to sit down and that she has tried to help but that the patient will not talk to her. Mrs X has mentioned that she has read that she can request a caesarean section and will not leave until this is confirmed.

The clinic is very busy, so, to avoid delaying the clinic, the consultant goes into the junior doctor's cramped room and sits on the couch. Mrs X is dressed in a smart suit with perfect makeup and a shiny clasped bag on her knee. She looks at the ground but starts to shout about how difficult the registrar is. She insists that the consultant confirm that she can have a c-section before she will speak. The consultant feels overwhelmed and asks her why she wants this, 'It's an unusual request in a gynaecology clinic and you seem very upset?' Her lip wobbles and tears snake down her cheeks. The consultant swaps with the registrar to the desk seat and offer a tissue.

She says that she just cannot consider a vaginal delivery. The tissue is twisted in her fingers and her knuckles turn white. She struggled to have sex and was a 'late starter', needing help from a private gynaecologist to use dilators and eventually Botox. She currently uses the combined oral contraceptive pill, condoms and spermicide. She cannot risk getting pregnant in case she is 'forced' to have a vaginal delivery. Sex is painful and tense and she does not enjoy it. Her husband is fed up with her rejections and wants a baby. He has sent her to the doctors and sits outside waiting for the verdict. All of their friends are having children and he wants them to be playmates. There is pressure from their families and she is not getting younger. Her friends seem relaxed and happy about childbearing and have shared their delivery stories. These are making her feel that a disaster is inevitable. She leans forward with wide eyes and says, 'I know it sounds stupid and I can rationally see that this is not the case but I think I will die if I have a vaginal delivery'.

Introduction

Tocophobia is an increasing presentation in both psychosexual and antenatal clinics. The prevalence is established at 14% (1). It is widely felt to be one of the more difficult consultations to manage in obstetrics and workshops to assist obstetricians in management of this condition are often oversubscribed. Patients frequently present requesting a caesarean section and, in the current financial climate of endeavouring to reduce costs, Care Commissioning Groups (CCGs) are setting key performance indicators (KPIs) to reduce caesarean sections. Additionally, operative birth is associated with higher morbidity (bleeding, infection, thromboembolic disease and visceral damage) and resulting mortality rates. This can leave the obstetrician conflicted with a wish to reduce fear and psychological harm to his patient versus risk reduction, litigation and funding.

Patients may present to primary care in a covert manner with contraceptive concerns, dyspareunia and non-consummation. Women often have a deep-seated fear of death in childbirth and so will do their upmost to avoid pregnancy at all costs. Anecdotally, psychosexual dysfunction goes hand in hand with primary and secondary tocophobia; in primary tocophobics, if questioned, the vast majority will describe difficulties with sex prior to conception or present as non-consummation because of fear.

Tocophobia is not just associated with antenatal psychological morbidity but also raised rates of postnatal depression, impact on the mental well-being of the baby for life, increased length of labour, lower birth weights and increased prevalence of admission to neonatal intensive care (8%) (2).

Background

Prevalence is perceived to be increasing (1) and this is thought to stem from an update of the National Institute for Health and Care Excellence (NICE) guidelines (7) where widespread media reports suggested that women could request a caesarean section as a birthing option if supported by their obstetrician. Women who may never have considered falling pregnant previously because of tocophobia began to present to antenatal clinics, often with a copy of the guidelines or at least referring to them. Background maternal request section rates were once in the order of 1% but have increased up to fourfold (2).

Many women will present saying that they would never have attempted to conceive had it not been for the media representation of the accessibility of lower segment caesarean section (LSCS) for maternal request. It is not uncommon to see women who are post-menopausal expressing regret that their fear has meant an enforced sexless/childless marriage to avoid exposure. There are even celebrities who are now confessing to this in the open press. Additionally, the advent of botulinum toxin use for vaginismus has meant successful consummation in some women without resolving psychosexual issues so that women will conceive but then struggle to manage the process of birth. Botox will relax the levator ani muscles (pelvic floor) temporarily (3 months or so) to allow consummation, but anecdotally this often returns following as the underlying cause has not been addressed.

'I know that there are two routes: vaginal delivery and caesarean. 'She then holds her hands over eyes like blinkers – 'but I can't even look down the other paths'.

Patient who had Botox to consummate but then chose caesarean section.

There is a cohort of women who have experienced child sexual abuse or sexual assault, causing their tocophobia. Psychosexual dysfunction and fear of childbirth are clearly exemplified in this situation where women fear the loss of their control over sex, and this is naturally transmitted onto childbirth. Interestingly, a study from Scandinavia into the success of labour and childbirth in these two groups showed a clear slowing of labour and increased medical intervention rate in those with adult sexual assault versus near normal labour length and vaginal delivery in victims of child sexual abuse (CSA) (3). Anecdotally, women who achieve vaginal delivery will often report better sex lives.

'You gave me back the part of my body that my father took away. My husband and I are now enjoying a healthy sex life for the first time.'

**Victim of CSA who achieved a vaginal birth after
initially requesting a caesarean section.**

Additionally, a large Scandinavian study identified a rate of 13% of tocophobia in Swedish men (2,4), which was associated with an increased rate of caesarean section requests and high anxiety at 1 year postnatal. Men can present with their often-mute wives requesting caesarean section. While this can be a presentation of male tocophobia, domestic violence should also be considered. It might be anticipated that witnessing traumatic childbirth could lead to sexual dysfunction in men, but they rarely present and there is little found in literature searches on this as a topic.

Tocophobia is categorised into *primary* affecting nulliparous women and *secondary* affecting multiparous women. Women with primary tocophobia typically start to exhibit symptoms in adolescence and prevalence can be increased twofold by web-based education on reproduction and childbirth. Typically, women mention graphic films at sex education. They may also have low self-esteem and may have a history of eating disorders. They perceive a lack of social support and may have friends or family with poor childbirth experience.

'I remember sitting on the floor in my mum's hairdresser's shop as a little girl listening to her repeatedly telling them how dreadful my birth had been and not a single woman had a good birth story. I can't imagine that it would be OK for me.'

Primary tocophobic unable to have unprotected sex.

Secondary tocophobics will have experienced a traumatic event in their previous birth. Risks are increased after stillbirth or pregnancies with congenital abnormalities. Prevalence increases with medical intervention and adverse events but women can also present with 'textbook normal vaginal deliveries'. In post-partum debrief women frequently recount dismissive attitudes from healthcare professionals in these cases. Secondary tocophobics may never manage to achieve penetrative sex and so may never present in pregnancy again. Lower levels of fecundity are clearly demonstrated after emergency LSCS – a factor that has been attributed to tubal disease but never demonstrated. Secondary tocophobia may well be the underlying cause. Excellent communication to women during labour and after delivery is essential and many of these cases recount lack of empathy in maternity staff as the cause behind their trauma.

'The doctor came in and looked between my legs – I was in stirrups and had been for hours – and said, 'Oh my god, it looks like the plate of meat that I left for my dog this morning'. Every time my husband tries to initiate sex I shut my legs – all I can see is a plate of dog food.'

Forceps delivery 8 years before – she had not had sex since.

Women with tocophobia are categorised by the 2015 *International Classification of Diseases, Tenth Revision, Clinical Modification (ICD-10-CM)* Diagnosis Code F40.9 *Phobic anxiety disorder, unspecified.* Women often have co-existing anxiety and depression and may suffer from obsessive-compulsive personality disorder. They have an increased risk of postnatal depression which can directly impact on their bonding with baby and have long-term implications for the mental health of their children.

Management

While there are currently few centres with expertise on tocophobia or designated teams (like the Aurora teams in Sweden), the evidence of support in the antenatal and peripartum period by healthcare workers (not specifically trained therapists) can increase uptake of vaginal birth to 86% in those requesting LSCS (2). There is no doubt for me that my psychosexual training has enormously helped in my management of these cases by enabling identification of fears in patients and allowing them to find their solutions, but any experienced maternity worker can help these women by listening, considered communication and support. Tocophobics need to feel in control of their choices and care.

As the predominate fear of women is loss of control: of the body changes of pregnancy, of the pain of childbirth, of their vagina in the maternity department and of their minds in the postnatal period, it is vital to allay their fears at the beginning of consultation by agreeing that you and another colleague (medico-legally advisable in maternal request LSCS) will agree to an elective LSCS if they are happy to take on potentially additional risks. Once this is offered, a complete change of demeanour is observed and women and their partners will then be open to discussing fears. If this is not the case, a continued 'battle' for LSCS will ensue where fears will not be openly discussed and often escalate to aggression or official complaints.

CASE 2

Mrs Y was referred by a normally calm colleague who had felt threatened by her anger and considered calling security into the clinic. Their referral was profoundly apologetic at sending over an aggressive and difficult patient. On arrival, Mrs Y asked why she had been passed over to another consultant 'like an unwelcome gift'. Tears of anger and frustration spat across the desk and she closed her arms across her chest: 'I'm not leaving till I get what I want – a caesarean'.

The doctor put down her pen and leaned forward, 'I'm happy for you to have whichever birth you want, it's your choice but one that must be made with all options discussed'.

Mrs Y let out a breath: 'At last, you are listening to me while others haven't, I cannot put my precious baby through this dark and dangerous cavern – it feels like she will fall from my cervix from my beautiful warm and safe womb over a cliff edge. She needs to be safe and I need to be in control to ensure that safety'. As she said this she deflated and shed tears.

On examination, her legs quivered at the effort of keeping her vagina closed but, with support, she eventually self-examined and shed tears of joy. It later transpired that she had been a victim of CSA and as a result felt totally out of control of her own vagina. She chose vaginal delivery in the pool.

Once women feel in control of their mode of delivery, it is sensible to ask them to write their birth plan with the help of their midwife, friends and family between consultations. In my previous Trust, we had a wonderful birth centre with a homely feel and experienced and caring midwives. As many tocophobics are also fearful of hospital/clinical environments, birth centres offer a bridge to the hospital that can be vital in women who are so phobic that they struggle to contemplate the operating theatre. In multiple cases women felt so supported that they wanted to and achieved delivery at the birth centre.

> 'I have decided that I will have a water birth in the birth centre. You have made me see that my biggest fear is doctors, their instruments and vaginal examinations. Doctors are afraid of birth centres and water – like cats – so I will be very safe there.'

This was a severely tocophobic woman who was a victim of CSA who initially requested LSCS and went on to achieve a water birth in the birth centre. I have to confess to smiling at this remarkable insight into the mindset of many obstetricians.

Additionally, if a patient feels very well supported by a particular member of staff in antenatal planning, I personally advocate them signing their birth plans as an agreement to support it unless the woman's life or that of her baby is endangered. I also add a proviso that says I can be contacted if there is deviation from the birth plan against the woman's wishes in the non-emergency situation. Contrary to popular belief, since I started this, I have never been called but have repeatedly been told that this assurance kept couples going through their labours and deliveries. I will also assure women that they can change their minds throughout labour and revert to a 'semi-elective' (emergency) LSCS within reason – depending on the workload in the maternity unit.

Preventing Secondary Tocophobia

Women with secondary tocophobia often benefit from a birth options appointment where an experienced midwife can sit and debrief by going through the delivery notes and answering questions as they proceed. A period of free speech where the patient describes their experience first and is listened to for a few minutes may demonstrate the pertinent points. As with all psychosexual consultations, the health professional is the mirror and having the patient's emotions expressed during their story reflected back to them can be very helpful in identifying the true fear and aid birth planning for the next baby.

It is common for many of these women to report issues with communication. Many midwives and obstetricians express dismissive attitudes towards women who exhibit signs of trauma after 'completely normal vaginal deliveries' when they see women with 'multiple life-threatening complications who are fine'. Maternity staff are not there to impose their views on what is traumatic for women but to treat each patient as an individual and support them in whatever way works.

> 'I know that I had a 'textbook normal water-birth' but can only see the midwife's face when I started to deliver. She looked terrified and kept muttering that 'she had never done this before' and wished that her colleague would come. It's made me terrified of a home birth again. I feel terrified when my husband cuddles me if it feels like it might progress to sex. I've lost all my confidence in my body.'

The quote above is from a woman with reduced libido and non-consummation since her home birth 2 years ago. She was denied an after-thoughts clinic appointment as she had a normal birth. A review could have brought some valuable learning points in communication for the junior midwife involved.

In a similar vein, a woman with multiple complications including a uterine inversion did not feel worried when a senior member of staff attended and instilled confidence, but developed a morbid fear of both sex and the birth related to a series of staff repeatedly saying to her perineum,

> 'Oh my god, what the hell is that?' 'I've no idea what to do' 'I've never seen anything like this before'.

Her support and planning towards birth involved a gradual progression towards driving near to the hospital, onto meeting a senior midwife in reception and multiple visits later to being in the delivery room. Debrief involved staff in person and via simulation of the experience in skills training. Additionally, she was given emergency access to the gynaecology services for checks of her perineum postnatally. She repeatedly assessed the doctor's reactions and comments as these were performed and, as she improved, visits became less and less frequent. Women should be encouraged to utilise whichever modality helps them (e.g. hypnobirthing).

Interestingly, evidence for 'after-thoughts' clinics has previously demonstrated an increased incidence of long-term post-traumatic stress disorder (PTSD) in those that are debriefed in such clinics. However, a recent Cochrane review demonstrates no benefit or harm with after-thoughts clinics (5). Evidence is based on debrief in the 6-weeks postnatal period rather than longer-term debriefing. Anecdotally, women are often exhausted and unable to process their feelings about delivery at 6 weeks and should be considered for later appointments when they feel ready. However, it is also vital that the delivering team reassures couples with an immediate post-delivery discussion of future birth planning (e.g. 'you could have a vaginal birth next time, your perineum is likely to heal very well').

Signs and symptoms of PTSD are said to occur in up to 10% of women postnatally. While many can be helped by the psychosexual approach, some will require more long-term and detailed counselling. There is an excellent PTSD centre at the Maudsley Hospital but more local assistance may come from eye movement desensitisation reprocessing therapy (6).

SUMMARY OF MANAGEMENT

FIRST CONSULTATION

- Offer caesarean section if requested
- Listen to patient/couple's fears
- Identify key points
- Suggest that they write a birth plan for spontaneous vaginal delivery and LSCS
- Consider a tour of the birthing unit
- Follow up with an experienced midwife/birth options clinic
- Consider a visit to the midwifery-led birth centre

SECOND CONSULTATION

- Discuss current feelings
- Talk through birth plan
- Consider referral to a second consultant obstetrician

USEFUL COMMENTS/QUESTIONS

- 'I would be happy to support you in the birth of your choice if you are aware of the risks and benefits'.
- 'If you decided to go for a vaginal birth, what would help you feel more in control?'
- 'If there was one thing you wanted to avoid what would it be?'
- 'We cannot do anything without your consent'.
- 'Have you considered the birth pool?'

Treatment Plans

Currently there are no recognised treatment pathways for women from national organisations, such as the Royal College of Obstetricians and Gynaecologists/NICE, bar brief mentions in perinatal health of tocophobia as a risk factor for postnatal depression. Obstetricians with psychosexual medicine training could be an ideal solution to caring for these women and, anecdotally, great improvement has been seen in both antenatal/peripartum and postnatal periods by using these types of consultation skills. Vaginal delivery should not necessarily be seen as the ultimate goal, but those women who feel empowered enough to proceed to labour and achieve vaginal delivery appear to benefit the most with more reports of feeling happier and improving sexual function.

Summary

Tocophobia is a common condition with both acute and chronic implications for the welfare of mothers and babies. It can impact on not only mental but also physical morbidity and needs a clear birth plan for the care of women that is guided by the woman and her specific fears. While the majority can be managed very effectively by engaged maternity staff, there should also be a low threshold for referral to specialist perinatal mental health (PNMH) or PTSD services as there are increased risks of postnatal depression. They can also present not pregnant with sexual difficulties and our training can help them greatly with managing their fears. There is currently no research to justify this but, anecdotally, women with tocophobia (particularly primary) describe sexual dysfunction – often vaginismus and non-consummation.

REFERENCES

1. O'Connell MA, Leahy-Warren P, Khashan AS, Kenny LC, O'Neill SM. Worldwide prevalence of tocophobia in pregnant women: Systematic review and meta-analysis. *Acta Obstet Gynecol Scand* 2017;96(8):907–920.
2. O'Connell M, Leahy-Warren P, Khashan AS, Kenny LC. Tocophobia – The new hysteria? *Obstet Gynecol Reprod Med* 2015;25(6):175–177.
3. Gottfried LW, Hallak LF. Inter-relationships between sexual abuse, female sexual function and childbirth. *Midwifery* 2015;31(11):1087–1095.
4. Hofberg K, Ward MR. Fear of childbirth, tocophobia and mental health in mothers: The obstetric-psychiatric interface. *Clin Obstet Gynecol* 2004;47:527–534.
5. Bastos MH, Furuta M, Small R, McKenzie-McHarg K, Bick D. Debriefing interventions for the prevention of psychological trauma in women following childbirth. *Cochrane Database Syst Rev* 2015;(4):CD007194.
6. Baas MA, Stramrood CA, Dijksman LM, de Jongh A, van Pampus MG. The OptiMUM-study: EMDR therapy in pregnant women with posttraumatic stress disorder after previous childbirth and pregnant women with fear of childbirth: Design of a multicentre randomized controlled trial. *Eur J Psychotraumatol* 2017;8(1):1293315.
7. National Institute for Health and Care Excellence (NICE) guidelines. 2014. https://pathways.nice.org.uk/pathways/caesarean-section#path=view%3A/pathways/caesarean-section/deciding-whether-to-offer-caesarean-section.xml&content=view-node%3Anodes-woman-requests-caesarean-section.

FURTHER READING

Cowan F, Frodsham L. Management of common disorders in psychosexual medicine. *Obstet Gynecol* 17(1):47–53.
Geissbuehler V, Eberhard J. Fear of childbirth during pregnancy: A study of more than 8000 pregnant women. *J Psychosom Obstet Gynaecol* 2002;23:229–235.
Greenfield M, Jomeen J, Glover L. What is traumatic birth? A concept analysis and literature review. *Br J Midwifery* 2016;24(4):254–267.
Lukasse M, Vangen S, Oian P, Schei B. Fear of childbirth, women's preference for cesarean section and childhood abuse: A longitudinal study. *Acta Obstet Gynecol Scand* 2011;90(1):33–40.
Lukasse M, Schei B, Ryding E; on behalf of the BIDENS study group. Prevalence and associated factors of fear of childbirth in six European countries. *Sex Reprod Health* 2014;99–106.
Pacik PT, Geletta S. Vaginismus treatment: Clinical trials follow up 241 patients. *Sex Med* 2017;5(2):e114–e123.
Raisenen S, Lehto SM, Nielsen HS, Gissler M, Kramer MR, Heinon S. Fear of childbirth in nulliparous and multiparous women: A population based analysis of all singleton births in Finland in 1997–2010. *BJOG* 2014;121(8):965–970.
Storksen HT, Eberhard M, Garthus-Niegel S, Eskild A. Fear of childbirth; the relation to anxiety and depression. *Acta Obstet Gynecol Scand* 2012;91:237–242.
Stroll K, Hauck Y, Downe S et al. Cross-cultural development and psychometric evaluation of a measure to assess fear of childbirth prior to pregnancy. *Sex Reprod Healthc* 2016;8:49–54.

20

Psychosexual Aspects of Sexual Preference and Gender Identity Issues

Susan V. Carr

Introduction

How It All Began

When I was a junior doctor in Glasgow, Scotland, in the early 1980s, the Head of Service, the indomitable Libby Wilson announced her retirement. I was summoned to her office. She announced I would take over her psychosexual clinic, then slapped five case-note files onto the desk.

> 'Your inheritance', she said, 'Transsexuals...and if you don't know what that is...look it up!'

This was the pre-instant electronic information era, so 'looking up' was not easy, and required multiple library visits. Over the next 20 years, as a medical professional working in a public psychosexual clinic, I did indeed learn, but mostly in the traditional institute way, from the patients, these individuals whose lives are so influenced by their minority sexual identity and orientation issues.

Historical Context

The clinical recognition of transsexualism was brought to the fore by the ground-breaking publication by Harry Benjamin in the United States in 1966, *The Transsexual Phenomenon*, citing the first transwoman in the United States, Christine Jorgensen, who had been treated in Denmark. This of course was a 'scandal' in America, but paved the way for increased recognition of the rights of transpeople to good quality clinical care and acceptance by society (1).

He wrote,

> For the simple man in the street, there are only two sexes. A person is either male or female, Adam or Eve. With more learning comes more doubt. ...every Adam contains elements of Eve and every Eve harbours traces of Adam, physically as well as psychologically.

It is precisely this 'doubt' with which psychosexual input can work within clinical consultation, reflecting back to the client the feelings which they have brought into the room, and the unknowing which only they can eventually know.

Fortunately, society is more able to recognise and accept these differences, and the scientific community has produced much useful data in order to inform the clinical care of such individuals.

The Psychosexual Consultation

Transsexuals, now more usually known as transgender, are individuals who, in simple terms, feel as if they are living in the wrong body.

Classically they will have memories as far back as the age of about 4 years old, which would support the current biopsychosocial origins of transgenderism. They will come into the clinic saying, 'I am a man' or 'I am a woman…but I have the wrong body'.

This, of course, can cause a lifetime of stress, and just being able to express their feelings about their mind-body incongruence can be an enormous relief.

We look at two relevant case histories, which clearly illustrate the major issues.

CASE 1: THE STORY OF GRACE

It was a Tuesday afternoon in autumn. The psychosexual clinic was part of the largest publicly funded sexual and reproductive healthcare setting in Scotland. There were multiple clinics running simultaneously providing a variety of services for contraception, medical gynaecology, genitourinary medicine and the psychosexual clinic. The waiting room was filled to overflowing. I picked up the case note on my desk and went to the waiting room calling for Grace. The room became silent as a very tall, heavily built individual stood up and crossed the crowded waiting area. Grace was wearing a man's beige overcoat, sandals and had bright red lipstick and with bright red polished fingernails. His mousey brown hair was thin on top and was pulled into a ponytail at the back. He looked uncomfortable.

I brought him into my consulting room, introduced myself as the doctor, and reflected back this clear feeling of discomfort, both Grace's and mine.

This must be difficult for you, I reflected. I also noted that despite the female name, I still was sensing a 'he' in the clinic. However as Grace relaxed in the room, I found myself referring to Grace by the female pronoun. I reflected back this ambivalence, which was, of course, coming from the patient.

Grace sat for a few moments before coming out with her story.

Grace was 62 years old, born and brought up in a small fishing village on the east coast of Scotland. Her father was a fisherman and her mother stayed at home looking after the family. There were three children, an older brother and sister, and the patient in front of me, baby John, who was now called Grace. It had been a traditional fisherman's home. The father's work was hard and sometimes dangerous in harsh weather. Church attendance was expected on a Sunday, the children were disciplined for bad behaviour, but enjoyed a sense of freedom playing with their friends in the village. The parents drank at the weekend, and at this point the children 'kept out of their way'. Money was tight, but they always had a hot meal on the table and there was a strong sense of community.

'It was a good childhood' said Grace, then she began to cry.

She then said since she was very small, and growing up, she just assumed she was a little girl, just like her older sister. When she was able, about the age of 3 or 4, to put on her own clothes, she would always take her sister's skirts and put them on. She did not understand why her mother always told her to wear trousers. One Friday when she had been playing in her sisters' room and was wearing a skirt, the father returned from drinking at the local pub. He dragged Grace upstairs, belted her and said never do that again. She was 4 years old and for the next 30 years was too terrified to dress in any female clothing, even when old enough to understand the taboo which had been breached in her family.

As Grace grew up, despite preferring girls' toys, clothes and games, and knowing that she was a woman but with a boy's body, she seemed to understand that this behaviour, although natural to her, provoked anger at home, and ridicule outside the home, so she suppressed her 'girl' feelings and tried to become as masculine as possible. She grew tall and strong, and did well at sports at school then, on leaving, joined the army. All this time she was trying to make herself 'more of a man'.

She soon found the powerful masculine environment too much to bear. She made her first suicide attempt, to be followed by two more over the next 2 years. There was psychiatric input at the time, but she never once mentioned her gender confusion, she was too afraid. This clearly ended her army career so she moved to the city and went into different employment.

As part of her craving for 'normality', Grace had married and had a son, but the marriage had ended quickly when the wife had caught her trying on her ladies' underwear. The only family member who had remained in touch with Grace over the years had been the sister, who had always been kind. The sister had recently died of cancer, and it was this loss which prompted Grace, after a lifetime of concealment, to try to become able to live the life she felt was meant for her.

Grace then went on to have gender reassignment hormonal therapy, surgery and counselling and proudly told everyone, in her case, life began at 70.

This brief summary of Grace's story is unique to her, but has elements of the stories of many transsexuals.

CASE 2: THE STORY OF LUKE

Luke is aged 27. He is small, stocky and has a beard and acne scarred skin. He speaks with a deep voice in a broad dialect. He came to the clinic saying that he was unable to have sex. He had been with his partner for 3 years, and had never had sex. He volunteered that he had a female partner, they wanted to get married and have children, but having sex was a problem. In that first consultation, he spoke at length about his job, his partner and his dog, all in a very positive light, and said he was determined to 'sort out' his sexual problem.

On the second visit, he chatted cheerfully about his partner and a recent holiday they had taken. I wondered aloud if they had sex? 'Of course not', he said. I was slightly puzzled, and offered to examine him. He suddenly stopped talking.

After a prolonged silence, he said, 'Yes, you can examine me', and went silently to the couch.

He was covered by the sheet, head turned to the side and eyes tightly shut.

I slowly washed my hands and put on gloves, preparing for the examination. There was dread in the room.

On drawing back the sheet, I was faced with unremarkable female genitalia, and paused.

Luke was a transman, a female-to-male transsexual who had so successfully blocked his acknowledgement of his female body to such an extent that, until clinical examination, it was totally concealed.

After that revelation, Luke was initially distressed, but by using these feelings we were able to continue working over the next few months to help him resolve some of his issues.

He then went on to talk about his early life, which was always as a tomboy, his leaving home and gradually fulfilling his ability to live as he felt comfortable. He had a difficult time at school, when he was bullied and called names, but then went on to college where he had taken drink and drugs in order to try to blot out what he felt was an impossible life situation. Following a depressive illness which interfered with his studies, he sought help and was eventually referred to a clinic where he was being prescribed hormones, and had formal assessments, but said he now wanted to explore his feelings and options for the future.

After many sessions of psychosexual counselling, he felt content in the meantime to opt for breast surgery, but to leave options such as phalloplasty for the future.

These short stories illustrate the full role of the psychosexual therapist in working with transgender people, using the same core principles used in any consultation. Good background knowledge, however, of the options for hormonal and surgical treatments for transgender people will increase the confidence of both patient and clinician, and enable the clinician to better comprehend the transgender experience, and engage with each individual in a meaningful way.

The Biological Basis of Gender Identity and Sexual Preferences

To date, the biological basis of both gender identity and sexual preferences is unclear, but there are many pieces of evidence which point increasingly to what used to be called a bio-psychosocial model of development. In 1994, John Money wrote that causality with respect to gender identity disorder consists of genetic, prenatal hormonal, postnatal social and post-pubertal hormonal determinants, but there is as yet no comprehensive and detailed theory of causality (2). Scientific research has progressed since then. There is increasing evidence that the influence of prenatal androgens on the foetus has a certain effect on male-type activity interests and engagement, however relatively minimal effect on gender identity (3). There have recently been shown differences in resting state patterns in brain functional connectivity in male-to-female transgender people which are different from both their assigned gender, and that to which they aspire (4). There is evidence that during hormonal treatment, dimorphic brain structures may partly adjust to the characteristics of the desired sex for some transgendered people. He states, however, that data are inhomogeneous and often not replicated, and concludes that disentangling correlates of sexual orientation and gender identity requires more high-quality research (5).

There have been mosaic pieces of evidence over the past few years pointing towards a biological basis for homosexuality. These theories include brain structure and hormonal influences, birth order, fingerprint patterns and right-/left-handedness. More recently and convincingly, the study of gene regulation through non-genetic changes in DNA packaging has led to theories of epigenetics influencing the development of homosexuality (6).

Therefore, to date, in scientific terms, this is still a developing area, where it is hoped that new understanding of the origins and development of gender development may help recognition of the issues faced by any individual who is struggling with their sexuality.

Diagnosis and Classification of Gender Dysphoria and Sexual Preference

Almost more relevant to those living with the day-to-day issues pertaining to gender identity and sexual preferences are the ethical issues surrounding treatment. Since the original descriptions of gender dysphoria in the medical literature, gender identity and disorders of sexual preference have been classified within the *International Classification of Diseases* (*ICD*) and Related Health Problems section of mental and behavioural disorders. Most individuals in either of these groups feel that they just need some professional help in order to be themselves, rather than change gender, and that they are just minority groups within society rather than victims of any clinical condition. Thankfully the scientific community has taken this on board, and consequently there have been recommendations for an integrated approach to issues related to gender identity and sexual preference, and their inclusion in the sexual health, rather than mental health areas. This new chapter on Conditions Related to Sexual Health should overcome the artificial mind-body separation which was inherent in classification *ICD-10* (7).

The mind-body model of sexual health has always been a cornerstone of Institute of Psychosexual Medicine (IPM) psychosexual therapy, and by changing international classifications, this should help the wider clinical community embrace these concepts.

Additionally, recommendations for terminology are constantly changing. A useful reference is GLAAD (8) (www.glaad.org/about) a website promoting acceptance and aiding discussion on lesbian, gay, bisexual, transgender, and queer (LGBTQ) issues.

Prevalence of Transgender People and Differences in Sexual Preference

Although psychosexual practice always focuses on the individual, it is useful to understand the prevalence of individuals in society with issues of minority sexual identity and orientation in order to keep the awareness of minority sexual groups in our minds, and not become unthinkingly heterocentric.

The published figures for the prevalence of transsexualism vary widely, from 4.6 per 100,000 individuals, being 6.8/100,000 for transwomen to 2.6 for transmen (9), but prevalence differed by 'case' definition and when self-reported figures were assessed the figure was higher at 355/100,000 (10), and a meta-regression of population-based probability samples suggested a current US prevalence of 390 adults/100,000 (11), perhaps indicative of the large number of transgender people not wanting to have physical input.

In relation to sexual preference, this is a far larger minority. In a large population-based survey, 97% of men and 96% of women identified as heterosexual; however, 9% of men and 19% of women reported some history of same-sex attraction or experience, experience not seemingly correlating with identification (12).

There are individuals who identify as non-gender, and there is a current trend towards gender non-specific toys, clothing and indeed everything. Working in a psychodynamic way with patients, our job is not to 'label', but to facilitate each individual to find their own identity and level of comfort in society.

All gender identities, whatever people choose to call themselves, should be treated equally and with respect.

Clinical Treatment of Gender Dysphoria

This chapter discusses both gender dysphoria, or transsexualism, and sexual preference. There is a huge difference between these two areas of human sexuality, as transsexual people may request multiple medical and surgical interventions to allow the individual to be comfortable in their daily life, whereas no clinical physical interventions are necessary, or indeed appropriate, for individuals who have same, asexual, or bisexual preferences. Both groups may need psychosexual or psychological help in order to cope with some overwhelming issues, but that is also true of many in the majority cisgender, where sense of personal identity and gender correspond with the birth sex, and heterosexual population.

This chapter therefore summarises some of the clinical interventions which are helpful to the trans individual.

The clinical treatment of gender dysphoria traditionally depends on diagnosis by two mental health specialists according to current UK Multicollegiate Guidelines. There is a strong body of both professional and consumer thought that this 'medicalisation' of the condition is inappropriate, and there are evolving models of informed consent as opposed to psychiatric diagnosis which offer an ethical framework, ensuring the patient's autonomy throughout their treatment (13). On taking this approach, the clinician must also be aware of exercising their professional duty of care to the patient, and ensuring all treatments are delivered safely. The World Professional Association for Transgender Health (WPATH) describes international standards of care for all transgender people, although service delivery clearly depends on available resources (14).

The aim of treatment of transgender individuals is to assist them to feel comfortable and complete in their bodies, and enhance their self-acceptance and their acceptance in the wider community. These are not cosmetic procedures, but for many transgender people are fundamental to their mental and physical well-being. This will usually take the form of hormonal and surgical input.

Cross sex hormonal therapy has been shown to have positive psychological and physical effects on the transgender person (15).

Male-to-Female Transition (Transwomen)

For males-to-females, or transwomen, the goal is to feminise the body. Oestrogen, either with or without anti-androgens, can be given, which will encourage breast growth, decrease body and facial hair and decrease muscle mass. It will also diminish penile erections. This treatment should be given according to local and international guidelines, in order to minimise any possible complications such as thromboembolism, osteoporosis and depression. There is no increased risk of breast cancer when compared to non-trans women (16). Unfortunately, feminising hormones have no effect on the voice, therefore speech therapy is usually very useful as a feminising strategy for speech.

Most transwomen feel disgusted by their male genitalia, and also form a powerful emotional barrier to recognising this genitalia as part of their own body. They sometimes report attempts to self-mutilate, and in extreme cases, attempting to cut off their penis and testicles at stressful times in their lives when the physical symbol of the gender they feel no akin to has become unbearable. Therefore, surgical removal of this genitalia is essential in the majority of cases to enable them to have the ability to live comfortably in the converse gender role. When gender change surgery is being undertaken, surgery in specialist units is recommended, where, if desired, neovaginoplasty will be simultaneously performed. The most common technique is to use the penile skin inversion technique to create a neovagina and vulva as close to a biological vagina as possible. When revision surgery is needed, intestinal segments are used to form the vagina. Neovaginal stenosis is the most common complication of both techniques (17). There has, overall, been a high rate of satisfaction with the surgical result despite reports of sexual dysfunction (18). Transwomen's quality of life improved considerably post-surgery, and emotional stability and self-esteem were enhanced (19). Although revision surgery was sometimes needed, there was a general reported satisfaction with the operation (20).

Unfortunately, although rarely, there are those who experience disillusionment with their gender aspirations, and express regret post-surgery. Although technically reversal to aesthetically acceptable cosmetic male genitalia can be achieved with surgery and implants (21), this clearly indicates flawed pre-surgical assessment of the individual, and would make one concerned about the emotional and psychological issues which triggered this behaviour, and the ongoing emotional and mental state of that particular individual.

Other appearance and presentation enhancements can be chosen, with hair removal, speech therapy and breast augmentation being most commonly requested. Makeup, clothing and deportment advice may be helpful and are very much up to the individual.

Female-to-Male Transition (Transmen)

Testosterone therapy is the mainstay of treatment for female-to-male transsexuals. It increases facial and body hair, coarsens the skin, strengthens bones and deepens the voice. It also stops menstruation and enlarges the clitoris, and therefore the physical together with the psychological changes tend to increase libido.

The potential negative side effects could be reduced high-density lipoprotein and increased triglycerides (22); however alopecia and acne, which are listed as negative, may be perceived as positive signs of masculinisation, welcomed by the patient, and therefore are not necessarily unwanted outcomes.

There is now a range of options for genital surgery for transmen. The ideal phallus looks realistic, has tactile and erogenous sensibility and permits sexual function and standing urination without post-surgical side effects (23). Sadly, this is not yet always the case, even in highly skilled specialist surgical units. In general, phalloplasty with radial forearm flap leads to good results, and despite scarring on the forearm is considered worthwhile by the patient (24). There are now good alternatives to this technique such as suprapubic phalloplasty, which even without urethroplasty offers a good option to those who felt stigmatised by having a donor site scar on their arm (25).

Double mastectomy, or 'top surgery' as it is sometimes called, comes as a great relief to many transmen who have used tight and uncomfortable binders to flatten their breasts in order to concord with their otherwise masculine appearance. The underlying muscle may need to be built up to produce a male, rather than a female mastectomised chest, as the confidence to appear and feel masculine while in leisure or sports attire is of prime importance to many men.

As a transgender person, the journey to acquire physical congruence with one's gender can be complex, challenging, complicated and costly, with overwhelming emotional impact, although, in the main, worthwhile. Sadly, there is the potential for many losses as well as gains. One issue which has been more recently brought to the fore, in light of scientific advances in the field, is fertility. Recent World Professional Association for Transgender Health standards of care for transsexuals, transgender and gender non-conforming people, recommend discussion of fertility options, as offered to the general population (26), although clinical procedures relating to assisted conception which may be necessary will require the transgender person to acknowledge the reproductive parts of their body, which they have emotionally rejected. They should, however, have their options discussed and explained pre-hormonal therapy when it is possible to achieve a meaningful outcome.

There are other losses and social changes which the transgender person and their family and friends have to face. The impact on their close circle can be enormous. Marriages break up, friendships crumble and a parent will mourn the loss of the son or daughter to whom they gave birth. Relationships which are strong before any trans change will be more likely to survive, and can be a great support during the transsexual journey, however many cannot cope with these dramatic life changes and social and family structures become distant and change. Financial issue losses are common in countries where there is little or no public provision of gender reassignment treatments. Discrimination at work is also an issue, but there are now companies which, by law or generally altruistic management, have policies in place to educate staff about gender differences, and to ensure a safe and non-discriminatory work environment for all employees.

In psychosexual practice, one may come across individuals who do not wish to have permanent gender change treatments, despite an unshakeable belief that they have been born into the wrong body. It is an ideal context in which to reflect the seeming ambivalence in desire for physical change back to the patient, in order to help them explore their reasons for this. It could be fear of surgery, possibly cultural fears, or a true ambivalence about their gender goals.

It is essential that each individual is fully informed and understands the implications of any irreversible treatment. It has often been said that informed consent is a process, not an event, and it is in this respect that reflective psychodynamic therapy can help.

As we have seen illustrated, the life of a transgender person can be seen as a journey, which is inevitably more complex than that of a cis-gender individual, that is one whose gender identity and anatomical sex are congruent at birth. The transgender community is like any other in that they are all individuals and will have different life stories and trajectories. Some very high-profile trans individuals can be excellent role models, but one of the most frequently used phrases in the clinic was, 'I just wish to be ordinary', the same as the man or woman down the road. As psychosexual medicine clinicians we can enable each individual to work out some of their psychosexual problems, and free them up to attain their personal goals.

Health Issues Relating to Differences in Sexual Preference

Individuals who are not primarily heterosexual, such as lesbian, gay, or bisexual to name the three most prevalent groups, do not need clinical intervention in their lives unless they have a specific problem with their physical, sexual or mental health just as the majority of the population. Same-sex couples and non-heterosexual individuals are just as likely to present at a psychosexual clinic as anyone else, and there are no differences in approach to treatment. The same reflective analysis of the health professional-patient relationship, the patient history and the feelings and thoughts which are present or absent in the room, have the same relevance as with all patients, and are unique to that individual.

It does help, however, to have an understanding of some of the issues with which the individual has had to contend which may have bearing on the sexuality issues presented on consultation.

It is well documented that the health indices of lesbian, gay, bisexual and transgender (LGBT) individuals are worse than that of the general population, despite gays and lesbians being more likely to have a graduate degree (27). The LGBT community was more likely to smoke than the general population, and the women were more obese than heterosexual women. They are also less likely to participate in breast and cervical screening cancer prevention programmes, despite being at risk. Binge drinking was highest in bisexuals, all of which contributes to a less healthy lifestyle than their heterosexual counterparts. Many disparities in chronic health conditions in the younger sexual minority population persist into older age, and other conditions, such as cardiac problems and asthma are more likely to be reported by older lesbians and gay men (28). These conditions may be linked to cigarette smoking, alcohol and unhealthy eating (29), much of which behaviours are comfort responses to stress.

Gay and bisexual men have higher rates of psychological distress, drinking and smoking than heterosexual men, and the findings for lesbian and bisexual women also demonstrated higher rates of chronic illness, smoking and heavy drinking than heterosexual women (30). Sexual minority men and women who have experienced homophobic discrimination have higher rates of mental health issues and substance misuse than their peers who have not experienced discrimination (31). Linked to this, we find that men who have sex with men are also noted to have a markedly higher risk of HIV, syphilis, gonorrhoea and other sexually transmitted infections than the heterosexual population (32).

Sexual minority groups are often reluctant to present for healthcare due to anxieties about potential discrimination (33), and clinicians may say that they would like to know more about the healthcare needs of these groups. It is recognised that better education is needed to increase knowledge, awareness and positive signalling in healthcare settings that minority groups are on equal footing with all the other patients, therefore encouraging the patients to feel confident in their sexuality.

CASE 3: THE STORY OF MELANIE

Melanie entered the clinic room with a shy smile. She was an attractive woman in her late 30s, dressed in a casual, but professional manner and was appropriately dressed for her job, which she explained was working in communications for a large advertising company.

She then said that she had come for help as she was unable to have sex with her partner – and, in fact, had never had full sex. She had never used tampons. Her upbringing on a country farm had been strict but loving, and she always felt very much loved. That is why she did not understand why she was unable to have sex.

On the second visit I offered to examine her. She became tearful but agreed. On the couch she clamped her legs shut, and tears came into her eyes.

She had primary vaginismus.

Melanie was lesbian.

CASE 4: THE STORY OF ALANA

Alana strode into the clinic room, initially seeming confident, but then just sat and stared at me. She was wearing denim jeans and a jacket. She was overweight, and poorly groomed. I introduced myself and she nodded. I reflected back to her that she seemed uncomfortable in the room, then kept silent. She eventually spoke…all in a rush.

She then said that she had come for help as she was unable to have sex with her partner, and, in fact, had never had full sex. She had never used tampons. Her upbringing on a country farm had been strict but loving, and she always felt very much loved. That is why she did not understand why she was unable to have sex.

On the second visit I offered to examine her. She became tearful but agreed. On the couch she clamped her legs shut, and tears came into her eyes.

She had primary vaginismus.

Alana was heterosexual.

These vignettes illustrate that we must never make assumptions about patients and work with each person as they present in the room. That is what makes each consultation unique and equally challenging.

Summary and Conclusion

Melanie and Alana were two women, with different lives, different partners, yet with similar presenting sexual problems. In the cases at the beginning of the chapter, Grace and Luke had complex issues of gender identity, but were still able to express themselves in a therapeutic way in the psychosexual clinic. Sexual, emotional and relationship difficulties may be experienced by anyone, no matter what their sexual orientation or sexual identity. Each individual, of course, has had their own specific life journey, and by listening to them in a professional way the consultation can be constructive.

In psychosexual consultation, the patient's stories are their symptoms, and the clinical signs, feelings and emotions are all in the room. The traditional techniques of reflection and interpretation of the doctor-patient interaction within the consultation are ideally suited to any patient's story. The 'coming out' of anyone with issues of gender or sexual attraction to those close to them can be one of the most difficult points of their lives, and an opportunity to explore their confusion, fears and even excitement with impartial professionals may be valuable.

Therefore, the complex histories of some of our patients with issues concerning gender identity, sexual orientation or both can very appropriately become part of the psychosexual doctors' practice.

LEARNING POINTS

- The origins of transgender states and sexual preference difference are unclear, but certainly have a biological element.
- Transgender individuals may have sexual and emotional needs, as well as medical input in relation to physical gender change.
- Gender fluid is a term which is used to allow individuals to define their own gender identity.
- People with sexual preference differences have worse health indices than their heterosexual peers.
- Psychosexual medicine is suitable for anyone with a sexual or relationship difficulty regardless of gender identity or sexual preference.

REFERENCES

1. Benjamin H. *The Transsexual Phenomenon*. New York, NY: Julian Press, 1966.
2. Money J. The concept of gender identity disorder in childhood and adolescence after 39 years. *J Sex Marital Ther* 1994;20(3):163–177.
3. Berenbaum SA, Beltz AM. How early hormones shape gender development. *Curr Opin Behav Sci* 2016;7:53–60.
4. Clemens B, Junger J, Pauly K et al. Male-to-female gender dysphoria: Gender specific differences in resting state networks. *Brain Behav* 2017;5;7(5):e00691.
5. Smith ES, Junger J, Derntl B et al. The transsexual brain-a review of findings on the neural basis of transsexualism. *Neurosci Biobehav Rev* 2015,59:251 266.
6. Rice WR, Friberg U, Gavrilets S. Homosexuality as a consequence of epigenetically canalised sexual development. *Q Rev Biol* 2012;87(4):343–368.
7. Reed GM, Drescher J, Krueger RB et al. Disorders related to sexuality and gender identity in the ICD-11: Revising the ICD-10 classification based on current scientific evidence, best clinical practices, and human rights considerations. *World Psychiatry* 2016;15(3):205–221.
8. GLAAD. Los Angeles, CA. Available from: www.glaad.org/about
9. Arcelus J, Bouman WP, Van Den Noortgate W et al. Systematic review and meta-analysis of prevalence studies in transsexualism. *Eur Psychiatry* 2015;30(6):807–815.
10. Collin L, Reisner SL, Tangpricha V et al. Prevalence of transgender depends on the "case" definition: A systematic review. *J Sex Med* 2016;13(4):613–626.
11. Meerwijk EL, Sevelius JM. Transgender population size in the United States: A meta-regression of population-based probability samples. *Am J Public Health* 2017;107(2):e1–e8.
12. Richters J, Altman D, Badcock PB et al. Sexual identity, sexual attraction and sexual experience: The second Australian study of health and relationships. *Sex Health* 2014;11(5):451–460.
13. Cavanaugh T, Hopwood R, Lambert C. Informed consent in the medical care of transgender and gender-nonconforming patients. *AMA J Ethics* 2016;18(11):1147–1155.
14. Wylie K, Knudson G, Khan SI et al. Serving transgender people: Clinical care considerations and service delivery models in transgender health. *Lancet* 2016;23:388(10042):401–411.
15. Unger CA. Hormone therapy for transgender patients. *Transl Androl Urol* 2016;5(6):877–884.

16. Tangpricha V, den Heijer M. Oestrogen and anti-androgen therapy for transgender women. *Lancet Diabetes Endocrinol* 2017;5(4):291–300.

17. Horbach SE, Bouman MB, Smit JM et al. Outcome of vaginoplasty in Male-female transgenders: A systematic review of surgical techniques. Aesthetic and functional outcome of neovaginoplasty using penile skin in male-to-female transsexuals. *J Sex Med* 12(6):1499–1512.

18. Buncamper ME, Honselaar JS, Bouman MB et al. Aesthetic and functional outcomes of neovaginoplasty using penile skin in male-to-female transsexuals. *J Sex Med* 2015;12(7):1626–1634.

19. Papadopulos NA, Zavlin D, Lellé JD et al. Male-to-female sex reassignment surgery using the combined technique leads to increased quality of life in a prospective study. *Plast Reconstr Surg* 2017;140(2):286–294.

20. Van der Sluis WB, Bouman MB, de Boer NK et al. Long term follow up of transgender women after secondary intestinal vaginoplasty. *J Sex Med* 2016;13(4):702–710.

21. Djordjevic ML, Bizic MR, Duisin D et al. Reversal surgery in regretful male-to-female transsexuals after sex reassignment surgery. *J Sex Med* 2016;13(6):1000–1007.

22. Irwig MS. Testosterone therapy for transgender men. *Lancet Diabetes Endocrinol* 2017;5(4):301–311.

23. Frey JD, Poudrier G, Chiodo MV et al. An update on genital reconstruction options for the female-to-male transgender patient: A review of the literature. *Plast Reconstr Surg* 2017;139(3):728–737.

24. Van Caenegem E, Verhaeghe E, Taes Y et al. Long-term evaluation of donor-site morbidity after radial forearm flap phalloplasty for transsexual men. *J Sex Med* 2013;10(6):1644–1651.

25. Terrier JE, Courtois F, Ruffion A et al. Surgical outcomes and patients' satisfaction with suprapubic phalloplasty. *J Sex Med* 2014;11(1):288–298.

26. De Roc C, Tilleman K, T'Sjoen G et al. Fertility options in transgender people. *Rev Psychiatry* 2016;28(1):112–119.

27. Lunn MR, Cui W, Zack MM et al. Sociodemographic characteristics and health outcomes among lesbian, gay and bisexual US adults using Healthy People 2020 leading health indicators. *LGBT Health* 2017;4(4):283–294.

28. Fredriksen-Goldsen K, Kim HJ, Shui C et al. Chronic health conditions and key health indicators among lesbian, gay, and bisexual older US adults, 2013–14. *Am J Public Health* 2017;107(8):1332–1338.

29. Caceres BA, Brody A, Luscombe RE et al. A systematic review of cardiovascular disease in sexual minorities. *Am J Public Health* 2017;107(4):e13–e21.

30. Gonzales G, Przeworski J, Henning-Smith C. Comparison of health and risk factors between lesbian, gay and bisexual adults and heterosexual adults in the United States: Results from the National Health Interview Survey. *JAMA Intern Med* 2016;176(9):1344–1351.

31. Lee JH, Gamarel KE, Bryant KJ et al. Discrimination, mental health and substance use disorders among sexual minority populations. *LGBT Health* 2016;3(4):258–265.

32. De Coul EL, Warning TD, Koedijk FD et al. Sexual behaviour and sexually transmitted infections in sexually transmitted infection clinic attendees in the Netherlands, 2007–2011. *Int J STD AIDS* 2014;25(1):40–51.

33. Knight DA, Jarret D. Preventive healthcare for women who have sex with women. *Am Fam Physician* 2017;95(5):314–321.

21

Internet Pornography: Addiction or Sexual Dysfunction?

Catherine White

Introduction

It is becoming more common in practice to encounter those whose sexual dysfunction has a familiar theme: pornography.

The patient may present in a number of ways:

- Acknowledging a clear connection between pornography and their loss of libido, erectile dysfunction, delayed ejaculation
- With overt concerns about sexual or pornography addiction
- Unaware of any connection at all

The contributory effect may only become evident as they progress through therapy.

Whether or not we feel it is within our remit to treat addictions, with the increasing prevalence, it is important to develop an understanding of some of the mechanisms linking sexual difficulties to pornography (porn). This will enable us to assess the patient comprehensively, without exclusion and to fully utilise the therapeutic relationship.

Pornography

Pornography, from the Greek meaning 'the writing of [or about] harlots', has no official definition. There are many descriptions but for the purpose of this chapter I use the legal interpretation taken from the UK 2008 Criminal Justice and Immigration Act Part 5, Section 63(3):

> An image is 'pornographic' if it is of such a nature that it must reasonably be assumed to have been produced solely or principally for the purpose of sexual arousal

You may ask why, when 'pornography' has existed for hundreds of years, is it a problem now?

Pornography has undergone a huge metamorphosis from early erotic imagery found in pamphlets, books and magazines, to professional or homemade films on DVD, to today's offerings. The latter includes an endless variety of easily accessible, free-streaming, high-definition, often real-time and interactive material. In fact, pornography is so commonplace that soon we will be unable to imagine a time when there were multiple obstacles to acquisition.

We are a species that has been shown to have tactile and somatosensory empathy. Diffusion magnetic resonance imaging (MRI) studies that measure brain activity in participants while they witness the sensations and the actions of others demonstrate this empathy by consistently showing vicarious activation in the corresponding cortices (1,2). It is for this reason that porn can be arousing to us. We can think of it perhaps as 'erotic empathy'.

It is not that long ago that sexual therapists would have suggested that a couple view some pornography as a means to stimulate their flagging libido, often assuming scenarios showing mutual tender intimacies. Today it is commonplace in pornography to see a lack of intimacy and often gratification from abusive scenarios. Positive erotic components are often missing and sex may appear simply as an act of transgression. Arousal patterns may be further intensified by the voyeuristic presentation of violent pornography, increasing susceptibility to escalation (3).

It would appear to be the transition in the method of presentation of pornographic material that has opened the doors for porn-related sexual dysfunction. Without today's variety, ease of access and anonymity, there would appear to be little problem.

Usage

We live in a world where there is an ongoing sexualisation of contemporary culture. It is worth considering the change in high-speed Internet availability that has occurred over the past 10 years: in 2006, only 50% of UK adults had home broadband with an average use of 36 minutes daily (4); 2017, 91% had home broadband, 99% of those aged 16–34 and 97% of those age 35–54 years had recently used the Internet, often for hours a day and many of them on mobile devices (5); 90% of those age 16–24 years have a smartphone (6).

Looking at these dates it would appear to be no coincidence that the porn industry in 2006 was astute enough to develop the free streaming of pornographic material so that as more people accessed faster Internet speeds, pornography became more mainstream.

We are well aware that puberty and adolescence stimulate a natural curiosity to learn about sex and it is second nature to 'Google it'. Playground pressure to look is mounting and the easy accessibility of highly explicit pornography can for some set up the potential 'norm' for a highly neuroplastic adolescent brain. A National Union of Students (NUS) 2015 survey of 2,500 young people revealed that one-third of them had used porn for sex education as teenagers (7). Average age for first viewing of porn in one survey was 11 years and a tenth of 12- to 13-year-olds surveyed feared they had an addiction to porn (8, p. 27).

These adolescents are potentially our clients of the future.

When in 2007 psychosexual therapists started to see healthy young men in their 30s reporting erectile dysfunction, the common factor noted was that they were working within the information technology industry and therefore had the most prolonged access to high-speed Internet, and as a result, online pornography. The Kinsey Institute in 2007 was responsible for the first research in pornography-induced erectile dysfunction (PIED) and pornography-induced low libido (PILL) (9). Since then, the difficulty explaining the sharp increase in the number of men under 40 presenting with difficulties of erectile dysfunction, delayed ejaculation, lack of satisfaction and loss of desire has encouraged the plethora of research into pornography and its effect that continues today. The bulk of investigation has concerned male pornography use, probably due to the willingness of subjects to seek help and the more easily measurable physical effects. However in the past few years this has expanded to include more work about women. There are some differences emerging and I consider this later in a dedicated section.

Neuroscience

The Reward-Motivation Pathway

How does our brain behave when faced with a stimulus, particularly one that contributes to our survival such as food or sex? The human brain is programmed through dopamine to incentivise survival behaviours through the reward-motivation pathway. See Figure 21.1 and Adinoff (54).

This dopaminergic system is modulated by various neurotransmitter systems, including cholinergic, opioid, cannabinoid, GABAergic (main inhibitory mediation) and glutamatergic (main excitatory

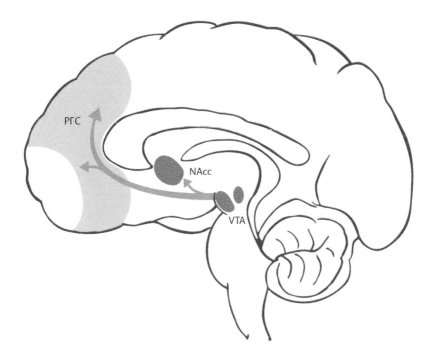

FIGURE 21.1 The brain reward circuitry projects from the dopaminergic neurons in the midbrain ventral tegmental area (VTA) to the nucleus accumbens (NAcc) in the medial prefrontal cortex (PFC) and to the associated limbic structures.

mediation). The route travelled backwards and forwards is known as the *mesocorticolimbic* pathway or *reward-motivation* pathway. Activation of this dopamine system mediates the rewarding effect not only of drug but also of non-drug or behavioural stimuli (10). There are many other additional contributing factors, and particularly of interest is the transcription factor deltaFosB, a Fos family protein, which can be thought of as the 'molecular switch' for addiction in its role as mediator of reward memory. Its presence and behaviour appear to be genetically determined, suggesting genetic susceptibility to addictive behaviour. It is known to accumulate in the nucleus accumbens following induction by chronic as opposed to acute exposure to drugs of abuse. It has also been shown to accumulate in the same area following chronic overconsumption of *natural* rewards, demonstrably running and sucrose drinking (consuming sugary drinks). This causes a state of sensitisation and increased incentive drive for the reward (11).

To simplify, we can think of dopamine as the main neurotransmitter driving both normal and addictive behaviour (reward, pleasure, fine tuning of motor function, compulsion, perseveration). The attractive and motivational property of a stimulus that induces further appetite for that stimulus is known as the reward. Anticipation of the reward stimulates the production of dopamine that then travels down the mesolimbic pathway. Its effect on the nucleus accumbens in the prefrontal cortex (PFC) determines the level of *wanting* or desire for the stimulus. This is known as incentive salience (31) (Figure 21.2).

Thus, dopamine can be seen not as the pleasure chemical that dictates 'liking' of a substance or behaviour, but the driver, *the fuel for craving*. The reward, as described, is the *prospect* of pleasure rather than the pleasure itself (12). Modification of the system occurs through the 'steady on' influence of neurotransmitters such as glutamate and GABA. However, these modifying influences can be overwhelmed when there is endless novelty available. Continuous stimulation of the system results in repeated spiking of dopamine levels, which then serves to reinforce the appetite. Just as in drug addiction where the exogenous drugs of abuse compete for certain dopamine (D2) receptor sites, so do endogenous neurotransmitters, produced by the positive emotional effects of 'natural' rewards. The pathways would appear to be shared (13). Reduction in the D2 dopamine receptors causes escalation as the subject tries to potentiate and recreate the high (14). Prolonged disruption of the neuronal pathways appears to cause a physical change and reduction of the neurofilament proteins.

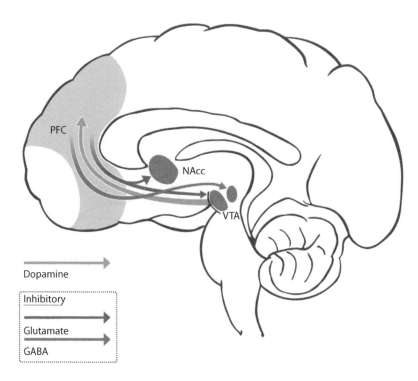

FIGURE 21.2 Incentive salience: the production of dopamine stimulates further neurotransmitters such as glutamate (1, excitatory) and GABA (2, inhibitory).

Hypofrontality and Addiction

The PFC, or anterior part of the frontal cortex is that part of the brain that mediates executive functioning: goal planning, internally guided behaviour and impulse control. All are necessary for countering urges and modifying risk-taking behaviour. The PFC is highly developed in the human but interestingly is an area whose development tends to lag behind that of other parts of the brain. It does not reach its optimal balance until our mid-20s. The adolescent is thus particularly vulnerable to the development of addictive behaviour when exposed to excessive dopaminergic stimuli (15,16).

Damage to the PFC has been studied in detail in patients following a stroke, with tumours and after trauma. Unsurprisingly, disruption to the area results in impulsivity, compulsivity, emotional lability and impaired judgement. Collectively this is known as hypo-frontal syndrome or *hypofrontality* (22).

It is easy to imagine from these characteristics that similar frontal abnormalities occur in those with drug addiction (opiates, cocaine and methamphetamine), and this has been demonstrated through MRI-based studies using voxel-based morphometry (VBM). Interestingly, the same frontal dysfunction is also associated with compulsive consumption of natural rewards, namely food and sex (17). This was demonstrated for the first time in 2009 in a preliminary study using diffusion MRI techniques, in patients unable to control their sexual behaviour (18).

The Coolidge Effect

A behavioural psychologist first described the Coolidge effect in the 1950s. It was titled in relation to a joke made by Calvin Coolidge, American president 1923–1929, when he and his wife were being shown around an experimental rooster farm. He responded to his wife's comment about the excessive mating frequency of the roosters noting that they at least were mating with a different bird each time (19).

Thus the Coolidge effect was the illustration through animal studies of a natural desire for sexual variety and new experience. Demonstration in rats showed greater reward circuit activity with exposure to a new sexual partner. It was observed that male rats when faced repeatedly with the same female partner showed progressively longer ejaculation time, post-orgasmic sluggishness and early cessation of activity. This was seen to be in stark contrast to those male rats to whom a different female rat was presented after each ejaculation: the male continued until completely exhausted, urged on by repeated surges of dopamine (20).

The reward circuitry is responsible for the cognitive processing of an experience, the positive reinforcement and subsequent trigger to perpetuate behaviour. This change in the neural circuitry is called *neuroadaptation*. It is facilitated by repetitive, high-emotion, high-frequency exposure (21,22). These are conditions that can easily be fulfilled by today's Internet use, including online pornography with its opportunity for rapid novelty just as the Coolidge effect.

Humans, although a species that tends to stay in pairs, experience a similar effect associated with sexual novelty. When exposed to sexually arousing novel female images, men produced larger volumes of ejaculate with higher motility and in less time (23).

Addiction?

There has been much debate around the terms *addiction* and *compulsion* when relating to sex and/or pornography use. Each term can be helpful in understanding the problem but equally has its limitations.

The question is still the same: why is it so easy to develop a problem with Internet pornography?

This can initially be answered by the three 'A's' described by researcher Alvin Cooper as the 'engine' of addiction – see Delmonico's work entitled 'In memorium to Alvin Cooper' (24).

- *Accessibility*: merely a smartphone
- *Affordability*: almost infinite free content
- *Anonymity*: no one need know what you access

The American Society of Addictive Medicine (ASAM)

> A primary chronic disease of brain reward, motivation, memory and related circuitry. Dysfunction in these circuits leads to characteristic manifestations (biological, psychological, social, spiritual), reflected in a pathological pursuit of reward and/or relief by substance use *or behaviour.*

The addiction is characterised by the following:

- Inability to consistently abstain
- Impairment of behavioural control
- Craving
- Diminished recognition of significant problems
- A dysfunctional emotional response

(See ASAM website for the full definition [25].)

It illustrates that in order for something to be an addiction it needs to have an associated negative impact.

As an alternative to addiction, some favour the term *sexual compulsivity*, although this does not appear to take into account the 'high' associated with sexual compulsion and the 'anxiety' usually felt with other compulsive behaviours where there is generally no reward (compare hair pulling, hand washing).

The condition of *hypersexual disorder* (26), was proposed in 2010 for the *Diagnostic and Statistical Manual of Mental Disorders, Fifth Edition* (*DSM-5*). The American Psychiatric Association (APA) repeatedly rejected this.

An abbreviated version of the proposed criteria for hypersexual disorder is as follows:

- Over a period of at least 6 months, recurrent and intense sexual fantasies, sexual urges and sexual behaviour in association with a number of criteria
- Clinically significant distress or impairment in social occupational or other important areas of functioning associated with the frequency and intensity of these sexual fantasies, urges and behaviour
- Sexual fantasies, urges, behaviour are not due to direct physiological effects of exogenous substances, a co-occurring medical condition or to manic episodes
- Individual is at least 18 years of age

This description certainly has features that without doubt describe aspects of the problem, but it also has some limitations as an umbrella for the 'addictive' behaviour concerning Internet pornography. Moreover, it suggests by its title that the person would be more likely to have a high sex drive, quite the opposite to the reality.

Since then, the APA has recognised *behavioural* addiction related to the Internet, specifically the addictive potential of Internet Gaming Disorder (2013 *DSM-5*). The World Health Organization *International Classification of Diseases* (*ICD-11*) published in June 2018 has added Internet Gaming Disorder within the addictions section as anticipated and although it has also extended the sexual dysfunction categories to include C672: Compulsive Sexual behaviour disorder, it has not classified Sexual Addiction as a distinct condition. This has already attracted much comment prior to publication and will no doubt continue to do for the foreseeable future (55,56). Perhaps something to take into account is that particularly in the United States the naming of a condition has significant implications for the medical insurance companies and their obligation to fund therapy and so the cynics would suggest that this may carry some weight. However, they are still using *ICD-10* and it is anticipated that they will not move to *ICD-11* for many years. For this chapter however I prefer to look at the practicalities rather than become overly distracted by classification.

What Happens in Practice?

Thinking back to the reward-motivation pathway when viewing pornography, we need to consider the 'fuel for craving'. The heightened arousal created by each click of a mouse or swipe of a page causes a surge of dopamine in anticipation of the reward. The search for novelty within the environment (Coolidge) activates the reward system, which is then repeatedly triggered by seeking (surfing) the endless and rapid variety of content.

The activity of using Internet pornography and its power to deliver unending stimulation is thought to constitute 'supernormal stimuli' (phenomenon first described by Tinbergen [28]). This ornithologist was jointly awarded the Nobel Prize in Medicine in 1973 for work around individual and social behaviour patterns. A *supernormal stimulus* was the term coined after demonstration that one could build an artificial object that was a stronger stimulus, or releaser for an instinct, than the object for which the instinct originally evolved. Thus for Tinbergen, one illustration was that birds would preferentially sit on plaster eggs that were larger with more defined markings or saturated colour than sitting to hatch their own eggs which were paler and dappled. Hilton refers to this phenomenon in porn where the person may show preference for two-dimensional but highly stimulating sexual imagery over human contact for sex, despite the evolutionary instinct of sex for procreation (29). Chronic overuse is highly stimulating. Recruitment of our natural reward system occurs at higher levels than encountered by our ancestors as our brains evolved, thus making it liable to switch into an addictive mode (30).

Escalation

The more the viewer seeks and masturbates to porn, the more dopamine is produced so that eventually the receptors and signals in the brain fatigue. The viewer is left still wanting, but unable to reach the desired level of satisfaction, and so becomes desensitised. For a man this may mean difficulty in maintaining an erection with imagery that would previously have provided reliable stimulation. Even with an erection they may find that ejaculation is delayed and ultimately may be absent as they struggle to reach the previous level of arousal. The viewer may experience their libido diminishing as pornography takes the 'sex' out of sex. They may even avoid ejaculation and practise 'edging', remaining at the point just prior to orgasm and ejaculation, for as long as they can tolerate. In this way they satisfy the craving for the 'seeking' behaviour for the maximum amount of time. When ejaculation occurs, they may feel deflated rather than satisfied as they know the activity or ritual is now over.

In order to escape this effect, the viewer may expand their tastes in the pursuit of novelty. Sexual images that cause anxiety, shock and disgust can stimulate adrenaline alongside dopamine just as in sex (31). The chemical combination is mistaken for pleasure as the disgust reflex is turned off. The viewers may find themselves masturbating to content that appears to them abhorrent and shameful when 'sober'. Desensitisation may equally induce a transition from viewing pre-filmed imagery to actual interaction, be it online in chat rooms or with webcams. Eventually visiting sex workers may be the only way to satisfy the craving. A sense of shame and need for secrecy will inevitably develop alongside concerns that their own sexual tastes and proclivities are unacceptable. When faced with a patient describing escalation it is important to be mindful of any mention of illegal or forensic activity.

Assessment

One of the aims of our assessment is to differentiate between pornography use and problematic pornography use.

Our patient may admit to use but it may not be causing them any problem at all; use may be purely recreational. Additionally, evidence has shown that Internet pornography usage may have had a number of positive impacts on the experience of individual sexuality, particularly among the youth, and more marginalised populations such as LGBTQ (lesbian, gay, bisexual, transgender, queer or questioning) and the disabled (32). Pornography consumption may merely empower by leading to an expansion of the 'established script' rather than an abandonment of usual sexual behaviours (33).

The past few years have seen a plethora of research into Internet use disorders, particularly gaming and gambling. With respect to pornography, a number of clinicians including Mark Griffiths devised the PPCS or problematic pornography consumption scale, based on his (2005) six-component addiction model (34). It used a rigorous set of screening questions to quantify the patient's usage and the impact it was having on their social, emotional and occupational well-being. The Internet Sex Screening Test (ISST) followed this and then in 2014 the problematic pornography usage scale (PPUS) aimed at developing further the core factors that were related (35).

However, the safe space that we provide where sex can be discussed with our patients in a non-judgemental and thoughtful manner is, I feel, enough for our Institute of Psychosexual Medicine (IPM) work. In an environment of acceptance, we can work to eliminate the shame so commonly felt and gain insight into the detrimental effects they may be experiencing, without employing a specific questionnaire.

What we are looking out for is an unhealthy relationship with a mood-altering experience. Some of the things to consider are as follows:

- Has something that started as the pursuit of pleasure become something the patient has to do in order to feel normal?
- Are they using it to anaesthetise themselves from feelings of loneliness, anger, anxiety or loss?
- Do they perceive their behaviour to be out of control? Where pornography is used to modulate emotion it is likely this will become the case.

- Do they find themselves spending increasing amounts of time thinking about, preparing for and viewing pornography?
- Has the type of material they are viewing changed to something that they would never have imagined themselves participating in and would not like to admit to now?
- Have they fetishised certain behaviours as a result of their viewing habits without which they are unable to engage in partnered sex?
- Are they struggling to become aroused with their partner in comparison to when using porn?
- Have they repeatedly tried to stop or limit their usage and failed?
- Have they had or do they have other addictions?

What Predisposes Our Patient to Addiction?

Internet pornography is readily available in an anonymous setting. Why then does every user not develop an addiction or compulsion to use?

There is a vast body of knowledge concerning addiction and what makes us susceptible. As IPM therapists most of us have some knowledge of, but not specialist training in, this field. It is an extremely complex topic and way beyond the scope of this chapter. However, it is helpful to be aware of some of the theories surrounding the subject.

Robert Miller in his *Feeling State Theory* of addiction believes that all destructive behaviours associated with impulse control have their basis in normal healthy desires. He sees the addiction as a result of the positive feeling that becomes rigidly linked with a specific behaviour or 'feeling state'. When this feeling state is triggered, the person will feel compelled to carry out the behaviour in search of the desired sensation. It is quite easy to see how this would apply to the search for sexual arousal (36):

$$\text{Intense desire} + \text{Intense positive experience} = \text{Feeling state}$$

$$\text{Feeling state} + \text{Triggering event} = \text{Desired feeling} + \text{Compulsive behaviour}$$

He advocates a rigid protocol of behavioural treatment using the impulse-control disorder protocol with eye movement desensitisation and reprocessing. Clearly this requires specialist training for the therapist.

Attachment, Trauma, Opportunity

When considering an individual's vulnerability to developing an addiction, there are particular categories that we can consider:

- Attachment induced, where the patient is more likely to look to an inanimate thing rather than a person for comfort, not having had the experience of 'safe' attachments in their early life.
- Trauma induced, which may be the result of early life experience or something more recent such as a death in the family.
- Opportunity induced, which in the case of Internet pornography could be as simple as having a smartphone. It is worth noting that in adolescence, the prevalence of peers sharing pornography in the playground may mean that exposure to material could be unintentional.

Understandably there is more often than not a crossover between the groups, but there is some evidence from support groups to show that 'opportunity' may be the most influential factor in online pornography addiction (37). It is helpful though to listen out for those things in a patient's story that may indicate any one of these vulnerabilities.

Unlike substance addiction where the negative effects may become evident very quickly, Internet pornography use can escalate and develop an addictive pattern with very few side effects over many years. It can alter the user's sexual template. In fact it may not be until the patient seeks out a partner and finds that they have no libido or are unable to maintain an erection when faced with a real-life situation that they realise they have a problem. They have often developed a series of convincing arguments for themselves such as their viewing is merely for relaxation, harms nobody, relieves loneliness or boredom and thus can have no negative impact. Escalation though may have a variety of negative consequences:

- Financial, if participating in paid-for pornography content (on multiple Internet links direct from the free content), use of escorts or even findom, the fetish of financial domination by an escort.
- Social, where they lack motivation to interact with their family or socialise with friends, becoming more reclusive.
- Occupational, where the constant distraction to check their phone, pull up a favourite page on the computer or pop out for a rapid encounter with nearby escort, renders them unable to concentrate on or complete tasks.
- Health, when they start to suffer from lack of sleep, anxiety or depression. It is not uncommon for a patient to have felt suicidal and present complaining that it has 'taken over their life' and that they are totally exhausted by it.

Young men who have had no sexual fantasy or arousal prior to their introduction to pornography may experience a whole host of difficulties when faced with 'real-life' partnered sex. They are likely to have conditioned their sexual arousal to solitary sex. They may have no concept of intimacy associated with sex and expect their partner to be able to perform like a 'porn star.' The physical sensations of sweat and the smells of bodily arousal may overwhelm them. Pornography after all does not smell. They are vulnerable to developing a negative body image as they do not meet the physical standards that they see online: a sense of inadequacy can result from comparing penis size, musculature or levels of sexual stamina; unrealistic expectations for young women to have 'perfect' breasts, neat labia and no pubic hair. The perception of what is normal can be altered for both self and partner creating unnecessary anxiety.

Converting the physical position they favour to masturbate into one where they can engage with a partner may feel impossible, similarly in older men where physical challenges may be more relevant. All the associations that they have fostered with sexual arousal, and for men erection and ejaculation, may be impossible to reproduce when there is another party present.

When a patient is at the stage of experiencing difficulties only with partnered sex there may be reluctance to admit that their 'satisfactory pornography driven sexual experience' may even be a factor. The temptation to retreat to a world of cyber-sex, when all libido experienced with their partner has dissolved, is a potent one. The trigger to address the problem may only occur when no amount of escalation of the type of images viewed or risks taken can produce sexual satisfaction.

CASE 1

I called Colin in from the waiting room. He had a diffident air, was tall and slim with work overalls and heavy boots. He had asked for a re-referral to our service having been seen 8 months earlier by a colleague but been unable to engage with therapy at that time.

There was little emotion and he had an air of detachment. He sat still but jiggled one leg in a repetitive motion while seeming to scan the floor. He said that he had a problem that needed fixing but he could not do it himself so he had come back.

Colin had just passed 30, which he saw as a milestone. He had two young children, a wife whom he said he loved but that he had no desire for her sexually at all. When they did have sex it was perfunctory, he struggled to keep an erection and he derived little satisfaction. He said he was not that bothered really as they were often tired but it was causing problems between them.

I wondered aloud with him whether this was all about their busy lives and young family or whether he knew of anything else that might be playing a part. His referral had mentioned his pornography use yet he had not mentioned it at all.

I asked him about masturbation. Did he use any pornography, and was his lack of desire only related to sex with his wife?

While staring at the floor he said that things might be easier if they were more adventurous sexually. He found that if he fantasised about some of the pornography he had seen online then he could usually maintain an erection with her despite his lack of desire. Had he talked to her about any of this I enquired?

The words came tumbling out. She had caught him masturbating to webcam girls online. 'I just can't see the problem' he said. 'It's normal. It's not hurting her. I've always done it – everyone does it'. The first bit of eye contact. There was an air of defiance. It felt like having my teenage son challenge a rule I had laid down. 'I just don't get why she's so upset. She's told me if I don't sort it out she's leaving'. I shared with him that his anger was palpable, and he nodded his head in agreement.

The next time I saw Colin, he appeared to be a little more relaxed. He looked me in the eye and volunteered that he had been reflecting on his pornography use. It had all started in his late adolescence during his first job. A couple of his colleagues had shown him magazines and lent him an occasional DVD. It had felt exciting. He visibly puffed up his chest as he described how it had made him feel good and turned him into a 'proper man'. Home had been difficult. His dad had often shouted at him for not doing well at anything and for being lazy and his mum had been wary of a close relationship, as his dad had said it was making him 'soft'. School had been a misery. He had felt like an outsider with few friends. He had been skinny and bullied then, but being able to banter with the lads at work about things he had discovered on the computer helped him to feel he belonged. He looked forward to retreating to his bedroom each evening and finding the images of the perfect girl in the perfect scenario. The sense of anticipation would begin in the late afternoon as he counted the hours.

Colin told me that over the next couple of years he had used pornography almost every day, and sometimes several times a day. It felt calming and reassuring despite his finding it more difficult to get aroused. He remembered meeting his first girlfriend and regaining that initial high and excitement that he had felt with the porn. He had tried to experiment with her, reliving the moves he had found so intriguing in porn but she was 'disgusted' with him and the relationship had quickly ended. He mentioned feeling ashamed and humiliated and vowed to himself to keep it secret. Almost immediately he had found solace by increasing the hours spent watching porn. His mates were experimenting with recreational drugs but he found nothing came close to the relief from any anxiety he felt after flicking to the sites he had saved on his computer.

As he spoke it felt as if he was discovering all of this for the first time. 'I can say it here and you're not judging me'.

At our third meeting he said that he had stopped looking at porn, and then qualified it with 'well, tried to'. His body language was more relaxed; he was able to meet my eye. He explained that it was not until he had been talking about it in our sessions that he realised just how much he relied on it to feel better, mainly to reduce anxiety. It had felt weird to him to realise this and he mentioned that he had been getting pretty sick of desperately waiting for his wife to go out each time he needed to 'calm down'. He had started to feel he was 'some kind of a pervert' and even resenting time that she and the kids were around. He disclosed the powerful urges he had felt to look since stopping, and how this felt the same as when he moved from images to films and then to chatting live online. He said he just did not understand why it was so compelling; if he knew why he was doing it maybe he could stop. I thought it was appropriate to explain to him a bit about his reward-motivation pathway. We talked about dopamine, and about the reinforcement that happened each time. I reflected some of the early life vulnerabilities that I felt were present and how they may have made him more susceptible to developing a problem. 'I've never been able to talk', he said. 'I always think people will laugh at me if I say how I feel. It's too risky'.

The session was ending and I suggested he looked at a couple of resources that are available online to further explain what was going on:

- *The Road to Brighton*, Web reference (38)
- *Paula Hall's 'Kick Start Recovery Kit'*, Web reference (39)

Two months later and Colin returned to see me. He was smiling for the first time and sat easily in the chair. He shared that he had been completely abstinent from porn and even felt that he was much less preoccupied by the urges to search online. He flushed as he recalled the thrill at managing to talk to his wife about it and share his understanding with her. They had come up with a plan for him to relinquish his laptop and downgrade his smartphone to one that would merely text and make calls. This had made it so much easier he said, and he felt she was involved and was starting to trust him again. His constant anxiety seemed to have dissipated. The final thing that he wanted to share with me was that he had started to see her as sexy again and they had resumed some physical contact with sensual moments. He wanted to take it slowly and savour all the feelings that he recognised had been almost numbed by the porn. He felt that she would be more likely to trust him this way as he knew that she still had anxieties about whether he would just go back to his old habits. They had not yet progressed to intercourse but he acknowledged that the relationship was so much better that this would happen eventually.

Colin finished by saying that he felt he did not need to come again: 'I feel liberated from porn'. The lack of desire that he had presented as his initial problem had become quite secondary. Briefly, it all felt a bit too good to be true. I found myself feeling a little anxious on his behalf.

Reassuringly however, his parting words were to express a degree of realism; he knew he was susceptible to going back, which for him right now was not conducive to a healthy sex life with his wife. He felt that the urges may never disappear completely and that he may never find a substitute for that early high he got from the pornography but for him right now communication was the key. He volunteered that he could not risk the negative spiral of shame that happened as a result of any secrecy. I discharged Colin with a caveat that he could return to the service within 6 months for a single follow-up appointment if he felt the need.

I wondered at the time which one of us I was attempting to reassure.

Discussion

The potential health risks of Internet pornography are not as well understood as those for tobacco, alcohol and drugs of abuse. It is increasingly socially acceptable and use of Internet pornography is seen as the norm. This may be why men can be slow to make the connexion between their pornography viewing and their sexual difficulties.

In 2016, a comprehensive review of the effect of Internet pornography on sexual function reinforced what so many of us have suspected. It found a number of studies that correlated pornography use with arousal, attraction and sexual performance difficulties, including difficulty orgasming, diminished libido or erectile dysfunction. The studies also noted a negative effect on partnered sex, and less sexual and relationship satisfaction. There was a preference for using Internet pornography to achieve and maintain arousal over partnered sex and greater brain activation to the former in those reporting less desire for sex with a partner (40). As mentioned earlier, the adolescent brain with its immature frontal cortex is more susceptible to pathological learning of the reward system. Worryingly there is therefore a greater risk of addiction in adolescence and studies have found a greater future use of 'deviant pornography' including bestiality and child pornography (41).

Women and Internet Pornography

Much of this chapter has focussed on the effects of Internet pornography use in men. This stems from the dominance of research which has concentrated predominantly on men, previously noted to be likely to the availability of subjects presenting with physical effects suffered around erection and ejaculation. However if we consider forums and online resources we find that there are many women who also suffer from compulsive and potentially addictive use of porn. An approximate figure taken from self-help group https://nofap.com, a community-based porn recovery site using peer-to-peer support (42), would suggest that 30% of female sex workers are in fact sex addicts, many of whom may have begun their journey through pornography use.

Several studies looking at gender difference in pornography use have revealed quite consistent results: it would seem that consumption by men is greater than by women; that men watch more hard-core rather than soft-core porn; that women tend to watch more often with a partner than alone (in contrast to men); that women reported greater subjective arousal if fantasising about a partner when watching explicit pornographic stimuli (43,44).

Context appeared to be more important for women than men, although interestingly in one study, eye tracking showed that women were initially more likely to look directly at genitals whereas men looked at female faces (45).

Women, like men, may present to us with reduced desire or reduced sensitivity to sexual arousal with their partner but this seems to be strongly correlated with many contextual factors including relationship, health and past sexual attitude (46). There is, however, an association with pornography consumption in women and more frequent, casual and risky sexual encounters (47). Therefore, when helping our female patients to untangle any compulsion for risky sexual encounters, we need to consider discussing their pornography use in addition to the associations with this behaviour with which we are more familiar. Women reported pornography being influential around their sexual practises, for example their participation in anal intercourse, despite the majority reporting the experience as a negative one. Thus when listening to our patient who is experiencing a loss of desire and reluctance to engage in sex, it is appropriate to enquire into their expectations around sexual practises and the influences on such (48). Women are less likely than men to volunteer a preference for using pornography for sexual arousal than for partnered sex and so when enquiring routinely about masturbation in the consultation we should remind ourselves to quantify whether this is satisfactory *without* pornographic stimulation, rather than assume this is so. Finally, an awareness of the susceptibility of young women to be negatively affected by being solicited for creating pornographic imagery, whether in adolescent sexting or the more organised introduction through 'modelling' to the porn industry, may help us in our work with them around sexual dysfunction (49).

Treatment

Research has shown that there are those who experience online sexual activities in a healthy manner. However, as previously described, there are a number of men and women who through a variety of susceptibilities will experience the negative consequences of problematic use of Internet porn.

Defining this as an addiction or a compulsion is not vital in order to decide on an initial treatment path. There is also a category of patients who may perceive themselves to have an addiction (SPPAs or self-perceived pornography addicts) but who would not fit the usual criteria for the same. This is something heavily influenced by the patient's religious beliefs and cultural norms and something for which further enquiry and sensitive explanation may suffice.

Several studies have looked at treatment in various forms: individual therapy, group therapy, pharmacotherapy and peer support. Encouragingly 'all studies (bar two*) reported positive impacts of treatment (i.e. an overall reduction in cyber-sexual behaviours) following the implementation of the

---

* The two studies not reporting reduction in cyber behaviour did however report improvement in mood and overall risk (51).

intervention, irrespective of type, but with behavioural treatments proving more beneficial in alleviating symptoms and thus negative consequences' (50).

Just as in other addictions, there is a strong argument for abstinence as a form of treatment (52). This may require very specialised help for some, but others may not require anything more than our support as we explore with our patient the likely other factors that play a role in their sexual dysfunction. Achieving abstinence (sobriety) can be complicated, however, as the ultimate aim is to have a healthy sex life (recovery) rather than abstinence and therefore absence of arousal and sex (contrast drug or alcohol addiction).

Sexual dysfunction recovery times seem to relate to pre-porn exposure to masturbation and sexual experience. They can therefore often be more rapid in the slightly older patient. If there has been a sexual template set prior to their compulsive pornography use then it can be re-awakened, as it will still exist within their limbic system memory. Those who have known nothing different however and who have begun their pornography exposure at a time when their brain was highly neuroadaptive may find that they require many months of abstinence before they regain any libido, erectile function or ability to ejaculate (53).

We may feel that it is in the patient's best interest for us to refer to specialised settings or signpost them to self-refer. There are a variety of options available:

- www.sexaddictionhelp.co.uk – A free online tool for sex and porn addiction recovery: Paula Hall Kick Start Recovery Programme
- https://atsac.co.uk – Association for the Treatment of Sexual Addiction and Compulsivity
- 12-step programmes: face-to-face, online, tele meetings:
  - Saauk.info – SAA (Sex Addicts Anonymous) UK
  - www.Slaauk.org – SA (Sexaholics Anonymous) UK
  - www.slaa.org – SLAA (Sex and Love Addicts Anonymous)
  - www.cosa-recovery.org – COSA (Compulsive sexual behaviour problems and partner support)
  - www.pornaddictsanonymous.org – Pornography Addicts Anonymous
- www.relate.org.uk – Relate, help with sex addiction, various centres with specialisms
- www.nofap.com – Provides useful community support and reassurance to those who wish to achieve abstinence; advocates total abstinence from masturbation to pornography and from sexually compulsive behaviour in an attempt to 'reboot' sexual desire and function but without the 12-step emphasis

Conclusion

When considering our patients I am not suggesting that the mention of pornography use should mean that we abandon our usual assessment and way of working and simply direct all our patients to 12-step groups or online forums. It is, however, important for us to incorporate awareness of the potential association of our patients' difficulties with Internet pornography in order to offer them a more thorough understanding of their problem. This way we will be able to differentiate between those with whom we can work successfully in an IPM fashion, and those who perhaps fit a purely addictive picture and would benefit from a more structured addictions model of therapy.

Unfortunately, therapy for behavioural 'addictions' is even more poorly funded than that for the more established addictions such as to drug and alcohol. Our role may thus be to signpost the patient to relevant self-help literature (see Useful Resources section in this chapter) and online options while we work alongside them. The potential outcome here is that as they eliminate the effects of the pornography use, we are there to work with them on the residual factors that may be contributing to their sexual dysfunction.

REFERENCES

1. Bastiaansen JACJ, Thioux M, Keysers C. Evidence for mirror systems in emotions. *Phil Trans R Soc B* 2009;364:2391–2404.

2. Keysers G. Expanding the mirror: Vicarious activity for actions, emotions, and sensations. *Curr Opin Neurobiol* 2009;19(6):666–671.
3. Templeman TL, Stinnet RD. Patterns of sexual arousal and history in a 'normal' sample of young men. *Arch Sex Behav* 1991;20(2):137–150.
4. Ofcom. *The Communications Market: Broadband.* Digital Progress Report 2007. London: Ofcom.
5. Ofcom. Connected Nations Report 2017. London: Ofcom.
6. Office for National Statistics. Internet Access: Households and individuals over 16, 2017. Available from: https://www.ons.gov.uk/peoplepopulationandcommunity/householdcharacteristics/homeinternet andsocialmediausage/datasets/internetaccesshouseholdsandindividualsreferencetables.
7. National Union of Students. Student Opinion Survey. November 2014. Available from: www.nus.org.uk/ Global/SRE%20Research%20Nov%202014.pdf.
8. Martellozzo E, Monaghan A, Adler JR, Davidson J, Leyva R, Horvath MAH. (2016) "I wasn't sure it was normal to watch it…"A quantitative and qualitative examination of the impact of online pornography on the values, attitudes, beliefs and behaviours of children and young people. Project Report. Middlesex University, NSPCC, OCC. 2016. http://dx.doi.org/10.6084/m9.figshare.3382393. Final accepted version (with author's formatting). Available from: Middlesex University's Research Repository at http://eprints. mdx.ac.uk/19989/.
9. Janssen E, Bancroft J. The Dual-Control Model: The role of sexual inhibition and excitation in sexual arousal and behavior. In E Janssen, (Ed.), Online Doctor. *The Psychophysiology of Sex.* Bloomington, IN: Indiana University Press, 2007, 197–222.
10. Bardo MT. The Mesolimbic Dopamine Reward System and Drug Addiction. In PM Miller, et al. (Eds.) *Biological Research on Addiction: Comprehensive Addictive Behaviors and Disorders.* Lexington, KY: University of Kentucky, 2013, Vol.2, 209–217.
11. Nestler EJ, Barrot M, Self DW. ΔFosB: A sustained molecular switch for addiction. *PNAS* 2001;98(20):11042–11046.
12. Berridge KC, Robinson TE. What is the role of dopamine in reward: Hedonic impact, reward learning, or incentive salience? *Brain Res Brain Res Rev* 1998;28(3):309–369.
13. Nestler EJ. Is there a common molecular pathway for addiction? *Nature Neurosci* 2005;9:1445–1449.
14. Trifilieff P, Martinez D. Imaging addiction: D_2 receptors and dopamine signalling in the striatum as biomarkers for impulsivity. *Neuropharmacology* 2014;76(Part B):498–509.
15. Yau YHC, Potenza MN. Gambling disorder and other behavioral addictions: Recognition and treatment. *Harv Rev Psychiatry* 2015;23(2):134–146.
16. Dahl RE. Adolescent brain development: A period of vulnerabilities and opportunities. *Ann NY Acad Sci* 2004;1021:1–22.
17. Fowler JL, Volkow ND, Kassed CA. Imaging the addicted human brain. *Sci Pract Perspect* 2007;3:4–16.
18. Miner MH, Raymond N, Mueller BA et al. Preliminary investigation of the impulsive and neuroanatomical characteristics of compulsive sexual behavior. *Psychiatry Res* 2009;174:146–151.
19. Johnson RN. *Aggression in Man and Animals.* Philadelphia, PA: WB Saunders, 1972, 94.
20. Fiorino DF, Coury A, Phillips AG. Dynamic changes in nucleus accumbens dopamine efflux during the Coolidge effect in male rats. *J Neurosci* 1997;17(12):4849–4855.
21. Holden C. Behavioral addictions: Do they exist? *Science* 2001;294:980.
22. Hilton DL, Watts C. Pornography addiction: A neuroscience perspective. *Surg Neurol Int* 2011;2:19.
23. Joseph PN, Sharma RK, Agarwal A et al. Men ejaculate larger volumes of semen, more motile sperm, and more quickly when exposed to images of novel women. *Evol Psychol Sci* 2015;1:195.
24. Delmonico DL. In memoriam Alvin Cooper. *Sex Addict Compulsivity* 2004;11(3):82–84.
25. American Society of Addictive Medicine. www.asam.org/resources/definition-of-addiction.
26. Kafka MP. Hypersexual disorder: A proposed diagnosis for DSM-V. *Arch Sex Behav* 2010;39(2):377–400.
27. NSPCC. Childline annual review 2015/16: It turned out someone did care. London: NSPCC. 2016. Available from: https://lfstest.nspxyz.net/services-and-resources/research-and-resources/2016/ childline-annual-review-2015-16-turned-out-someone-did-care/
28. Tinbergen N. *The Study of Instinct.* Oxford, UK: Clarendon Press, 1989.
29. Hilton DL. Pornography addiction—A supranormal stimulus considered in the context of neuroplasticity. *Socioaffective Neurosci Psychol* 2013;3:20767.
30. Toates F. *How Sexual Desire Works: The Enigmatic Urge.* Cambridge, UK: Cambridge University Press, 2014.

31. Barlow DH, Sakheim DK, Beck JG. Anxiety increases sexual arousal. *J Abnorm Psychol* 1983;92:49–54.

32. Harper GW, Serrano PA, Bruce D et al. The internet's multiple roles in facilitating the sexual orientation identity development of gay and bisexual male adolescents. *Am J Men's Health* 2016;10(5):359–376.

33. Weinberg MS, Williams CJ, Kleiner S et al. Pornography, normalization, and empowerment. *Arch Sex Behav* 2010;39(6):1389–1401.

34. Bőthe B, Tóth-Király I, Zsila Á et al. The development of the problematic pornography consumption scale (PPCS). *J Sex Res* 2018;55(3):395–406.

35. Kor A, Zilcha-Mano S, Fogel YA et al. Psychometric development of the problematic pornography use scale. *Addict Behav* 2014;39(5):861–868.

36. Miller R. The feeling-state theory of impulse-control disorders and the Impulse-Control Disorder Protocol. *Traumatology* 2010;16(3):2–10.

37. Hall P, Recovery K-S. *Sex Addiction Help. Initial Questionnaire Analysis*. Paula Hall & Associates. Available from: www.paulahall.co.uk/.

38. YouTube. *A mindmap for sex and porn addiction*. Paula Hall & Associates. Available from: https://youtu.be/1BHAREf9zmU

39. Kick Start Recovery. Available from: Sexaddictionhelp.co.uk; https://thelaurelcentre.co.uk/sex-addiction-recovery-courses.

40. Park BY, Wilson G, Berger J et al. Is Internet pornography causing sexual dysfunctions? A Review with Clinical Reports. *Behav Sci* 2016;6(3):17.

41. Seigfried-Spellar KC, Rogers MK. Does deviant pornography use follow a Guttman-like progression? *Comput Hum Behav* 2013;29:1997–2003.

42. NoFap. Available from: https://www.nofap.com/forum/index.php.

43. Carvalho J, Gomes AQ, Laja P et al. Gender differences in sexual arousal and affective responses to erotica: The effects of type of film and fantasy instructions. *Arch Sex Behav* 2013;42(6):1011–1119.

44. Hald GM. Gender differences in pornography consumption among young heterosexual Danish adults. *Arch Sex Behav* 2006;35(5):577–585.

45. Rupp HA, Wallen K. Sex differences in response to visual sexual stimuli: A review. *Arch Sex Behav* 2008;37(2):206–218.

46. Hartmann U, Philippsohn S, Heiser K et al. Low sexual desire in midlife and older women: Personality factors, psychosocial development, present sexuality. *Menopause* 2004;11(6 Pt 2):726–740.

47. Harkness EL, Mullan B, Blaszczynski A. Association between pornography use and sexual risk behaviors in adult consumers: A systematic review. *Cyberpsychol Behav Soc Netw* 2015;18(2):59–71.

48. Rogala C, Tydén T. Does pornography influence young women's sexual behavior? *Women's Health Issues* 2003;13(1):39–43.

49. Smith PK, Thompson F, Davidson J. Cyber safety for adolescent girls: Bullying, harassment, sexting, pornography, and solicitation. *Curr Opin Obstet Gynecol* 2014;26(5):360–365.

50. Griffiths MD. Internet sex addiction: A review of empirical research. *Addict Res Theory* 2012;2:111–124.

51. Griffiths MD. A systematic review of online sex addiction and clinical treatments using CONSORT evaluation. *Curr Addict Rep* 2015;2:163–174.

52. Pitchers KK, Balfour ME, Lehman MN et al. Neuroplasticity in the mesolimbic system induced by natural reward and subsequent reward abstinence. *Biol Psychiatry* 2010;67:872–879.

53. Cash H, Rae CD, Steel AH et al. Internet addiction: A brief summary of research and practice. *Curr Psychiatry Rev* 2012;8(4):292–298.

54. Adinoff B. Neurobiologic processes in drug reward and addiction. *Harv Rev Psychiatry* 2004;12(6):305–320.

55. Prause N, Janssen E, Georgiadis J et al. Data do not support sex as addictive. *Lancet Psychiatry* 2017;4(12):899.

56. Potenza M, Gola M, Voon V et al. Is excessive sexual behaviour an addictive disorder? *Lancet Psychiatry* 2017;4(9):663–664.

USEFUL RESOURCES

Carnes P. *Out of the Shadows (Revised Edition)*. Center City, MN: Hazeldon, 2001.

Griffin-Shelley E. *Adolescent Sex and Love Addicts – In Clinical Management of Sex Addiction*. Abingdon, UK: Routledge, 2002.

Hall P. *Understanding and Treating Sex Addiction*. Abingdon, UK: Routledge, 2013.

Hall P. *Sex Addiction: The Partner's Perspective*. Abingdon, UK: Routledge, 2015.

Hall P. *Confronting Porn, A Comprehensive Guide for Christians Struggling with Porn and Churches Wanting to Help*. London: Care/Naked Truth, 2016.

Lewis M. *Memoires of an Addicted Brain*. New York, NY: Public Affairs, 2011.

Steffens B, Means M. *Your Sexually Addicted Spouse: How Partners Can Cope and Heal*. New York, NY: New Horizon Press, 2009.

Weiss R. *Cruise Control – Understanding Sex Addiction in Gay Men*. New York, NY: Alyson Publications, 2005.

Wilson G. *Your Brain on Porn – Internet Pornography and the Emerging Science of Addiction*. Kent, UK: Commonwealth Publishing, 2015.

For websites in specialist addiction settings, see list in text.

FURTHER TRAINING FOR PROFESSIONALS

Diploma in Sex Addiction Counselling, ISAT (The Institute for Sex Addiction) training. E-mail: info@ theinstituteforsexaddictiontraining.co.uk.

22

Non-Consensual Sex and Psychosexual Problems

Sally Soodeen

Introduction

Sexual problems arise for many different reasons, as can be seen from the preceding chapters; but sadly, for a significant minority of patients presenting to a psychosexual clinic there will be a history of sexual trauma.

This is an area of psychosexual medicine that is crucial to reflect upon if we are going to be of use to those who seek our help. The history may be clearly detailed in the referral letter; something that the subject has sought help for previously and actively struggled with for many years; or it may come to light as together you begin to unpick this person's particular story and difficulty. Even then it may never become explicit but merely be sensed in the room like a ghost or a shadow that is present but not ready to show itself to the light.

Sexual Abuse and Its Sequelae

Non-consensual sexual contact includes any situation where full consent for whatever activity of a sexual nature that occurred was withheld or could not fully be given for whatever reason. It has been defined as 'where a person(s) uses force or other means so that they can do sexual things to you that you did not want them to do or where a person uses force or other means to make you do things you did not want to do' (1). One of the sequelae may be a sexual problem.

Both sexual assault (SA) and childhood sexual abuse (CSA) are considered here. The victim may be of any age or gender, sexual preference and from any social group. Disturbingly, male rape was only recognised in law as late as 1994 (2).

It is not uncommon to receive a referral detailing there has been trauma in the past but this is fully resolved and definitely not the cause of the problem presenting today; thus, issuing a warning signal 'don't go there'. That may well be true and the history in question might not be relevant at all; but it is our job to sensitively assess whether the background needs some gentle exploration and acknowledge that a line had been drawn. Conversely, the opposite may occur and the history of sexual trauma is presented so openly it can feel like an impenetrable blanket around which any other work must be negotiated, when in fact it is acting as a barrier, smothering the underlying and often unrelated problems and stopping us from working effectively.

We are talking about a common problem; figures widely vary but it is conservatively estimated that 12% females and 8% males were sexually abused in childhood (3), and 20%–33% women (over the age of 16) have experienced sexual assault (4). There has been much less research done regarding male victims. A British study of 930 homosexual men reported that just over a quarter had been subjected to sex without consent (1).

Figures are higher in attendees of genitourinary medicine clinics or gynaecology outpatient settings (5), many initially presenting with physical problems especially pain or symptoms relating to possible infection. We know women with a history of sexual trauma are more likely to experience pelvic pain (6). Sexual problems post-CSA are extremely common; one source quotes as high as 94% (7).

Other psychological and physical negative health outcomes are common after sexual trauma including

- Anxiety and depression
- Post-traumatic stress disorder
- Substance misuse
- Suicidal tendencies
- Chronic pain
- Chronic muscle tension
- Gastrointestinal disorders
- Cardiac symptoms (5,8,9)

Stories can sometimes be difficult to hear for those trusted with the disclosure. Once heard, it can be hard for the practitioner to assimilate and absorb the pain and distress. The work can be messy, especially if the trauma occurred at a young age and the perpetrator was a primary caregiver. Other forms of childhood abuse such as emotional abuse, physical abuse or neglect may be relevant.

As Gill Wakley writes; '(they may) need support from a doctor who doesn't get overwhelmed by the story' and 'there will be a need for reflection and repair for the doctor'.

The importance of the individual story must be emphasized; avoiding making assumptions. 'Listening to find out what the problem is for that particular patient and not allowing distraction by the awfulness of sexual abuse is the most important skill that can be offered to the patient' (9). This has been emphasised in other parts of this book.

Sexual abuse and assault involve creating or exploiting a power imbalance. The victim is left with a sense of shame, guilt and powerlessness (9). This needs careful recognition in the consultation. The Institute of Psychosexual Medicine (IPM) teaches us to approach a problem in a spirit of mutual ignorance and shared endeavour. 'The professional needs to avoid taking control; which can reinforce the sense of helplessness. They should…remain safe unshockable, unaroused by the excitement of the revelation/drama' (9).

Working with Patients Who Have Suffered Abuse

The practitioner/patient relationship is the cornerstone of our work. While working with victims of sexual trauma there will, however, be times when we struggle to build a strong therapeutic alliance. There may naturally be a fear of intimacy (7) and possibly a need for the survivor to remain in control within relationships to feel safe from harm. At times this dynamic can be played out during the consultation. The power imbalance that inevitably occurs when someone visits your consulting room, often after several months wait, to seek your advice for a very personal intimate problem may invoke a defence. The consultation risks being experienced as a re-creation of the abusive situation. There are times when you might begin to feel like a perpetrator. This is most likely during a genital examination. Asking someone to undress, expose their genitalia and possibly permit penetration by a swab or speculum in an environment which makes them feel uncomfortable to begin with could re-create some very distressing feelings. However, it may be something totally unpredictable that triggers a disturbing reaction, something that is not even identifiable to the patient and unrelated to the previous trauma.

The need for reflective case discussion with appropriate colleagues, ideally as supervision, cannot be emphasized highly enough.

> As the young woman took her seat after what had been to my mind, a perfectly normal examination with a chaperone present; I asked her if she was OK. She stared absently into the distance and spoke with quiet controlled anger. 'I feel violated' she said. I felt chilled, and the strength seemed to drain from me. Yet I was totally unable to unravel what had caused her to feel this way; there was nothing specific about what had just occurred that either of us could identify to have triggered this reaction. It was only in discussion with my training group that I was able to question whether she may have previously been sexually abused.

Similarly, there could be situations where damage inflicted on the patient causes them to relate to you in learnt roles that oscillate between presenting as a victim and a perpetrator.

The 'victim' is helpless and vulnerable; making you into a 'rescuer' and hence reinforcing their inability to help themselves. The 'perpetrator' could be experienced by you as abusive, temporarily making you into a victim who is thus paralysed from doing the work needed in the room (adapted from Karpman) (10). You are, after all, probing much relied upon defences and the threat of danger that arises may provoke a hostile response. The pivotal factor in this situation is to be able to recognise what is occurring and try to reflect the feelings, thus enabling the patient to begin to understand their own struggle. Uncomfortable as it may feel; these interactions could be massively therapeutic.

There will be times where it becomes clear that the trauma remains unprocessed or too overwhelming to address and the clinician must make the decision to stop psychosexual work and allow this other work to happen. This could be, for example, with trauma-focussed cognitive behavioural therapy or eye movement desensitisation and reprocessing (11). We need to accept that this point of recognition is a valid outcome for brief psychosexual therapy. The patient may choose to return to think more about their sexual difficulty at a later time.

> Classification of the severity of trauma is unhelpful in this setting. Hudson-Allez writes 'It is unhelpful to classify abuse into mild or severe as each individual experiences their trauma differently irrespective of the classification of the event (3)'. It is far more important to think how much past events are affecting the present than to trawl through what actually happened.
> Once again, the individual story is paramount.

CASE 1

Anya was 36. Sex had been painful since the birth of her second child 6 years ago. She was small and slightly built with an easy smile and deep-set eyes. There was something childlike about her as she followed me in from the waiting room. She was in a loving relationship with Aron and they had sex about five or six times a year, but she had no spontaneous desire and described a feeling of distance during intimacy, as if disconnected from her body. There was now little pleasure during sex, and occasionally she would have flashbacks to the abuse she had suffered as a child which was hugely distressing for both of them. Aron was affectionate and patient. He did not pressure her and she appreciated that.

Anya had been sexually abused by her uncle from the age of 9 to the age of 12 when she told her mother. The family moved after this and subsequently she never saw much of him. Her teenage years had been difficult and she had sought sexual partners as a refuge, acknowledging that it made her feel better about herself.

Her brother had in some ways blamed her for the fragmentation of their close extended family. He had developed a drug problem in his teens. Anya carried a huge amount of guilt for what had happened but had undergone counselling in her early 20s and felt that the issues around the abuse had fully resolved. She had met Aron at 26 and their sex life was exciting and fulfilling at first, which is why she could not understand what was happening now.

I offered to examine her and she agreed willingly, maybe a little surprisingly considering how painful she had found previous examinations. She lay neatly on the bed, with a sense of being terribly compliant. I reflected this, a picture of someone who did as she was told, to please others?

Anya looked thoughtful. She said she did see herself as someone who needed to please other people to maintain her own self-esteem. I wondered if this was what was happening in sex, that she felt she needed to keep Aron happy and strengthen their bond as a family.

Anya returned next time looking more adult. She said she had realised that by choosing to continue having sex but in a detached dissociated way it prevented her from feeling any enjoyment or pleasure. It was like she was opting to put herself in a position similar to continued abuse, rather than allow herself to have needs and feel pleasure. She was then able to talk about how the sex with her uncle, although it revolted her and was painful had sometimes felt physically pleasurable and how ashamed she felt about it. She had coped by pretending she was not really there. On becoming a mother herself, these feelings of guilt and shame were re-awakened.

Over the next few sessions she was able to establish that the sex with her husband was different and ground herself in the reality of the here and now. The flashbacks became less terrifying as she did this, and she concentrated on developing coping mechanisms.

Anya craved affection but really struggled when the affection was seen a prelude to sex. Deep inside was a huge sense of guilt and responsibility for the break-up of her family. She had grown up with a sense of feeling she needed to be a 'people pleaser' to justify her own self-worth. As a young adult, she had used this desire to please others sexually, and the excitement of a new relationship with Aron allowed enjoyable sex in the early days, along with a very strong desire to create a stable family structure. Sex helped to reinforce her bond with him.

However, she had always approached sex with a slight sense of detachment. Sexual pleasure triggered feelings of self-blame and shame; therefore any feeling of arousal became linked with guilt and distress. Even anticipating sex triggered painful emotions so this became extended to sexual approaches, even foreplay or affection. She developed a fear of losing control during sex, which she saw as re-creating a sense of powerlessness.

Bob Foley writes; 'Adult perpetrators are very good at convincing victims that they are at fault. Sometimes they are left feeling that deep down they wanted the incident to happen' (12).

Foley visualises guilt as something survivors often carry around like a physical burden, unable to find any relief from the heavy load. He asks us to imagine it like a pile of bricks sitting on a table; what a weight to burden yourself with, to pick up those bricks each morning and load them into your backpack. Freedom from this guilt means learning that there is a choice, that it is possible to walk away unburdened, leaving the weight on the table.

'Only the survivor can put the bricks in his backpack, although others will try' (12). Many victims feel judged by those around them and may need help and support to put that burden back on the table. IPM work involves examining or at least acknowledging those bricks.

It is not uncommon for the sexual problem to be triggered after the birth of a child, especially if that child is female. Likewise, when a child nears the age when the abuse in the parent began, problems might begin. There may be deep-seated anger towards their own mother for not protecting them. If the mother was the abuser it hits the child hardest (3). Childbirth itself places a woman into a state of powerlessness and may be traumatic, especially if prolonged or complicated with multiple medical interventions and invasive examinations.

In Anya's case some understanding of her difficulty was gained from thinking together about how the examination affected her. Genital examination is a very powerful tool in working with survivors of sexual trauma. It may bring to light previously unacknowledged body unease. Castellini writes; 'Subjects reporting a history of childhood sexual abuse represent a population of patients with profound uneasiness, involving body perception, as well as sexual functioning' (13).

The very act of penetration by the examiner's fingers or speculum, however gently done with full consent and explanation may invoke a phobic or aversive reaction as it somehow triggers memory of the previous unwanted abusive intrusion. There are times when this can help to gain a further understanding of the difficulty, but as Bass describes, 'body memories' with no pictures attached might be triggered, allowing little understanding of where they originated (14).

At this point, in the room with someone whom you suspect may have been abused, it may be wise to be wary of a temptation to start digging for repressed memories; Hudson-Allez cautions that psychological splitting occurs to help cope with trauma. This allows the person to forget it, burying it deep in the subconscious. She believes this is functional, and repressed material will emerge when the person is able to cope with it (3). After all, identifying as a 'victim' implies something soiled or damaged. A gentle question will usually suffice to leave the door open if they are ready to talk about it.

Jehu (7) in 'Beyond Sexual Abuse' writes about coping skills training. This would be individualised to fit the particular difficulties, with the emphasis on the patient learning to recognise early signs of distress or threat and react to them with coping responses rather than avoidance or panic, i.e. 'Don't think about how bad you may feel, think about what you can do about it'. Appropriate coping skills might be relaxation training, or thought and image stopping techniques such as reality orientation. This is where the victim concentrates on the immediate environment and learns to describe in meticulous detail the people and objects around them. Jehu suggests working out in advance a specific 'coping plan' to use in particular situations where a threat is perceived. These techniques have been shown to work well where a specific trigger is identified such as a sexual advance or the prospect of a genital examination.

The sexual problem does not always manifest at the start of a relationship. While things are not too serious and full of novelty, sex may well be enjoyable and problem free. But relationships with the abuser may have been a complex web of emotions, particularly if it was someone closely connected to the child such as a family member or authority figure. Jehu writes 'the more intimate a relationship becomes the more likely it is that it will recapitulate the earlier traumatic experience with the offender who was emotionally close to the victim' (7). This at times leads to the inability to have an affectionate and sexual relationship with the same person, reflecting the craving for affection from the offender who reciprocated by imposing sexual demands either instead of, or in addition to, affection (7).

It may be difficult to predict what will trigger feelings of powerlessness, self-blame or depression. The most innocuous sexual advance or feeling can trigger a flashback or distressing memory or bodily sensation. Even self-examination may feel like an intrusion. Bass talks of flashbacks as ghosts (14). The memory might not be associated with any pictures but may be a distressing 'body memory'.

It is not surprising how much easier it is then to disconnect from your body during a sexual experience, even if it is loving and consensual. The ability to dissociate is likely to be what helped the child to cope with the abuse but is now what is precipitating or perpetuating the hindrance for the adult. Similar phenomena occur after sexual assault. Recognising this and why it is happening with time to talk it through is crucial, allowing the patient to have the choice to reconnect with his or her body. An example of this is the patient who presents with 'no sensation' in their genitals. On testing neurologically everything appears to be normal but they are unable to perceive any stimulation; as one woman put it 'it depends whether it is on or off today', as if referring to something totally separate to a part of her own body. Jehu refers to this as 'genital or sexual anaesthesia' (7). Bass talks about taking your body on a first date; learning to make love to your own body (14). If touching the genitals is too difficult, she advises choosing a patch of skin somewhere on your body that is unlikely to provoke dangerous sensations and take care of it, rub lotion into it or touch it with a sensual fabric. Reconnecting with physical sensation without dissociating away could be a step towards being able to tolerate sexual activity. Sensual is sometimes a way to access sexual.

A lack of sexual arousal or libido is distressing, as if withholding from a partner who may be loving and caring. Rather than challenging the patient about wanting to restore libido, it could be easier to think of a willingness to begin to think about sex, which may be a more accessible legitimate entry point if not experiencing any sexual desire (14).

CASE 2

For the last 5 years, Harry was struggling to maintain his erection. Now in his late 40s, he had been abused by a teacher at his Catholic boarding school. Many years later the teacher had served time in prison and there had been a court case generating media interest which had been very difficult for him. He worked in marketing and was, at times, very successful but was also prone to heavy drinking and periods of deep depression. Like many victims of sexual abuse he suffered nightmares, anger problems and anxiety. Harry identified as gay and he would regularly use social media to meet men for sex, which gave him some physical pleasure but was often regretted. He expressed that what he really wanted was to have a loving partner. He enjoyed receiving anal sex but would love to be able to have an erection that allowed him to achieve penetration as well. Ten years previously he had been sexually assaulted in a park after binge drinking but not gone to the police for fear of not being taken seriously. When he was alone he could masturbate easily and generally maintained a good strong erection.

He was an attractive man and was often sought by others for sex. Harry's general practitioner (GP) had previously given him Viagra which gave him an erection but he described himself as being able to 'sabotage' its effects in the presence of a partner and the erection was soon lost. He saw himself as someone who overthinks things and would easily get overwhelmed by negative thoughts and the expectation of failure.

Harry was lively and chatty with a tendency to bite his nails while talking to me. He found it hard to sit still. The room seemed to fill with nervous energy as he entered, and our appointments would often over-run. A large built man with white blond hair, now flecked with silvery grey, he took great care with his appearance, always looking as if he had thought about what to wear for an appointment. There was something that made me reflect he never quite seemed to feel good enough, as if there was always something to prove.

I asked if I could examine him and he consented, but as he lay on the bed he almost looked as if he was apologising for his genitals. I reflected on the discrepancy between how other men saw him as sexual and how he might be feeling about himself. He began to speak about the abuse. As a child adults would tell him he had angelic looks, and the abusing teacher made him feel as if Harry himself had initiated the sexual contact between them. His involvement with the teacher had afforded him some special privileges at school. The guilt he felt was magnified by worrying about how, during the abuse, he had easily got an erection when he was touched, even though inside he was sickened and afraid. He told me one of the reasons he had not reported the assault was because he was erect and he worried he would not be believed as it had taken place in a park where it was known that men meet for anonymous sex.

I reflected that it seemed as though his erection was linked with fear and danger, not pleasure and he agreed. We talked about how potency could have the power to do harm as well as to share pleasure. Harry never returned for a follow-up appointment.

Harry's abuser had made him feel as if he initiated the sex between them, and despite a successful prosecution of the offender, he had never managed to lose the guilt and shame leaving him with periods of depression and self-destructive behaviour. He struggled with becoming intimate, choosing sex which was physically satisfying but where he did not feel at risk of emotional exposure. It may have been this fear of intimacy which meant he did not attend a follow-up appointment after we had uncovered some of his defences. By choosing to engage with sex that he knew he would later regret, he was on the brink of conducting a re-enactment of his victimization, as if self-harming.

He was not able to feel comfortable with himself as a confidently powerful male; the idea of him being able to penetrate someone else with his erection was not something he was ready to live with. Male identity in our society still prises the characteristics of independence, competence and power (2). Harry's abusive past had prevented him from being able to nurture his positive masculine selfhood. He frequently felt needy, weak and powerless.

Repeated victimisation reinforced his feelings of vulnerability; as Foley writes (12); 'survivors picture themselves going through life with a target painted on their backs'. In fact, boys who suffer abuse as children are more likely to be the victims of sexual assault as adults (1).

It is known that there is a significant association between CSA in boys and risk of alcohol abuse and self-harm in adulthood (1). Overall, however there has been less research done regarding sexual trauma in males than females and some of the work historically focussed on the possibility of victims becoming perpetrators themselves as adults (1).

We know there is huge under-reporting of sexual crimes against men. If the victim does not identify as MSM (a man who has sex with men), there is a fear of being labelled gay and he may struggle with his sexual identity. There is little research into male victims of sexual assault by females. A myth still exists that in a sexual assault a terrified male victim would not become erect or ejaculate. This is a view that at times has been shared by lawyers (2). However, high levels of physiological arousal can lead to involuntary erection and/or ejaculation, even in terrified men (2). Male survivors may be left with huge guilt if they feel their genitals did respond, despite their explicit lack of consent.

There is another myth that men should be strong and able to defend themselves. We know that perpetrators commit sexual assault in order to show control over others rather than for sexual satisfaction (2). Not all sexual assaults on males are committed by men who would normally choose to have sex with men; the intention being to dominate and humiliate. The response of a terrified man to an assault may include 'helpless and passive submission' (2) which can add to his feelings of fractured masculinity.

In time, when he is in the right place and with the right help, Harry may be able to build his sexual self in a secure and positive framework free from guilt and shame.

CASE 3

Bryony was 20. She had been referred by the nurse at her GP practice because attempting to take a swab test had been very painful. When asked if it hurt during sex Bryony had become tearful. The nurse had noted that she had attended the GP surgery several times over the past couple of years complaining of discharge and had been treated for thrush. She missed her first psychosexual appointment but the GP wrote requesting another, saying her problems were continuing.

Sitting in the waiting room behind thick makeup, with a large fringe of hair covering one eye, she found it hard to meet my gaze as I called her. She was clearly very nervous. I asked how I could help, but she said she was not sure why she was here, just that her GP asked her to come.

Gradually we pieced together a story of sex that was painful with no expectation of any pleasure for her, and a feeling of being contaminated with infection despite repeated negative swab tests. When I suggested an examination she looked reluctant saying no one had ever found anything. On asking why she finds examinations so difficult, she complained about the speculum being 'shoved up there'. That sounds horrible, I commented, even violent. She allowed me to gently wonder if she had ever been hurt, or had any harmful experiences with sex.

Bryony started to cry. Two years ago she got drunk at a party and a boy whom she vaguely knew offered to walk her home. He raped her in a park next door to the party and left her there. He had then told others that she had invited him to have sex with her and even one of her friends believed him. A couple of people had even made jokes about it, implying she was a sexual predator herself. Bryony was left feeling dirty and humiliated, unable to defend herself or protest. Her demeanour reflected her sense of utter powerlessness.

During the assault she described how she had become floppy and passive; although she had clearly not consented, she now berated herself for not having resisted more and felt guilty for this.

I suppressed my instinct to reassure, to become motherly and tell her it was not her fault, even to encourage her to report him to the police. I was worried he will do this again.

Instead I asked how she felt about her body. 'It feels disgusting'. She went on to describe how distressed she felt when she noticed vaginal discharge on her underwear. Since then she had never been able to tolerate the feeling of being sexually aroused and had totally 'shut off' from her genitals. She never masturbated and had not been able to put a finger inside her vagina.

Bryony allowed me to empathise with her feelings of powerlessness and contamination, as well as exposure. I then attempted to encourage her to see her symptoms in the light of these very powerful feelings, and she was able to see the link. I did however, reassure her that the 'flop' response to trauma is a very well-recognised part of the flight, fight, and freeze or flop response which is an inbuilt survival technique, not a sign of acquiescence.

She returned for two further sessions; although sex was not any more enjoyable for her, she made no further mention of the discharge and her confidence in her body began to grow.

Bryony was suffering from low self-esteem and possibly underlying depression after her trauma. It did not seem surprising that she was unable to get aroused and enjoy sex. The cruelty and injustice of what happened to her had made it difficult for her to grow into her sexual self as she might otherwise have done. She was also afraid of being perceived as too sexual which society views as a negative trait, especially for girls; so, she effectively shut down her sexual response. Sexual shame is higher in victims of sexual trauma (15).

Her focus on the vaginal discharge gave her a reason to seek help, even though she had been unable to directly ask for the help she really needed. Repeated reassurance that the discharge was physiological did nothing to address her deep feelings of contamination and self-disgust and may have actually made her feel more alienated.

Victims often present with physical symptoms. As Gill Wakley writes (9), 'powerlessness makes you manipulative; unable to ask for things directly for fear of repeated pain and rejection'. This also applies to sexual needs, especially if sexual pleasure is linked to guilt or feelings of self-disgust. Bryony had no expectation that sex would give her any pleasure.

Self-blame and self-disgust are very common after sexual assault, and all aspects of sexual functioning may be affected. Bryony may choose to react by avoiding sexual contact for a while, which may be exactly what she needs as there will be less risk of her triggering negative thought patterns. However, if this avoidance is prolonged it may eventually deny her the chance to be exposed to positive, loving and therefore corrective sexual experiences, thus maintaining her sexual difficulties (16). Meanwhile, she will hopefully be able to continue working to restore her self-esteem and feelings of self-worth while learning to enjoy her body sexually without provoking shame.

Conclusion

Not all those presenting with sexual problems have been abused, and not all those who have experienced sexual trauma will present with sexual dysfunction, but our sexual selves evolve out of a web of our past life experiences. In those who are affected, any aspect of sexual function may be impaired. The severity of the abuse is much less relevant than the individual experience of it. Shame, guilt and powerlessness are overwhelming emotions that stunt the growth of a healthy sexual self. Brief intervention psychosexual therapy, particularly involving a psychosomatic genital examination, is an invaluable tool in helping survivors of sexual trauma overcome sexual difficulties.

REFERENCES

1. Coxell A, King M, Mezey G, Gordon D. Lifetime prevalence, characteristics, and associated problems of non-consensual sex in men: Cross sectional survey. *BMJ* 1999;18:846–850.
2. Coxell A, King M. Male victims of rape and sexual abuse. *Sex Marital Ther* 1996;11(3):297–308.
3. Hudson-Allez A. *Time Limited Therapy in a General Practice Setting.* London: Sage, 1997.
4. Ashby BD, Kaul P. Post traumatic stress disorder after sexual abuse in adolescent girls. *J Paediatr Adolesc Gynaecol* 2016;29(6):531–536.
5. Cichowski SB, Dunivan GC, Komesu YM et al. Sexual abuse history and pelvic floor disorders in women. *South Med J* 2013;106(12):675–678.

6. Petrak J, Doyle AM, Williams L et al. The psychological impact of sexual assault: A study of female attenders of a sexual health psychology service. *Sex Marital Ther* 1997;12(4):339–345.

7. Jehu D. *Beyond Sexual Abuse; Therapy with Women Who were Childhood Victims*. New York, NY: John Wiley and Sons, 1988.

8. Schliep K, Mumford S, Johnstone E et al. Sexual and physical abuse and gynaecologic disorders. *Human Reprod* 2016;31(8):1904–1912.

9. Wakley G. *Sexual Abuse and the Primary Care Doctor*. London: Chapman and Hall, 1991.

10. Karpman S. Available from: http://karpmandramatriangle.com

11. Post-Traumatic Stress Disorder; management; Clinical guideline CG26; March 2005. Available from: www.nice.org.uk.

12. Foley B. *The Death of Innocence: Surviving Trauma*. Bob Foley, 2002.

13. Castellini G, Lo Sauro C, Lelli L et al. Childhood sexual abuse moderates the relationship between sexual functioning and eating disorder psychopathology in anorexia nervosa and bulimia nervosa. *J Sex Med* 2013;10(9):2190–2200.

14. Bass E, Davis L. *The Courage to Heal: A Guide for Women Survivors of Childhood Sexual Abuse*. London: Vermillion, 1988.

15. Pulverman C, Meston C. Sexual dysfunction among women with a history of childhood sexual abuse: The role of negative appraisal of genital arousal and sexual shame. *J Sex Med* 2016;3(6):S240–S241.

16. Kelly E, Gidycz C. Mediators of the relationship between sexual assault and sexual functioning difficulties among college women. *Psychol Violence* 2017;7(4):574–582.

23

Vaginal Dysmorphia

Clare Gribbin

Introduction

This chapter explores the psychological, psychosexual and psychosocial issues that some women encounter relating to the structure and appearance of their genitalia and vaginal anatomy. This is a growing issue in Western society and particularly for young people including adolescents. Psychosexual doctors and allied health professionals are increasingly seeing patients with significant concerns about the appearance of their genitalia and consequential psychosexual dysfunction.

It is important that those working in psychosexual medicine have a thorough understanding of some key definitions, diagnoses and related topics in order to have an informed approach to any client's individual issues. In our practice we may have clarity about what psychosexual medicine is and is not, but our patients do not arrive with a pre-determined label or problem. Our knowledge must be up to date and broad enough to ensure that we work within appropriate ethical and legal frameworks. We also have a duty of care to inform our patients of options and signpost them to the right service if they need alternatives. The pathway for people requesting female genital cosmetic surgery (FGCS) now includes counselling. It is therefore essential that healthcare professionals practising psychosexual medicine are equipped to see these patients. They may or may not have a declared sexual issue.

The chapter therefore describes and discusses female genital and vaginal morphology, vaginal dysmorphia, FGCS including labiaplasty and briefly comments on body dysmorphia, medically indicated genital and vaginal surgery and female genital mutilation (FGM) for context and completeness. Ethical issues and the law are described where relevant. Psychosocial influences and current controversies are highlighted. These areas are essential to our knowledge base if we are to be effective psychosexual practitioners.

The final part of the chapter centres on what the psychosexual practitioner has to offer. Much of this detail is covered in other chapters and therefore it is presented in summary form. A case history and other patient examples are included to illustrate client issues and psychosexual practice.

This chapter aims to equip readers with the knowledge and background to confidently explore psychological, psychosexual and psychosocial issues relating to clients' perceived anatomical concerns about their genitalia.

Normal Female Genitalia: What Does This Mean?

There is a wide variation in the external genital appearance in women. In Westernised nations, the modern ideal appearance of the vulva is flat, hairless and with no protrusion of the labia minora or clitoris (1). The media and Internet portray female genitalia as non-protuberant and women use these sources to benchmark themselves against perceived normality (2). The Internet gives access to images not previously available – images chosen/put on there by questionable sources, i.e. not clinicians. One could argue that the images are pre-pubertal and that the majority of women from adolescence onwards could perceive themselves as abnormal in comparison to the public images available to them. Herein lies the issue. The labia minora, the clitoral hood and the clitoral body are portrayed publicly as ideally hidden within the labia majora. For the majority of women post-puberty, this is not the case. Many women are therefore at risk of perceiving their genitalia as abnormal. This abnormal perception leads some to seek medical help and others to live with psychological torment, low self-esteem or perceived vaginal dysmorphia. There is no doubt that there has been a steady increase in requests for genital surgery for perceived abnormal appearance (3).

The challenge of what is 'normal' is compounded by a lack of knowledge within some healthcare practitioners as well as a lack of published literature. There have been some studies on labial size, but the numbers are small (4). Some have defined a stretched labial width of 6 cm as being abnormal and therefore a justification for surgery. Others have different criteria. There is no agreed and consistent consensus on this. Labial hypertrophy remains a poorly defined diagnosis with no clear diagnostic criteria. What is clear is that women's genital and vaginal anatomy is very varied and often asymmetrical (as with other body parts). What is 'normal' is wide ranging. If medical practitioners are unsure of normality this can lead to unnecessary referrals to tertiary care or private facilities which further reinforces and medicalises the issue. Healthcare practitioners should familiarise themselves with normal variance and gain confidence in exploring this with clients. Many clients could be reassured without the need for referral on to counsellors, medical practitioners or surgeons.

What Is Vaginal Dysmorphia?

The *Oxford Dictionary* defines *dysmorphia* as follows: 'deformity or abnormality in the shape or size of a specified part of the body' (5). This relates to any part of the body including the vagina. In this chapter, the term *vaginal dysmorphia* is used to describe a deformity or abnormality in the shape or size of the female genitalia or vagina. This may be real (actual) or perceived by the woman.

Vaginal dysmorphia as defined in this chapter is not a psychiatric condition (see section Body Dysmorphia: Body Dysmorphic Disorder). It is however a relatively new and frequent presentation to psychosexual and medical services in Western society. In the majority of cases referred, the problem relates to perceived deformity or abnormality or simple dislike of the genitalia and is therefore psychosocial and/or psychosexual in nature. However, in a minority, actual deformity or abnormality may found. The vaginal examination will reveal these cases during the consultation.

Female Genital Cosmetic Surgery Including Labiaplasty: What Is It and Why Are Requests Increasing?

The Royal College of Obstetricians and Gynaecologists (RCOG) defines FGCS as follows: 'FGCS refers to non-medically indicated cosmetic surgical procedures which change the structure and appearance of the healthy external genitalia of women, or internally in the case of vaginal tightening' (6).

There are a range of procedures under the umbrella of FGCS including labiaplasty (labial reduction), vaginal rejuvenation, hymenoplasty, revirgination and clitoral hood reduction. Radman (7) was one of the first to publish in the medical literature on labiaplasty. Liao et al. (8) published a review of the literature showing that it was not a commonly requested procedure until about 15 years ago and there is a paucity of papers published in the literature. It is a relatively recently developed surgical option in Western society.

The reason why FGCS is becoming more popular is a complex and extensive subject and an in-depth analysis is beyond the scope of this chapter. In brief, there are many companies marketing FGCS as a solution to better sexual experience, a younger body, being more attractive and being more youthful. Many make claims with no evidence base and omit discussion of the potential complications. Advertisements make claims such as: following FGCS you will feel better about yourself, feel body confident, no longer feel embarrassed or isolated, feel restored. These claims are very attractive and appealing with little or no regard for the whole story. Adolescents are a particularly vulnerable group. They compare themselves to their peers and want to 'fit in'. Sex education in schools has made significant advances for boys in educating them that male genitalia are very varied. However, sex education has done little to reassure girls that the female genitalia vary in shape, size and symmetry. The fact that FGCS is on the rise and particularly in the private sector means that we must be equipped to deal with the requests and understand what is offered as well as the issues and the consequences for our clients.

Labiaplasty is probably the most commonly requested and offered FGCS. It is therefore worthy of explanation in this chapter. There are different types of surgery for labiaplasty which might be offered. These claim to have different complications associated with them. However, due to multiple factors there is no good research to date which gives reliable data on outcomes.

One surgical approach is to use a straight or slightly curvilinear incision (Figure 23.1); this is also known as 'edge resection'. Edge resection is reported to be the simplest procedure with the quickest recovery and with the least complications. Those describing the surgery mention that the labial edges can be replaced by scarred suture lines that cause chronic irritation and discomfort. They also report that with this method the natural contour of the labia can be compromised.

An alternative incision is the 'wedge resection' (Figure 23.2). Some report that this is more likely to preserve the normal contours of the labia and reduce the amount of exposed scar tissue. A reported disadvantage is that it is associated with more swelling, possibly due to lymph drainage issues.

Other modifications of the wedge resection are described where several smaller V-shaped wedges of labia are removed to try to improve outcomes. These are described as modified wedge, Z resection or M resection.

The labia minora play an important role in sexual response and function. At their edges there is dense nerve innervation and the presence of oestrogen receptors. At their base there is erectile tissue which becomes engorged during arousal. There is no good research on sexual function following labiaplasty. There are, however, numerous patient accounts of sexual dysfunction following FGCS. Clearly this

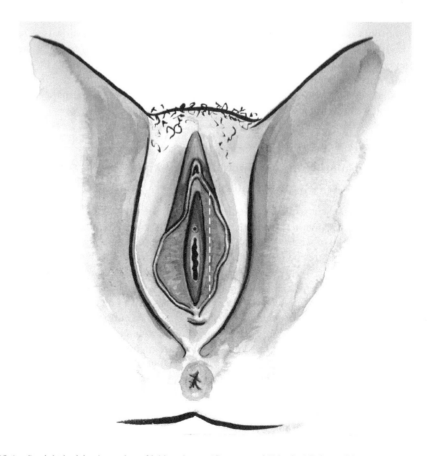

FIGURE 23.1   Straight incision/resection of labia minora. (Courtesy of Sidonie AR Brough.)

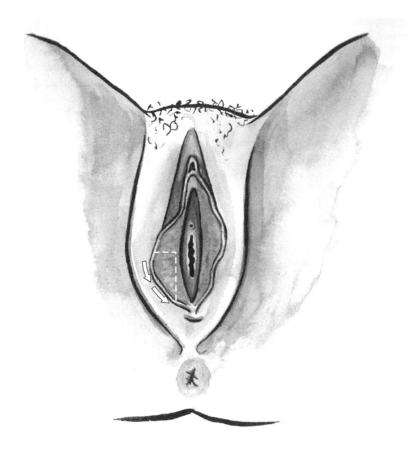

FIGURE 23.2   Wedge resection of labia minora. (Courtesy of Sidonie AR Brough.)

needs to be set against the potential bias that patients whose sexual function has improved will not seek medical attention. Reliable research into surgical and sexual outcomes is lacking. Liao concludes that surgery appears to have been offered on demand, justified by verbal reports of physical and psychological difficulties that were not formally evaluated pre- or post-surgery.

FGCS is promoted by television programmes and the media. Procedures are publicised as 'safe' and without complications or side effects. Possible short-term complications include bleeding, infection and wound dehiscence. Longer-term complications include sexual difficulty, dyspareunia, vulvodynia, chronic pain, scarring, pruritus, skin discolouration, asymmetry and continued dissatisfaction following surgery. Obstetric effects include a likely increase in the need for episiotomy and request for caesarean section.

The overriding messages from the media, the private sector and advertisements are to promote surgery and abnormality among women rather than acceptance of normal genitalia. In contrast, the medical community is concerned about regulation of procedures, standard setting and information giving for cosmetic procedures. Much debate has been generated and the Department of Health published a review of the regulation of cosmetic interventions in 2013 (9). Healthcare practitioners should help women understand that their expectations regarding results following labiaplasty are often unrealistic and unachievable due to false information and claims from those promoting it (10). The RCOG in its Ethical opinion paper 2013 (6) clearly states that 'There are as yet no controlled or prospective studies investigating the clinical effectiveness, risks or long-term outcomes of labiaplasty'. To my knowledge this situation remains unchanged.

The rise in demand and availability of FGCS is evidence of an increasing psychosocial issue in Western society. The combination of psychological factors and the modern social environment including social media have impacted on some individuals' physical and mental well-being as well as their ability to function. The National Health Service in most areas has stopped funding FGCS. This has created a demand for private-sector surgery which is largely unregulated and has no evidence base.

One clear and consistent message that all health practitioners should promote is that if FGCS is to be undertaken, it should not be performed on anyone under the age of 18. This is because the labia minora are still developing and complications, such as asymmetry, could easily occur as the labia continue to develop and change. The younger the person is when they undergo FGCS the greater the potential problems (6). There is also concern that sexual sensation could be more affected by surgery at a young age.

Increasing numbers of adolescents present with unrealistic expectations about what their genitalia should look like. Increasingly young people are exposed to pornography and many young women have had partners informing them that they do not 'look normal' after benchmarking against Internet pictures which are distorting reality. Adolescents have a strong desire to fit in with their peer group. They are more vulnerable than adults to the media and peer pressures to conform.

There is no good evidence base to justify labiaplasty as a clinically effective procedure. Consumer satisfaction should not be confused with clinical effectiveness (8).

Medically Indicated Female Genital and Vaginal Surgery

There may be medical justifications for some types of female genital and vaginal surgery, e.g. physical pain and hypertrophy due to rubbing on clothing or pain in participating in certain activities such as horse riding or cycling. Patients presenting with these physical issues are in the minority among those presenting and requesting surgery in today's Western culture and society. They are usually relatively easy to distinguish as they concentrate on verbalising physical symptoms and may have physical signs. There is usually an absence of body image issues, and they are often in a stable long-term relationship. They may report sexual discomfort depending on the physical issue. This contrasts with those requesting FGCS whose presenting complaints are focussed on appearance. Commissioning of services varies by region. In some areas these clients may fulfil criteria for surgery: female genital surgery, not female genital cosmetic surgery (as their issue is not primarily cosmetic). It remains important to discuss surgical risks and potential changes in sexual pleasure in order that the client can make a fully informed decision about options including all the risks and benefits.

Body Dysmorphia (Body Dysmorphic Disorder)

It is important for the psychosexual practitioner to have some knowledge and understanding of body dysmorphic disorder (BDD) and to have clarity that it is distinct and different from the term *vaginal dysmorphia* used in this chapter.

BDD is characterised by time-consuming and excessive appearance-related preoccupation with non-existent or slight defects in physical appearance, such that patients believe that they look abnormal, unattractive, ugly or deformed, when in reality they look normal. The preoccupation with perceived flaws leads to repetitive behaviours which are difficult to control and not pleasurable. BDD causes distress and/or impaired functioning and is often associated with suicidal ideation and behaviour. Compulsions are a core feature (11).

Body dysmorphia or BDD is an important and clearly defined psychiatric diagnosis. It is diagnosed according to the American Psychiatric Association's *Diagnostic and Statistical Manual of Mental Disorders*, Fifth Edition (*DSM-5*) (12).

The *DSM-5* diagnostic criteria for BDD include the following:

- Preoccupation with at least one non-existent or slight defect in physical appearance (e.g. thinks about the perceived defects for at least 1 hour per day).
- Concerns about appearance lead to repetitive behaviours (e.g. mirror checking, excessive grooming or skin picking) or mental acts (comparing one's appearance with that of others) at some point during the course of the illness.

- Clinically significant distress or psychosocial impairment resulting from the appearance concerns.
- Appearance preoccupations are not better accounted for by an eating disorder.

The majority of patients with this condition first present to non-psychiatric services requesting treatment. The most common request is for surgery for their perceived physical defect. Phillips (11) states that these treatments are ineffective for these patients and can be risky for clinicians to provide. By contrast, pharmacotherapy (e.g. selective serotonin reuptake inhibitors or clomipramine) and/or cognitive behavioural therapy tailored specifically to BDD are often efficacious.

Women presenting to medical and psychosexual services with concerns about their vaginal appearance could have BDD specific to the vagina. There are various screening tools and alerting factors such as a client who has already had one or several previous cosmetic surgeries. Psychiatric referral should be made if there is suspicion of BDD to ensure that patients get the best assessment and management. Psychosexual work may be undertaken if appropriate after psychiatric assessment and/or treatment.

KEY POINT

BDD is a psychiatric condition and its first presentation may be to psychosexual services rather than psychiatric. It is important that if BDD is suspected that the patient is referred to the right services for appropriate assessment and help. Vaginal dysmorphia is not a psychiatric diagnosis but may include clients with BDD or other psychiatric conditions.

Female Genital Mutilation

A chapter about vaginal dysmorphia and FGCS would be incomplete without reference to FGM and the ambiguity and blurred boundaries in some areas that exist between them.

The World Health Organisation (WHO) (13) classifies FGM as follows:

Type 1: Partial or total removal of the clitoris and/or the prepuce (cliteroidectomy)

Type 2: Partial or total removal of the clitoris and the labia minora, with or without excision of the labia majora (excision)

Type 3: Narrowing of the vaginal orifice with creation of a covering seal by cutting and appositioning the labia minora and/or the labia majora, with or without excision of the clitoris (infibulation)

Type 4: All other harmful procedures to the female genitalia for non-medical purposes, for example, pricking, piercing, incising, scraping and cauterisation

There are clear similarities between FGCS and FGM but also some key differences.
Similarities between FGCS and FGM

- Both may involve partial incision of female genital tissue for cultural reasons.
- Both drive a perceived need for surgery that is based on cultural expectations of how female genitalia ought to look.
- In both, the drive for surgery may be motivated by aesthetics, shame and/or conformity/ belonging (or any combination of these).
- Most FGCS procedures compare anatomically with type I or II FGM in respect of the amount of tissue removed.

Differences between FGCS and FGM

- FGM is condemned in many countries and against the law in the United Kingdom. FGCS is unregulated and is permissible within the law in the United Kingdom.

- FGM is described by the WHO as ethically and morally wrong. FGM is recognised internationally as a violation of the human rights of girls and women. FGCS is not described as a violation of human rights.
- FGM is nearly always carried out on girls under the age of 18 and without consent. FGCS is recommended on women over the age of 18 and with consent.

The Female Genital Mutilation Act of 2003 (14) states that 'A person is guilty of an offence if he excises, infibulates or otherwise mutilates the whole or any part of a girl's labia majora, labia minora or clitoris'. The act also states that 'no offence is committed by an approved person who performs a surgical operation on a girl which is necessary for her physical or mental health'. It is this second statement that justifies FGCS in the United Kingdom on the basis that the female genital cosmetic surgery is necessary for the mental health of the client.

The comparison between FGM and FGCS is illuminating. It is possible to see the ambiguity and areas of potential interpretation to the law that could be argued. It is essential that anyone offering FGCS keeps detailed records of conversations and consent. It is possible to anticipate how a client undergoing FGCS could seek to accuse her surgeon of committing FGM if she chose to do so. It is also possible to anticipate how someone requesting FGM might argue their case on the basis of their mental health and well-being. Inevitably there will be grey areas when exposing the definitions, law and practice of real cases.

What Does the Psychosexual Practitioner Have to Offer?

Psychosexual practitioners who perform vaginal examinations have a unique role in clients with vaginal dysmorphia. The vaginal examination and exploration of the client's beliefs and fantasies about their external genitalia and vagina are key in both interpretation and client insight. Physical examination is also essential to exclude pathology or explore medical grounds for surgery (as opposed to cosmetic requests).

The following is a summary of consultation options used in psychosexual practice in relation to clients presenting with vaginal dysmorphia. Not all aspects will be appropriate for all clients.

KEY POINTS

- Listening, observing, feeling, thinking, and interpreting (LOFTI) as sometimes summarised in the Institute of Psychosexual Medicine (IPM) approach
- Exploration to determine if there are sexual issues relating to the client's story
- Exploration of significant events or experiences which relate to the current problem
- Vaginal examination to exclude pathology and explore perceptions, fantasy and feeling about genital appearance
- Education about the varied appearance of the normal vulva
- Picture or mirror work relating to the individual and/or varied vulval appearance
- Comprehensive information sharing about the pros and cons of surgery if the focus of the client centres on a request for surgery or a desire for surgery becomes apparent
- Reflection and interpretation are central to psychosexual work; they will always be dependent on what the client brings or leaves out of the consultation

---

Recommendations for counselling are integral to many referral pathways for vaginal dysmorphia or related issues. Regions differ in the type and range of counselling that is offered. Many colleagues trained by the IPM are seeing this patient group and offering an excellent service to the growing number of women with significant issues in today's society and culture.

Summary

The psychosexual practitioner needs to be informed and knowledgeable regarding the differential diagnoses and the controversies and debates surrounding vaginal dysmorphia. A clear understanding of FGCS, female genital surgery for medical indications and FGM is essential in order to work within General Medical Council regulations, understand ethical issues and work within the law.

There are increasing numbers of women presenting with anatomical concerns and sexual difficulty relating to the appearance of their genitalia and vagina. Psychosexual practitioners are ideally trained in counselling and examination to assess and help these clients with their issues. Psychosexual doctors are also ideally placed to signpost a minority of clients who might need the expertise of an alternative specialty rather than psychosexual counselling. Psychosexual doctors are well placed to distinguish between primarily cosmetic and primarily physical complaints where surgery may need cautious consideration.

CASE 1: MISS J: REQUEST FOR LABIAPLASTY

Miss J was a 19-year-old referred to the psychosexual clinic by a consultant gynaecologist following her unsupported labiaplasty request. She had been told by the gynaecologist that she was 'normal' and did not need surgery. However, she had left the gynaecologist's clinic in tears and so a referral was made to the psychosexual clinic.

Miss J was strikingly attractive, slim with dyed black hair, several body piercings and laced-up long black boots. She was confident and made immediate eye contact on entering the consulting room. Her opening conversation was 'I am not what I look like' and 'I am not what you think'. I did not say much initially except to say that I was here to listen.

She began to recount her story of being refused labial surgery which she felt was essential to all aspects of her happiness in life. She slightly aggressively informed me that she had only come as I was her last hope for getting the surgery which she felt she really needed. Despite her prickly and defended entrance, I really warmed to her and wanted to help. I felt myself being drawn in to her rather desperate need and genuine belief that something surgical must be done.

Miss J was brought up, along with her younger brother, by her mother. She recounted how they bathed together in their early years and this had felt normal and fun. She had her first sexual experience at the age of 14 at a house party. She had locked herself in the bathroom with a boy she had known quite well. They had enjoyed foreplay and she had hoped they might become an item. On entering school a few days later, a group of boys started to make jokes about the size of her clitoris and labia. At this point in the consultation she became tearful and quiet. Her sadness was palpable. I reflected back how the sadness was all consuming. She went on to say that she had several other attempted relationships and that each time she had been ridiculed personally and publicly regarding the size and shape of her genitalia. She had been verbally told that she looked like a boy. She now felt so unhappy with herself she could not live like this. She would not go swimming or wear tight shorts for fear that her anatomy would be exposed. She had not made any attempts at relationships for the last 2 years for fear of further ridicule. She was clearly desperate, sad and very compelling in her need for a 'solution'. I felt as though I wanted to offer her surgery to 'make it all better' even though I knew this was not likely to help her and would have the potential to make things worse.

Of note, she had no other history of cosmetic surgery or acknowledged concerns about body image. She seemed comfortable with her body, her outward appearance and self-esteem until it came to her genitalia.

I offered to examine her, and she agreed. She was clearly anxious about getting on the couch and exposing herself. I was anxious about what I would see. I had fully bought in to her description of abnormally large and protruding labia and clitoris. How was I going to reassure her if they were really large? When she finally allowed me to look with her, she had a very ordinary vulva.

The clitoris was just visible and the labia minora were not visible until I parted the labia majora to examine her vagina. My own relief felt exposed, though I do not think she was aware as she was too awkward and afraid. I asked her what she was afraid of and she was able to articulate her great fear that I would say that she was 'normal' and does not need surgery.

After the examination we discussed her fear, my findings and her perception of her genitalia. We agreed that her genitalia looked 'normal' to other people but that they did not look 'normal' to her. We explored again the reasons for this and the feelings she had about her genitalia. She visibly relaxed when she could see that I understood what she was saying and not arguing with her as other clinicians had. She verbalised that she did not believe that she could change the way she saw herself by talking about it. She was fixed in her position and I could not help her move forward in that consultation. We discussed relationships and how difficult it was for her to trust anyone sexually again. She verbalised that I had been the first person who really listened but that I was of no help if I could not support her request to have surgery. She had no money to go privately. She left the consultation very downcast. I offered her another appointment, but she did not take it up. I left feeling sad that I could not help her unlock her perception that her genitalia were manly and grossly abnormal.

Reflection

I have shared this case as one of the unsolved. There are many young women that I have counselled with labial issues where they are significantly helped by our IPM methods, examination and interpretations. Sometimes one consultation is enough to simply educate and help a patient change their perception of their genitalia. Some women come back for several appointments before they make significant progress. Miss J was not obviously helped in her consultation with me in that she did not get what she hoped for. I was full of empathy, drawn in by her clear distress at certain points and tempted to believe that surgery may help as I wanted to 'do something'. It remains a fact that surgery has no clinically proven benefit in such cases and that it has the potential to make Miss J's situation worse. I have counselled a number of patients where their perceptions of their genitalia have been made significantly worse and more difficult to manage post-labiaplasty. It is also important to acknowledge that we do not actually know what may or may not have changed for our clients once they step out of our consulting room.

REFERENCES

1. Bramwell R. Invisible labia. The representation of female external genitalia in women's magazines. *Sex Relat Ther* 2002;17:187–190.
2. Crouch NS, Deans R, Michala L, Liao LM, Creighton SM. Clinical characteristics of well women seeking labial reduction surgery: A prospective study. *BJOG* 2011;118:1507–1510.
3. Liao LM, Creighton SM. Requests for cosmetic genitoplasty: How should healthcare providers respond? *BMJ* 2007;334:1090–1092.
4. Lloyd J, Crouch NS, Minto CL, Liao LM, Creighton SM. Female genital appearance: 'Normality' unfolds. *BJOG* 2005;112:643–646.
5. *Oxford Living Dictionaries.* Available from: https://en.oxforddictionaries.com/definition/dysmorphia.
6. Royal College of Obstetricians and Gynaecologists. *Ethical opinion paper. Ethical considerations in relation to female genital cosmetic surgery (FGCS).* London: RCOG Ethics Committee, 2013.
7. Radman HM. Hypertrophy of the labia minora. *Obstet Gynecol* 1975;48(Suppl 1):78S–79S.
8. Liao LM, Michala L, Creighton SM. Labial surgery for well women: A review of the literature. *BJOG* 2010;117:20–25.
9. Department of Health. *Review of the regulation of cosmetic interventions.* Final Report. London: Department of Health, 2013.
10. Bramwell R, Moorland C, Garden AS. Expectations and experience of labial reduction: A qualitative study. *BJOG* 2007;114:1493–1499.

11. Phillips KA. Body dysmorphic disorder: Epidemiology, pathogenesis, and clinical features. UpToDate. Topic last updated 24 May 2016. Available from: www.uptodate.com/contents/body-dysmorphic-disorder-clinical-features.

12. American Psychiatric Association. *Diagnostic and Statistical Manual of Mental Disorders, Fifth Edition (DSM-5)*. Washington, DC: American Psychiatric Association, 2013.

13. World Health Organisation. Female Genital Mutilation. Available from: www.who.int/topics/female_genital_mutilation/.

14. Female Genital Mutilation Act. 2003. Available from: www.legislation.gov.uk.

24

Psychosexual Problems Approaching the End of Life

Marian Davis

Introduction

A young healthy person in their teens and 20s feels immortal, but the passing of the decades and/or serious illness means that in later life, contemplating the end of that life may become unavoidable. This inevitably affects one's sense of self and the way that relationships are experienced. One's sexuality is an integral part of both of these and as the end of life approaches, the change in one's sexuality may present as a psychosexual problem, either overtly or covertly.

The ageing process, illness and facing the imminence of death means that the term *future* has a completely different meaning. There is a stripping away of the extraneous, of the non-essential; and a person may become focussed on the critical aspects of who they are and what they want from life. They live in the present, reflecting on the past, and this may lead them to want to make up for lost time and to re-evaluate relationships.

CASE 1

Vic was referred to the psychosexual clinic at the age of 71, with a year's history of erectile dysfunction. Exploration of his feelings enabled him to talk about his long-held sense of being transgender. He wanted to be known as Sheila. Sheila had harboured these feelings all her adult life, but had never spoken about them. She had had a successful career as a solicitor, had married and had four children. The landmark of retirement had led her to look both backwards and forwards. Sheila felt that she had done her duty and wanted to live out her remaining years being true to herself. She was prepared to risk the fallout of disclosure. The doctor was able to help Sheila to tell her wife and family and to put them in touch with local support organisations. The feeling of time running out led to Sheila's overwhelming need to be true to herself. The presenting erectile dysfunction was indicative of Sheila's sense of the incongruence of her situation.

This reflection may be triggered by retirement, when the person no longer has responsibility for their professional self, or after children have left home, chosen their own paths, and come to terms with their own sexuality. These life changes can confer the freedom to explore one's own sexual needs.

CASE 2

Natalie was a 65-year-old woman, referred with vulvodynia. She had been happily married for over 30 years with a grown-up family. She had retired from the bank a few years previously and had become involved with a charity – doing their accounts. She went to a weekend meeting in another part of the country, got on well with the like-minded people at the charity, and after a few drinks on the final night had unprotected sex – the first time in her life she had ever had sex with anyone apart from her husband. She had not been in touch with the man since but had been unable to have sex with her husband because of superficial dyspareunia. Natalie had been tested for infections and was all clear, but was convinced that something was wrong. She had tried all kinds of creams and lotions but nothing helped. The pain was a symptom of her guilt and the doctor's role, as described by Casement (1), was to 'contain' this guilt, which dissipated over a few sessions. She was then able to have pain-free sex with her husband.

As at other stages of life, the sexual problem presented is a symptom of the underlying distress. For many people nearing the end of life, this stage is associated with deteriorating health and life-limiting illness. This chapter considers the possible impact of diagnosis, treatment and nearing end of life on the sexual function of both the patient and their partner.

Initially, possible barriers to discussing psychosexual problems in this group of patients will be considered.

Defences in the Doctor and the Patient

Various defences have been considered in other chapters, so here only those relevant in this context are considered. A number of issues may prevent a doctor talking about sexual function with an elderly patient or a patient who has a life-changing or life-limiting illness and vice versa. Retreating into reassurance or focussing on the physical and psychosocial may be a way of avoiding talking about the psychosexual.

Age

The doctor may assume that sex is not important to an elderly patient. The patient may remind the doctor of a parent or a grandparent or other relative. However, no matter how old they are, they might have concerns about sexual function. For patients of a certain generation, it could feel totally inappropriate to talk about their intimate lives with a doctor or other healthcare professional so it is up to the professional to facilitate this.

CASE 3

An ophthalmologist saw Henry, an 81-year-old patient with glaucoma, for review. She had seen him several times before. His appointments were usually quite brief – Henry was the sort of man who did not want to be a bother and was always aware of the other patients in the waiting room. His drops had been changed at the previous appointment from ß-blockers to latanoprost. The doctor examined him thoroughly and all was well. She was ready to wind things up, but Henry looked uncharacteristically reluctant to leave.

'Is there anything else you would like to ask me?' she said.
'It may be a silly question, but could these new eye drops give me erections?'

He went on to explain that for many years he had been unable to have intercourse with his wife. This had been a loss for both of them, but since his eye drops had been changed, his erections had returned. Unfortunately, his wife had died about a year previously.

Henry would not have raised the subject because he did not link his sexual difficulty to his medication. Although she knew that ß-blocker eye drops cause serum levels equivalent to oral medication, the younger female doctor did not consider that this 'delightful' older gentleman might have sexual needs.

With younger patients, at a time of their lives when they might be expected to be enjoying the physical side of their relationships and planning their future, having a life-limiting illness can feel very unfair. In the face of these losses, it can be very difficult for the doctor to start a conversation about psychosexual issues. However, in this situation also, the patient may also struggle to raise the subject, so the doctor should give the patient the opportunity to voice any concerns.

LEARNING POINT

Wherever we see patients, at whatever stage of their life, they may have a concern about their sexual function.

Inappropriateness of Subject Matter

Talking about sex may be seen as trivial compared with the medical issues at hand. For example, after a myocardial infarction, the doctor's concerns may be related to secondary prevention, to controlling blood pressure, reducing cholesterol, or checking renal function. In contrast, the priority of the patient or their partner or both may be the fear that if they have sexual intercourse, they might have another heart attack, or worse that they may die.

In a hospice setting, where the doctor and other members of the team will discuss all aspects of a patient's life including their symptoms, home circumstances, relationships, hopes and fears, and their spiritual beliefs, it may feel inappropriate to raise the subject of the patient's intimate life. Middleton-Green and Ward (2) developed an audit tool and analysed the notes of 15 patients in a hospice. An assessment of psychosocial needs had been carried out in 14 patients; psychosexual concerns had been explored in none, in spite of risk factors for sexual problems having been identified. Yet in a relationship that may go back decades, the physical side of that relationship might be very important, and the patient and their partner may want guidance on what is possible, what harm could be done or even what could help with an existing problem.

The Doctor's Own Life Experience

As in other interactions, the doctor must be aware of how their own personal experience impacts on their ability to fully be alongside the patient. Serious illness or death of a close relative may still impact on the doctor, or they may have difficulties with relationships in their non-professional lives. The doctor needs to own these feelings, and then to put them to one side so that they do not intrude on the consultation or the space between the doctor and patient, where they will both puzzle about the cause of the patient's problem.

Diagnosis and Treatment

In other chapters of the book, emphasis has been placed on the individuality of the patient experience and of the doctor-patient relationship (DPR), and at this life stage it is no different. While the physical treatments we prescribe for our patients are evidence based, the effect of the diagnosis and the impact of the treatment are individual to that patient. A patient loses the certainties that they held, they lose the plans they have for the future – at least temporarily. A patient may feel shame, anger, loss or guilt and these universal feelings may impact on an individual patient in a variety of ways, including affecting their sexual function.

Diagnosis

The impact of receiving a life-limiting or life-changing diagnosis, such as cancer, cannot be overestimated. The following examples show different ways that a serious diagnosis can result in a psychosexual problem.

CASE 4

George was a 75-year-old man, very well turned out in a jacket and tie with highly polished shoes. He was very traditional in his manner; he was used to providing for his wife, Mary, and family and when challenges arose, he was used to dealing with them. He had suffered from erectile difficulties since he received his diagnosis of metastatic lung cancer, 6 months previously. Exploring his reaction to the diagnosis revealed his impotent anger. He had been referred for magnetic resonance imaging 2 years previously because of back pain. A diagnosis of degenerative disease had been made. When the films were reviewed after his diagnosis, a potentially operable tumour could be seen. Two years on, his disease was only suitable for palliative treatment. George was consumed with anger at the failure of the doctors to spot this and his powerlessness to put this right for himself and Mary. He could not express this anger either with his wife or with the professionals who were treating him. The psychosexual clinic offered safe space to explore these feelings.

A patient may keep their fears about the implications of a diagnosis to themselves. This can lead to a distancing from their partner, whether out of a desire to protect them or because of the overwhelming nature of the fears they are carrying.

CASE 5

Sheila was a 53-year-old woman who came with loss of libido. A year previously, she had been given a diagnosis of ovarian cancer and had undergone surgery and chemotherapy. However, the disease was still present. It was a matter of pride that Sheila had never shed a tear since receiving the diagnosis. However, she and her husband, John, had drifted apart, and they had not made love for several months. The doctor noted the absence of feeling after such a devastating diagnosis and was able to explore with her the subconscious need to protect her partner from his potential loss. Her loss of libido was a way of avoiding the pain of separation. Sheila and her husband had not shared their private fears of what the future held, including that she might die, and this had prevented them being close in the present. In the consulting room, Sheila was able to talk about her fears and losses with the doctor. This was then something that she could replicate at home, allowing her husband to share his feelings. Following this, Sheila and John were able to become emotionally and physically close again.

The shock of a diagnosis may affect a patient's partner as well, resulting in a psychosexual problem. A partner may feel guilt at the diagnosis – even worrying that they might have caused the illness, e.g. in cases of HIV or carcinoma of the cervix, or that they might make it worse by further sexual activity. Having erectile dysfunction in this situation may be a subconscious attempt to protect the partner.

Sometimes the situation may be even more complex. For example, a patient presents with loss of libido following a serious diagnosis. When the doctor explores this, it transpires that she has been sent by her husband. He is something of a bully and has demanded regular sex throughout their marriage. She has felt obliged to comply although it has not been fulfilling for her for many years. The diagnosis now gives her an excuse to say no. The doctor's role may be just to validate her decision.

Treatment

The treatment for cancer can be disabling, disfiguring and disempowering. An autonomous person who has their place in society is transformed into a patient with a list of appointments, with things being done to them rather than by them. They no longer have a say in the day-to-day running of their lives.

A husband and father who has taken pride in providing for the family, who has defined himself by his professional role, who has been used to controlling and making the decisions in all areas of his life, finds that his life is reduced to a three-weekly cycle of chemotherapy. Decisions are made by others, depending on the results of his bloods. He finds himself divided – partly hoping the treatment will go ahead, partly hoping to postpone it because of how awful it makes him feel. He has lost the certainties of his life. He no longer knows how to define himself as a man.

A home-making mother who has endless calls on her time, who takes pride in being the carer, the centre of her family, the go-to person when there is a problem, finds herself instead the focus of everyone's concern. She hates being dependent on others, being the centre of attention. She has lost her identity.

The treatments themselves can lead to sexual problems. This may be a direct physical effect, e.g. hormone treatments for prostate cancer can cause erectile dysfunction, surgery for vulval cancer may mean that sexual intercourse is no longer possible. However, it can also be because of the psychosexual impact they may have. Chemotherapy can lead to hair loss. Gynaecological cancers may involve surgery that results in loss of fertility. Surgery, such as mastectomy or orchidectomy is potentially disfiguring. All these may remove a patient's sense of femininity or masculinity.

In addition, the treatment may cause significant side effects – exhaustion, nausea, pain. All of these factors can have an impact on the way that a patient feels about themselves as a sexual being, or on the way that their partner feels about them. For example, a partner may present with the psychosexual problem as a surrogate for the patient – the patient's reaction to the disfigurement of a mastectomy for example, leading them to reject the advances of their partner.

In addition, the partner may find themselves in a caring role – perhaps even providing personal care. This can be difficult to reconcile with their role as a lover and may lead to a loss of libido.

LEARNING POINT

Every patient (and their partner) will have an individual reaction to diagnosis and treatment of a life-limiting illness and so such an illness will have an individual impact on their sexuality.

CASE 6

Mary, a 53-year-old woman, had been having treatment for cancer for 4 years. At the time she was seen, she was in remission. She had been referred to the psychosexual clinic with 'recurrent thrush', (negative swabs), and dyspareunia. Outwardly, she was an attractive, cheerful woman engaging and engaged with the consultation and optimistic about the future. The doctor felt that she was getting nowhere, apart from noting a glimpse of frustration at the failure of the doctors to treat Mary's thrush. Aware of the block, she suggested an examination. Immediately, as Mary moved towards the curtain, the atmosphere changed. Mary submissively folded her clothes and put them on the chair, climbed onto the couch with a long sigh and lay there in a weary, resigned manner. The doctor ventured: 'It seems as though you have no say in what happens to you, as though the doctors have taken control'. Mary replied: 'I used to be so confident and then this happened – I just want to have my life back'. There was a very bleak silence. After the examination, Mary came and sat down, still very thoughtful. The examination had enabled Mary to get in touch with deeper feelings and, after further reflection, was the key to resolving her problem.

LEARNING POINT

A listening examination, starting from the moment it is suggested or avoided, can often be the key to understanding a patient's problem.

In addition to addressing the psychosexual issues, the doctor can prescribe treatments to mitigate against side effects of treatment – phosphodiesterase inhibitors for men who have erectile dysfunction following treatment for prostate cancer and topical oestrogens for women on tamoxifen for breast cancer. The latter will need reassuring about the safety of using oestrogens – the patient information leaflet lists breast cancer as a contraindication but the absorption and impact are negligible. This should be discussed with the patient's oncologist.

Palliative Phase

As a patient enters the palliative phase of their care, they and their partner and families have to adjust to the reality of a life-limiting illness. In accepting that there will be no cure, the patient and/or their partner may relinquish the language of 'fighting the illness', of being in a struggle. This may lead to them being more accepting of the likely outcome or it might increase their sense of powerlessness. The importance of the concept of future diminishes and this can be liberating for some – enabling them to truly live in the present. For others, the loss associated with the knowledge of being robbed of the plans they have made for themselves and their loved ones is hard to bear.

Taylor (3) found that in this situation, as well as the patient, the couple's relationship is dying. Becoming-apart-as-a-couple can be experienced as a psychosexual problem for either patient or partner or both.

The role of the doctor is primarily to relieve symptoms such as pain and breathlessness, to establish a preferred place of death and to provide emotional support to the patient and the family. It can be very difficult to raise the subject of their psychosexual concerns amid all these competing priorities. Yet physical intimacy and touch may be very important for the patient and their partner – or they may not. Either way, the patient should be given as much of an opportunity to talk about this aspect of their life as others. Avoiding this will result in an unmet need.

Even if the subject has been raised, the DPR may feel very different; a doctor was asked to discuss loss of intimacy with a male patient. She found it impossible to suggest a psychosexual examination. When she reflected on this she was aware of feeling that it would breach a perceived inviolability of the hospice patient.

Creating the opportunity for some privacy for a couple, in the midst of all the visits from medical and nursing staff, may be very important. Allowing a partner to share a bed in a hospice or hospital can help a couple maintain their intimacy. A young couple, who got married after her diagnosis of metastatic breast cancer, shared a double bed downstairs in their first home together. Her husband took leave of absence from work and the team looking after them knew that if there was a note on the front door, they should come back later.

As seen previously, the reaction to any life event is individual and nearing the end of life is no different. Some patients withdraw from intimacy, already separating themselves from their loved ones. For others, their physical condition may make sexual intercourse an impossibility, either because of surgery or because of symptoms such as bone pain. It may be appropriate for the doctor to give permission not to have intercourse and to explore other ways of being intimate. Touch of any kind can be very important – holding hands, gentle massage, brushing hair can all achieve intimacy and be a significant component of quality of life. In Taylor's (3) terms, it can achieve 'becoming-closer-as-a-couple'.

For the partner, they may feel sidelined in the relationship with their loved one by all the professionals who are providing personal and other care and making decisions with the patient about symptom control, preferred place of death, etc. The paraphernalia of equipment and the hospital bed may also be a barrier to getting close. They may feel that their home has been invaded by a long list of therapists, nurses and other professionals.

CASE 7

Derek was referred to the psychosexual clinic with erectile dysfunction. He was 45 and his wife aged 39 was dying of breast cancer. They had three children, two boys and a girl. The general practitioner (GP) said that Derek wanted to try alprostadil. The urgency was communicated right down the line, from the GP letter, through the GP secretary, to the clinic administrator who slotted him into a cancellation. The doctor found herself caught up in the mission to try and help him to make love to his wife before it was too late. Having made sure that there were no contraindications to using alprostadil, she found herself walking up and down the corridor outside her room waiting to see if the medication would work. Suddenly it dawned on her that the alprostadil and all the frantic activity were a defence to prevent everyone looking at the tragedy of this couple and their family. She tentatively knocked on her own door and went in. The medication had not worked. They sat down and began to talk. Derek's wife was gravely ill. He was worried about hurting her if they made love and the doctor explored with him other ways of being close. He talked about how she had changed physically because of the illness and because of the surgery and how that had affected their relationship. He talked about his fear of losing her, of how he would manage being a single parent, of how he could not possibly fill her shoes. His daughter was 11 – how would he be able to manage when her periods started, when she had boyfriend troubles, when she was planning her wedding, having a baby? He worried that she might carry a breast cancer gene, but had not felt able to discuss this. It all felt overwhelming. The doctor felt powerless to do anything but listen. She felt incredibly moved by the enormity of what Derek was facing. After a while he fell silent. The doctor sat there with the silence. He looked up and there were tears in his eyes. 'Do you know what is more frightening than anything else? The thought that this is it. That I am going to be by myself, not know love or have someone who really cares about me for the rest of my life'.

The doctor's role in this case was (again) to be a container for Derek's feelings. She heard him and did not judge him and shared his loss and his guilt and his fears. He was then able to go back and be there for his wife and children. He did not need a follow-up appointment but asked for a review appointment about 8 months later. His wife had died and he was able to look back and see that he had done all he could. He and the children were still grieving, but he no longer felt that things were unmanageable. He could see a way forward and had a sense of the future.

Addressing the physical side of their relationship, during a partner's final illness can be of great comfort to the bereaved. If a couple can talk about intimacy and achieve intimacy in a way that is compatible with their situation, it enables the patient to have some privacy at a time when the medicalisation of their lives leaves little space. It gives them some control where they have little say in what is happening and it puts them in touch with the relationship they had before the illness. This can contribute to the bereaved partner's sense of having done everything they could in accordance with their loved one's wishes.

LEARNING POINT

Addressing the psychosexual needs of a patient with life-limiting illness and/or their partner can have important benefits for their final days and help the grieving process for their partner.

The Bereaved

The death of a partner means the loss of intimacy. People often describe that they feel the loss most keenly at nighttime, when they go to bed. Beyond the normal grieving process, bereavement can have a profound effect on a person's medium- and long-term ability to form relationships. If a person has lost a partner, it can be very difficult to allow themselves to care for a subsequent partner; to allow themselves to be vulnerable; to risk being abandoned again. This can present as loss of libido, dyspareunia or erectile difficulties.

Sometimes the psychosexual problem can be caused by more complex emotions. The role of the doctor is to listen in a non-judgemental way, to create safe space for difficult emotions to be held, and to enable the patient to make sense of them.

CASE 8

Michael was a 45-year-old man who presented with erectile difficulties. He had been suffering from this since his father died, 2 years previously. At first, he described an idyllic childhood, living on a farm, and a father whom he had adored. The doctor felt a profound sense of loss which she shared with the patient: 'You must really miss him'. At the second appointment, Michael had just about closed the door before he burst out: 'I hated my father'. There was a release of extreme emotion as he angrily described a man who had been a bully, both to himself and to his mother. He had never had the courage to stand up to him in life and now it was too late. This anger had never previously been expressed. The doctor felt quite shocked at this outpouring, and said very little as Michael described his childhood. He had felt powerless and now it was too late. The doctor tentatively linked these feelings with his sexual problem, but Michael saw no connexion. When they met a few weeks later, Michael revealed that he no longer had a problem – he credited a Mediterranean cruise.

Conclusion

Death is an inescapable reality for all of us. The impact of impending mortality on a person's sexuality and intimate relationships, especially in the context of the diagnosis and treatment of serious illness can be profound. The patient and their partner can feel overwhelmed by events; trying to preserve the physical side of their relationship can be very difficult or seem trivial, compared with other concerns.

In addition to addressing psychosexual problems which are covertly presented, the professional has a responsibility to explore the sexual and intimate aspect of a person's life as part of the holistic care being given. A simple question such as 'How are you able to feel close to your partner?' may help to open up that conversation. After a serious diagnosis, helping a patient and their partner to maintain some intimacy in the face of all the potential losses can significantly enrich the patient's final days and hours and ease the pain of bereavement for their partner.

LEARNING POINTS

- Wherever we see patients, at whatever stage of their life, they may have a concern about their sexual function.
- Every patient (and their partner) will have an individual reaction to diagnosis and treatment of a life-limiting illness and so such an illness will have an individual impact on their sexuality.
- A listening examination, starting from the moment it is suggested or avoided, can often be the key to understanding a patient's problem.
- Addressing the psychosexual needs of a patient with life-limiting illness and/or their partner can have important benefits for their final days and help the grieving process for their partner.

REFERENCES

1. Casement, P. *On Learning from the Patient*. London: Routledge, 1985, 154–155.
2. Middleton-Green L, Ward A. Sexual healing: Is there something we are missing? *BMJ Support Palliat Care* 2016;6:406–407.
3. Taylor B. Experiences of sexuality and intimacy in terminal illness: A phenomenological study. *J Palliat Med* 2009;28(5):438–447.

25

Measuring Efficacy in Psychosexual Medicine

Philipa A Brough

Introduction

Efficacy is defined as 'the ability to produce a desired or intended result'. In today's world of financial constraint and ensuring interventions are carried out because there is good evidence to do so, it is essential to have information supporting all elements of healthcare to be delivered. However, in order to measure efficacy, the desired result needs to be understood and clarified. Concerning sexual problems one could ask is the desired result that the patient has an understanding of why the problem existed, the 'cause' or is it that the problem has been treated or gone? Most patients coming for psychosexual therapy would perhaps want both and therapists will report that happening for many, but for others it can be merely gaining insight into the problem alone which subsequently benefits their sexual lives. If we therefore simply use an objective figure to judge efficacy, outcome studies will not reflect patients' own perception of the effect of therapy. In Tom Main's book (1), *The Ailment and Other Psychoanalytical Essays*, he describes psychoanalysis as having 'liberating effects on the patient' but that would seem insufficient a reason to advocate psychosexual therapy based on Institute of Psychosexual Medicine (IPM) approaches alone.

This idea of the relevance of patients' views of how they have been helped by particular healthcare interventions has been explored in recent times with the promotion and use of patient-recorded outcome measures (PROMs). These assess the quality of care delivered to patients from the patient perspective, asking about symptoms, function and how quality of life is affected as the main criteria. Black in his paper on how PROMs could help transform healthcare (2) cites Hahn (21) and states 'the reliability of PROMs is similar to that of clinical measures such as diastolic blood pressure or blood glucose'. PROMs can be specific to a condition or generic. One advantage of PROMs over clinician-judged efficacy is that they avoid observer bias. Clinical procedures using PROMs include the operations of hip and knee replacements, where in the UK National Health Service (NHS), gains after these surgical treatments are evaluated using pre- and post-operative questionnaires. Information on health status is collected at a single point in time, before and after the procedures and provides an indication of the outcomes or quality of care delivered. Because of the large numbers of patients, the data produced can help assess effectiveness of the treatments on a patient's life in a way that is more meaningful than a clinical judgment.

When researching efficacy, one of the difficulties in understanding the benefits of psychosexual therapy is how to interpret DNA (did not attend) figures. If patients drop out of therapy is it that the problem has resolved or that therapy is not working? In her study auditing DNA questionnaires Davis (3) suggests that for some, DNAs may occur if the sessions are reaching the nub of the problem and for some this may be too traumatic or they are not ready to contemplate this. For patients who DNA and subsequently re-attend, is it because they think the therapy is helping? These postulated explanations illustrate the complexities in calculating how the effective psychological treatments work, but although the reasons for DNA may be different, examining efficacies of physical treatments should also include an understanding about what is happening here.

Effectiveness or 'the degree to which a desired result is produced' is measuring success rate. Again, we would hesitate as clinicians or therapists to decide for a patient how well their sexual lives have been helped by any therapy or indeed treatments. (A well-described phenomena is the partner whose very satisfactory sexual life of occasional sex in later life has been ruined by the invention of PDE5 inhibitors such as Viagra.)

It is impossible to research the efficacy as one would for pharmaceutical interventions as the gold standard double-blind, randomised, controlled study cannot be done when therapy is based on emotional understanding of subconscious thoughts and feelings. Qualitative research is more applicable in these situations as it values the importance of looking at things from the patient's perspective. This informs our understanding of what patients see a result to be, rather than the view of a clinician or researcher. Qualitative methods can be particularly useful in areas where little research exists and there are now increasing numbers of such studies published as acknowledgement of the best way to study biopsychosocial conditions. In their paper on qualitative research in urogynaecology, Doshani (4) states, 'There is increasing recognition that what matters to most women with chronic illness is how well they are able to function and how they feel about their day-to-day lives', and 'understanding patients concerns, expectations and requests is important for the measurement of healthcare quality, the delivery of health services and the costs of care'. This emphasises that without qualitative studies, even in the treatment of physical conditions, the healthcare we deliver is substandard. If we only use objective assessments to define cure in the group of patients in the previous study we would miss the most important outcome, that of improved quality of life and symptoms rather than total continence.

In their book *What Works, for Whom* (5) Roth and Fonagy summarise research studies evaluating psychotherapy efficacy (not specifically sexual), and we learn that it is not so much the therapy type that is significant in the outcome, but 'the ability of the individual practitioner to deliver a specific therapeutic intervention tailored to the needs of the client'. IPM therapy mimics this approach as clinicians do not use prescribed psychological interventions or formats but based on what they see and hear from individual patients are themselves the catalysts during this interaction. This approach brings relevant emotional and subconscious items to the surface or conscious level, to be acknowledged and understood.

Case studies over the last 40 years published in the IPM journals and elsewhere can be regarded as qualitative evidence of effectiveness, despite lack of objectivity. The clinicians writing about their observations have felt able and compelled to report the change in many of these patients and case reports of physical treatments are often the stimulus for further work proving the efficacy, if possible. These observations are based on clinical experience and observation which seems to have been given less credence in recent times.

Things, however, may be changing. In her paper on evidence-based medicine (EBM) Greenhalgh (6) argues that we now need to refine our use of EBM to enable meaningful interventions to patients. She advocates the inclusion of research based on case-based discussion to help formulate what may be best for an individual patient. She emphasises the need for 'broader, more imaginative research that includes the study of the patients experience of illness' not to replace EBM but to enhance it and individualise it for patients. This inevitably means that research questions and design have to be broader and less prescriptive to be able to capture the relevance of patients' views about efficacy and effectiveness of their treatment.

Outcome Studies

An early look at the benefits of psychosexual medicine therapy was published in the *British Journal of Obstetrics and Gynaecology* (BJOG) in1983 by Bramley et al. (7). This prospective study looked at the treatment of unconsummated marriage by 16 doctors trained by the IPM. The mean duration of symptoms in 159 couples admitted to the study was 4.2 years; 60% of them had consummated by 6 months and 72% by 24 months. Other improvements in sexual function occurred even among those failing to consummate. And 135 couples had previously consulted 253 other agents. The average cumulative length of treatment at the 6-month review was 3 hours. Partners attending alone did as well as couples who attended together.

This study was also included as part of an analysis of research into psychosexual medicine by Draper (8). She analysed three papers she herself had been involved in using the following criteria:

* Why? The precipitating stimulus for researching
* How? The reasons for the design of the study
* What? The value of the study

For this particular study the stimulus for doing it was proving efficacy as requested by the local health authorities (NHS) who were now funding the clinics. Previously the Family Planning Association (FPA), a charitable body, had run them. This is perhaps the first attempt to measure efficacy in psychosexual medicine therapy and ensure clinics were cost effective. The design of the study was subject to numerous discussions and considerations of questionnaires and grids specific to sexual well-being but ultimately it was simplified to identifying one specific symptom which engendered itself to observation of an outcome, i.e. non-consummation of marriage. A control group was considered and hotly debated, the lack of one threatening funding for the work. Eventually the impossibility of having a valid control group due to ethical concerns (of not treating a patient who presented with the problem) was argued and accepted by the foundation funding the study and it went ahead. Objectivity of the interviews with the patients before and after treatment was attempted by employing a psychiatric social worker to administer these before and after treatment. The authors argue that the study demonstrates 'comparison with other methods from the fact that of the 147 couples 135 had previously consulted 235 other agents and 72% of those who had failed to benefit from previous treatments were able to achieve penetration'. While there are flaws in this argument, for instance it is unknown exactly what treatments had been tried or whether the same treatments had been attempted on the patients who did not achieve penetration, it is often the case that patients are helped by attending psychosexual clinics after various other treatments, including physical, have been tried to no avail.

One of the earliest attempts to measure elements of efficacy in patients presenting with widespread sexual problems was published in 1996. The IPM journal published a study aiming 'to assess the acceptability and usefulness of an outcome and satisfaction measure in sexual medicine' (9). Postal questionnaires were sent out to clinic attenders with four questions including one asking for their view on whether their condition had improved. The satisfaction measure was stated as 89% but the response rate was only 42%. There was a comprehensive discussion with two case examples as a basis for comparing an objective successful outcome measure of only 24%, compared to the higher patient satisfaction figure. This again demonstrates that patients' views of the 'success' of interventions are often different to that of clinicians and reinforces the need to consider PROMs when judging efficacy and effectiveness.

Wilson et al. (10) examined 100 consecutive patient records of psychosexual clinic referrals and found 55% to be improved or greatly improved after their therapy, using IPM methods based on what was reported in the records. The patients presented with a wide range of sexual difficulties and were male and female. It is again acknowledged that there are challenges in this methodology of subjectively assessing the outcome of the sessions but it did demonstrate the brevity of the interventions: the average number of sessions patients attended was 2.38.

One of the challenges in measuring outcomes is to use an appropriate tool that is also validated. Hobbs et al. (11) used the MYMOP2 (Make Yourself Medical Outcome Profile) questionnaire in a pilot study to look at effectiveness in a psychosexual medicine service. This tool, which is problem specific, had been used in primary care and can be employed to look at the most important symptoms patients themselves want to address, rather than those their clinicians feel are significant. Two-thirds of patients demonstrated a meaningful change in their symptoms using the MYMOP2 scoring system. In the second wave of the study, which was presented at the IPM Annual Scientific Meeting (12), similar findings of improvement were found in a larger group of 89 patients.

In a sexual and reproductive health service, Brough (13) in 2015, looked at patient-recorded outcomes using two different methods: a pre- and post-treatment questionnaire developed originally by the IPM and a simpler visual analogue used at every consultation. Due to difficulty collating a meaningful number of post-treatment results the visual analogue was also used to look at progress during sessions. The numbers were small but all patients reported an improvement in their problem at discharge in 1 year and over a 3-year period 87% of 23 paired patient questionnaires reported the problem was improved post-therapy.

Usually lots of small studies can be more significantly analysed when put in a meta-analysis, and this has been attempted by Fur (14) looking at psychological interventions for sexual dysfunction: they looked at 20 randomized clinical trials comparing a psychological intervention with a wait list as well as some studies without a wait list. The overall post-treatment effect size for symptom severity had a *d* value of 0.58 symptom severity and 0.47 for sexual satisfaction. Psychological interventions were shown to particularly improve symptom severity for women with hypoactive sexual desire disorder and orgasmic disorder. The type of therapy however, was varied and included cognitive behavioural, psychodynamic, systematic desensitisation and marital therapy.

Can Psychological Interventions Prevent Unnecessary Surgical Interventions?

In a small retrospective case review (15), the investigation and management of sexual pain disorders in a district gynaecology department looked at the patient management outcomes when seen by an IPM-trained gynaecologist compared to a non-IPM trained gynaecologist in an out-patient clinic. In the IPM group, none of the attenders had surgical procedures for the pain but were helped by therapy, education, lubrication and hormone treatments. In contrast, 61% of the other group had had laparoscopies at the time of the study with 47% of these being negative and 41% showing only a possible aetiological pathology. More evidence is necessary to demonstrate efficacy of psychosexual medicine but in parallel with studies on psychodynamic therapy for other conditions there are increasing arguments supporting its efficacy and therefore potential benefits for patients. Yakeley (16) argues that psychodynamic psychotherapy is as effective as other treatments such as cognitive behavioural therapy, in her article summarising the recent evidence from high-quality outcome studies. She proposes a model for psychodynamic psychotherapy research based on attachment theory, which may subsequently help develop psychodynamic therapy tailored for specific conditions.

Measuring Outcomes

Despite challenges, various attempts at measuring efficacy have been attempted using a variety of validated and non-validated measures. Some tools are based on psychological treatments per se (or for any condition/problem) and some are more designed for sexual problems.

1. MYMOP2 tool (17). As mentioned earlier, the MYMOP2 tool has been used in a pilot and follow-up outcome study with psychosexual clients. This patient-generated tool was developed by the University of Bristol and measures quality of life but also can examine specific symptoms: physical, emotional or social. It is brief and simple to administer and validation studies have included patients of both orthodox and complementary practitioners. The structure and scoring make it easy to chart the scores of individual patients over time making it especially useful in case studies and changes in symptoms. However, the creators point out that due to the individualised nature of MYMOP it is unsuitable as a basis for economic evaluations.

2. A jointly developed outcome questionnaire is being piloted as a multi-society project. This tool was presented at the IPM Annual Scientific Meeting in 2017 in Liverpool (18) and is available to use in the United Kingdom. It is currently being evaluated to ensure that the team analyse how best to interpret the results and to assist this a large database has been set up. Forms are given to patients ideally before every intervention, and these ask for scores on quality and the importance of respondents' sex lives currently, as well as any associated distress. As we know, this is not always possible in some settings as it cannot be reliably predicted when a psychosexual interaction is going to happen but if used after the session there will have already been a therapeutic intervention and the results will not be comparable. This limits the usefulness of the tool for spontaneous ad hoc therapy but for specialist services it may add to our knowledge about efficacy.

3. At the European and World Sexual Medicine Conference in Lisbon 2018 a questionnaire was introduced by Frost (19). This sexual and relationship distress scale (SaRDs) was designed to

assess the effect of sexual problems and the distress caused within a relationship. Reliability and validity have been examined with a sample of 1,192 patients and the authors are encouraging therapists' coordinated use across the globe to try and enable meaningful comparisons of efficacy using a standardised tool.

Cost-effectiveness

Psychosexual medicine therapy is intended to be a brief intervention and this is illustrated in several studies; in the Bramley study (7) 46/71 couples consummated after only two visits to an IPM-trained doctor and the average number of sessions patients attended in other studies is similar (10,13).

> **We know the relationship between sexuality and infertility is complex and IVF treatment is particularly costly both emotionally and financially. Elstein (20) observed that infertility may cause sexual dysfunction, sexual problems may present in disguise as infertility or there may be coincidental sexual disturbance in the infertile couple. We also know that a proportion of patients referred for infertility have not consummated: patients undergoing infertility treatments may have primary sexual dysfunction as a cause or factor in the subsequent infertility. Those women with severe vaginismus for example may not even be able to undergo the necessary initial investigations such as a transvaginal scan or be unable to manage the introduction of a catheter for intra-uterine insemination. Therefore it would seem cost effective to screen and provide psychosexual therapy before costly infertility treatments begin.**

> **Psychosexual doctors often see patients who have had many other ineffective physical, pharmaceutical and other psychological treatments beforehand, with associated financial and emotional costs. One study showed 39% of patients had had pharmaceutical treatments prescribed and 7% surgical procedures performed including cystoscopies and laparoscopies before it was determined that the problem was psychological and the patient referred for therapy. (13)**

What of the patients who were reviewed in the Davies/Frodsham study (15)? The authors (tantalisingly, in a cash-strapped health system) suggest costs to the NHS and morbidity in surgery could be reduced if gynaecology doctors were IPM trained. Unfortunately psychological therapy and counselling sessions currently do not receive reimbursement in the same way as surgical and pharmaceutical interventions, despite that in the long run these options would save money in a system that has finite resources.

It is clear that two or three sessions with a psychosexual clinician are cheaper than any operative procedure and most likely pharmaceutical treatments too when clinician prescribing consultation and time are taken into account.

What is most important, however, is the cost to the patient in terms of continuing to suffer from a problem that may be responsive to and helped by psychosexual medicine 'interventions' but not having that option. Inevitably, patients will continue to try and access the help they need by knocking on other doors and it is these hidden costs that should be factored in when deducing whether or not the provision of psychosexual medicine is cost effective.

Conclusions

We can see that there are many hurdles to measuring efficacy in psychosexual medicine but it can be done. It is important to remember that psychological interventions have some major advantages over pharmaceutical treatments; they do not have physical side effects and they can increase sexual satisfaction over and above simply helping the original symptom, i.e. patients often report a better understanding of their problems and as a result the benefit of how to manage issues that may arise in the future in addition to relief of their current symptoms.

In psychosexual medicine it is important to consider the concept of shifts/understanding in the patient rather than 'cures'. Since the problem is a subjective one and is unique to the patient, this aim can be deemed appropriate, as the desired result cannot always be fully understood by the clinician or indeed the patient. A change may happen in the patient, that although objectively may appear to be a slight one, is enough to alter the sexual function and pleasure for the patient and subsequently their partner. This differs from traditional or physical efficacy where a universal outcome can be measured in all. We rarely hear how patients actually view the therapy. One patient of mine summarised it as follows: '(talking in the clinic) shakes everything around and things come bubbling up to surface that are significant'.

Tom Main states (1), 'Psychoanalysis is first an investigation, next a body of knowledge and last a treatment for neurosis'. If we apply that statement to psychosexual medicine we can see that the clinician interacting with the patient, 'analysing' is the investigation and the creation of a 'body of knowledge' with the patient during this interaction. The final part of the definition which is 'a treatment for neurosis' may be regarded as the reason for practising in an outcome-driven consultation, but it is the only part that we can realistically measure which perhaps highlights the limitations of traditional outcome measures, even psychological ones.

Finally what the patient records as a successful result should ultimately be the aim, if as clinicians we truly pride ourselves on being able to help patients with sexual problems. As Greenhalgh argues (6), 'in the educational field, it is time we extended the evidence base for integrated curriculums that promote reflection and case discussion alongside the application of evidence'.

REFERENCES

1. Main T. *The Ailment and Other Psychoanalytical Essays.* London: Free Association Books, 1989.
2. Black N. Patient reported outcome measures could help transform healthcare. *BMJ* 2013;346:f167.
3. Davis M. Facts from figures – A DNA audit. *Institute Psychosex Med J (IPMJ)* 2008;48:30–34.
4. Doshani A, Pitchforth E, Mayne C, Tincello DG et al. The value of qualitative research in urogynaecology. *BJOG* 2009;116:3–6.
5. Roth A, Fonagy P. *What Works for Whom? A Critical Review of Psychotherapy Research*, 2nd ed. New York, NY: Guilford Press, 2005.
6. Greenhalgh T. Evidence based medicine: A movement in crisis? *BMJ* 2014;348:g3725.
7. Bramley HM, Brown J, Draper KC, Kilvington J. Non-consummation of marriage treated by members of the Institute of Psychosexual Medicine: A prospective study. *BJOG* 1983;90(10):908–913.
8. Draper K. Research in psychosexual medicine. *IPMJ* 1995;9:2–5.
9. Stainer-Smith A. Dare we measure patient satisfaction? *IPMJ* 1996;12:11–14.
10. Wilson J, Mansour D. How effective is psychosexual counselling? Results of an 18 month audit. *IPMJ* 2012;61:7–11.
11. Hobbs R, Muir W. Use of MYMOP to measure effectiveness in a psychosexual medicine service. *IPMJ* 2014;66:16–18.
12. Hobbs R, Muir W. 'MYMOP', *Presented at the IPM Annual Scientfic Meeting, Southampton*, March 2018.
13. Brough P. Psychosexual therapy in an integrated Sexual Health service: Patient demographics, referral patterns and patient reported outcome measures. *IPMJ* 2015;68:17–21.
14. Fruhauf S, Gerger H, Schmidt HM, Munder T et al. Efficacy of psychological interventions for sexual dysfunction: A systematic review and meta-analysis. *Arch Sex Behav* 2013;42(6):915–933.
15. Davies JC, Frodsham LCG. Sex: What a pain! The investigation and management of sexual pain disorders in a district genecology department [Abstract]. In *Abstracts of the RCOG World Congress 2013*, 24–26 June. Liverpool, UK. BJOG. 2013. Pages 490–491.
16. Yakeley J. Psychodynamic psychotherapy: Developing the evidence base. *Adv Psychiatric Treat* 2014;20(4):269–279.
17. MYMOP2. Available from: http://www.bris.ac.uk/primaryhealthcare/resources/mymop/.
18. Hood C. Outcome tool presented at 2017 ASM NSOG development group.
19. Frost RN, Donovan CL. Sexual and relationship distress scale. In RR Milhausen, T Fisher, CM Davis, W Yarber, JK Sakaluk, (Eds.), *Handbook of Sexuality-Related Measures* (4th ed.). New York, NY: Taylor and Francis Group, in press.
20. Elstein M. Effect of infertility on psychosexual function. *BMJ* 1975;3(5978):296–299.
21. Clinical Significance Consensus meeting group, Precision of health related quality-of-life data compared with other clinical measures. *Mayo Clin Proc* 2007;82:1244–1254.

26

Services

Philipa A Brough

Introduction

Sexual problems occur in all groups, communities and sexualities, as our cases have demonstrated and are not rare, as borne out by research. We have seen all through the book that sexual problems present ubiquitously throughout the clinical environment and this can be quantified by the findings of the latest (3rd) Natsal (National Survey of Sexual Attitudes and Lifestyles) study (1):

- Problems with sexual response were common (41.6% of men and 51.2% of women reported one problem or more).
- Self-reported distress about sex lives was much less common (9.9% and 10.9% respectively).
- For individuals in a sexual relationship for the past year, 23.4% of men and 27.4% of women reported an imbalance in level of interest in sex between partners.
- It was found that 18% of men and 17.1% of women said that their partner had sexual difficulties.

Doctors and healthcare professionals realised many years ago there were patients unable to be helped by physical treatments, hence the initial interest by family planning doctors in sourcing training and guidance in the subject, resulting in the formation of the Institute of Psychosexual Medicine (IPM) in 1974. In more recent times other organisations have also tried to fill the gaps in provision in order to address the problems presented to them by their patients.

The provision of psychosexual care within sexual health settings is considered an essential component of good clinical practice (2). The advent of PDE5 inhibitors may have distracted somewhat from what are likely to be psychological factors in sexual dysfunction by the nature of the placebo effect. As reported in a newspaper article on Viagra (3), 'One executive said that in PDE5 studies 20% of the men taking a sugar pill placebo reported "rip-snorting erections".' We know that Sildenafil does not improve sexual function in men without erectile dysfunction but does reduce the post-orgasmic refractory time (4). This may be an acceptable and cost-effective short-term way for some male patients to address erectile difficulties but what about options for addressing the underlying causes?

Encounters with sympathetic, knowledgeable healthcare practitioners (HCPs) in primary or community care settings may be enough in a number of patients and we have heard cases and vignettes where brief interventions have helped, but for the patients needing more or who have not moved forwards during initial discussion, what of their options?

Service Provision

Sexual healthcare commissioned by local authorities (in England) encompasses all aspects of physical and psychological sexual health well-being. This includes for psychosexual care, 'the sexual health aspects of Psychosexual counselling' (5). 'Non-sexual health aspects', which some areas have interpreted to mean physical causes of sexual dysfunction that need physical treatments, are commissioned by local clinical commissioning groups and can include erectile dysfunction clinics where pharmacological treatments are prescribed.

These definitions are unhelpful when considering patients who attend with problems and has meant psychosexual therapy clinic services across the United Kingdom are inconsistent. Some areas have no National Health Service (NHS) specialists, for instance, or if there is one, long waiting times. Furthermore, this arbitrary split can result in increased costs for the NHS as there is further delay for patients who are trying to access appropriate help.

Although clinicians have realised for many years that providing sexual healthcare does not mean solely fitting an intra-uterine device or treating a chlamydial infection for instance, commissioners and policymakers are now agreed that holistic care is necessary and cost effective. This should include sexual dysfunction management and the provision of 'psychosexual care' either by recognition or signposting.

Surprisingly, men with erectile dysfunction are invariably referred to urology departments and although the condition can occur after urological procedures as described earlier, it is not strictly a urological one per se. It is generally accepted that erectile dysfunction is in most cases a symptom of microvascular cardiovascular disease or psychological dysfunction but this has not altered the habitual referral pathway.

Therefore, in areas where psychosexual care is not provided for by sexual health or other services, help for patients can be patchy or non-existent. What happens to the patient who says they have no desire or libido where the doctor has tried all manner of hormonal or contraceptive pill formulations to try and help resolve the problem? These patients would have no option but to try private therapy or relationship services once they have undergone lengthy and unnecessary blood tests and other costly investigations.

This inequity is despite the provision included in sexual health service specifications, guided by the national specification in integrated sexual health services (6). When services have been out to competitive tender there has been confusion among commissioners as to what the mandate to provide 'sexual health aspects of Psychosexual counselling' actually means. Local authorities now commissioning such services have a learning curve in this new landscape not helped by confusing language and terminologies. Patients consequently have to resort to private, possibly unregulated and unproven therapists which can be costly, emotionally and financially. The patient may also be left with the problem. That is not to say that many counselling and other services, e.g. Relate, Samaritans and private counselors, are not helpful since being able to air and share problems in a safe environment can be supportive. However, this is not equivalent to psychodynamic therapy, which examines subconscious factors to determine possible causes of the problem. IPM clinicians utilise the latter and are also able to appropriately use a psychotherapeutic physical examination. Diagnosing those rare cases of a previously undiscovered physical condition is an additional benefit, as it is vital to exclude physical disease.

The South West Sexual Dysfunction Expert Advisory Group has written a comprehensive description and definition guidance document on sexual dysfunction which informed the Sexual Health Board annual report (7). This detailed document is designed to help commissioners from the Clinical Commissioning Groups (CCGs) and local authorities plan and develop services. It also makes specific recommendations for organisations and policy makers at local and national levels and describes a gold standard service delivery in addition to recommended minimum standards for smaller units with referral onwards if necessary.

As psychosexual medicine work combines physical and emotional doctoring, it is mainly represented by doctors and other HCPs working in both physical and psychological medicine.

Of course, work is done in many different settings and these are summarized below.

Where is Psychosexual Medicine Practised?

Doctors and HCPs practising in their chosen medical field while simultaneously seeing patients with psychosexual problems enables physical problems to be recognized if these have not been noticed beforehand. But it also means the emotional impact of dealing with the complex feelings of patients is more easily managed as the work is interspersed with other problems requiring usually less mentally draining input (albeit possibly physically more challenging, e.g. surgical procedures).

General Practitioners

General practitioners (GPs) as clinicians are trained to diagnose and manage the whole spectrum of physical and mental health, as well as promote and deliver preventative care. Their training includes emphasis on communication skills and the relationship they build with their patients. GPs will have patients whom they know need help psychologically or emotionally, but who come to them repeatedly with physical complaints. Many of these presenting problems are not indicative of an underlying sexual problem but it is likely some of them will be. GPs trained in psychosexual medicine often report that their ability to recognise and manage other psychosomatic presentations improves, and there is an increasing awareness of how common this is. If a patient has an underlying sexual problem, a sensitive GP consultation can go a long way toward helping this problem; sharing the issues and feeling acknowledged can have a considerable positive influence on the patient. Those with more developed skills can often move a patient forwards in one or two consultations and many GPs are aware that although time-consuming, this investment can prevent patients returning again and again with other issues when the true problem has not been aired or addressed. This can be seen as 'brief intervention'.

Healthcare Practitioners

The first port of call for patients is often primary care nurses. The caring and welcoming atmosphere that is usually created in these consultations, coupled with time to address issues (although this is changing as there is more pressure on workloads) means that patients often feel they can raise their sexual issues here. It is, therefore, a welcome step that nurses can now undertake IPM Diploma training, for those who are interested. In addition they are able to genitally examine patients, particularly those with skills and interests in sexual and reproductive health, which is a compulsory requirement to be able to embark on IPM training. This is also true of specialist physiotherapists, who have already gleaned that examining the pelvic floor of women, particularly those who have had traumatic deliveries, often leads to intimate and sexual problems being shared.

Specialist Services

A variety of provisions for sexual problems exists; there are different types or schools of therapy, different providers and lack of uniform standards of care. There have been attempts to standardise with service specifications, but these concentrate mainly on standards in access and waiting times. There is, however, recognition that sharing good practise can be achieved and will undoubtedly benefit patients. There is increasing collaboration with other therapy methods, e.g. cognitive behavioural therapy practised by College of Sexual and Relationship Therapists (COSRT) and recognition of the benefit of joint learning events as well as shared outcome measurement, as described in Chapter 25, to demonstrate effectiveness.

The IPM, although a training organisation, not a service provider, does provide a list of trained IPM therapists on its website. Currently there are 44 doctors listed, with 80% based in NHS services which some may find surprising as it is commonly thought that patients have to have access to private clinics for this type of therapy.

Services may be combined, offering physical treatments too. This can be appropriate but possibly tempts clinicians to jump to pharmacological remedies and devices first, especially if the emotional avenue is too challenging or stressful, the 'opening a can of worms' scenario subconsciously feared by many clinicians. Patients can feel angry and unengaged if they had not been expecting to look at emotional causes or have been encouraged to have expectations about physical treatments. Even with physical symptoms, e.g. pain or itching, there will be feelings attached to these and there may, in fact, be no appropriate physical treatments to offer.

Various practitioners offer psychosexual therapy:

- IPM clinicians in sexual health, gynaecology and genitourinary medicine
- COSRT practitioners
- Psychological therapists

- Psychiatric doctors
- Urology nurses
- Physiotherapists
- Cancer nurses

A referral system has to be focussed and specific to ensure inappropriate patients are not mis-referred, e.g. patients who are psychiatrically unwell, or have forensic issues or personality disorders. These do not normally fall under the domain of a psychosexual service and most therapists would not be trained to provide help for these conditions. The majority of services do not accept self-referral to ensure the most appropriate patients are seen but will accept referrals from doctors and nurses who have recognised the patient to have a psychosexual problem. To aid accurate referral, education activities and networking with local health communities is essential, as well as feedback to referrers outlining the patient's progress or condition at discharge, as in any other area of medicine. This is sometimes difficult when patients do not want information to be shared with other agencies. In practise, even if patients allow this, it is not essential to share detailed analysis of what was disclosed in the consultation, but a general diagnostic overview of progress made will usually suffice.

With specialist referral clinics it is usual to require return of an opt-in questionnaire, standard in many psychological services, and important to explain to the patient through leaflets and website information what to expect: the term *psychosexual* can spark an array of different meanings for a patient and may possibly make them feel hesitant about attending if not explained adequately, especially if their problem feels so physical, e.g. if they have pain. However, attendance behaviour can also inform the therapist about the patient: those who did not attend (DNA) can inform about patients' lack of readiness to deal with trauma. In the current financial climate those who DNA may seem unjustified and have to be managed appropriately which must be taken into account.

In contrast with other therapies, the practise of psychosexual medicine cannot occur without facilities to examine the patient. A talking therapy it may be, but as we have heard, the psychotherapeutic examination of the patient is the diagnostic tool unique to the specialism, often illuminating key causal factors of the sexual problem. A cosy clinical environment may help the patient relax, but an adequate examination couch is also necessary.

Individual or Couples?

As the practice of psychosexual medicine is based on the therapist studying the interaction between himself or herself and the patient, consultations do not usually involve the patient's partner. The training does not include the management of relationship issues although the patient's relationship with their partner may feature. If a partner attends, it is important for the therapist to consider the relevance of this. It may be a misunderstanding of what is expected of the therapy but equally, it could be one of the patient's defences from the HCP who they fear will delve into their innermost thoughts and fears. This is an important differentiation from other forms of sexual therapy where the relationship is usually the focus as is described later.

Discussion about Value and Health Economics

The value of providing psychosexual services is discussed in Chapter 25 but it is important to acknowledge what currently happens in many areas. Limited or no provision often results in patients being referred to a variety of mainly acute hospital departments for potential 'treatments'. These can be the obvious ones like gynaecology or urology but also can be dermatology for an itch, endocrinology or even psychiatry for lack of libido thought to be due to 'hormones' or mood.

Patients can be seen in secondary care for many months or even years, unsatisfying for the doctor as well as the patient, while trying to find an answer to their symptoms before being discharged back to their

GPs with 'no abnormality found'. There is therefore, a good case for healthcare professionals to have an understanding in not only psychosexual problems but also in psychosomatic presentations and how to help patients whose emotional problems in the words of Suzanne O'Sullivan 'generate a physical illness'. In her book (8) O'Sullivan, a neurologist, describes how difficult it is for doctors to consider that symptoms may not be due to underlying physical disease. She says, 'to consider a psychological cause for serious illness, it is vital that we believe such a thing is possible. Maybe if we understood better the way our own bodies lose control, triggered only by a feeling inside, then more extreme reactions might not seem so unacceptable'. She uses laughter to illustrate emotional release that cannot always be under control. 'If we can collapse with laughter, is it not just as possible that the body can do even more extraordinary things when faced with even more extraordinary triggers?' But she laments the lack of skills in clinicians in dealing with psychosomatic illnesses.

Training is covered in the next chapter but we know it is often patchy and inconsistent. One study of consultants in associated specialties found that although most encountered patients with sexual problems, very few had had training (9) and there was an admission of ignorance about how to recognise or manage patients with sexual difficulty.

The outcome from failing to recognise a sexual problem may be expensive treatments and surgical procedures, when we know that not only is the length of therapy generally brief as described above, often only two to three consultations, but a brief intervention with an IPM HCP unexpectedly within a consultation can have illuminating and meaningful results for the patient. Unfortunately, these outcomes will rarely be measured but the clinician will be often aware that there has been a shift in the patient's position that may have long-lasting benefits. This feeling is immensely satisfying.

It is important for all practitioners and services to have robust data about the provision; waiting times, outcome data and satisfaction studies are minimal.

Future

It would be beneficial for clinicians with psychosexual therapy skills to be part of a spectrum of services as discussed. Identification of patients is most likely to bring benefit from brief interactions crucial to their well-being and consequently prevent a drain on other services and unnecessary interventions.

For this to happen medical and clinical training programmes need to ensure they cover psychosexual problems as undoubtedly clinicians will encounter these issues. In this way, early recognition of a problem will ensue, which is essential, as well as being ultimately cost effective.

REFERENCES

1. Mitchell KR. Sexual function in Britain: Findings from the third national survey of sexual attitudes and lifestyles (Natsal-3). *Lancet* 2013;382(9907):1817–1829.
2. Department of Health. A Framework for Sexual Health Improvement in England [pdf]. 2013. Available from: www.gov.uk/government/uploads/system/uploads/attachment_data/file/142592/9287-2900714-TSO-SexualHealthPolicyNW_ACCESSIBLE.pdf.
3. Andrews A. Viagra: The little blue pill that revolutionised our sex lives. *The Guardian Newspaper*, 3 December 2017.
4. Mondaini N, Ponchietti R, Muir GH, Montorsi F, Di Loro F, Lombardi G, Rizzo M. Sildenafil does not improve sexual function in men without erectile dysfunction but does reduce the post-orgasmic refractory time. *Int J Impot Res* 2003;15:225–228.
5. Commissioning Sexual Health Services and Interventions. *Best practice guidance for local authorities.* London: Department of Health and Social Care, 2013.
6. Integrated Sexual Health Services: National Service Specification, 2013. Available from: www.gov.uk/dh.
7. www.southglos.gov.uk/documents/SW-Office-for-Sexual-Health-Annual-Report-2016/17.
8. O'Sullivan S. *It's All in Your Head.* London: Chatto and Windus, 2015.
9. Brough P, Batra S, Pilkington A. Psychosexual dysfunction – Do secondary care specialists feel equipped to manage it? *IPMJ* 2017;71:9–11.

27

Training in Psychosexual Medicine

Jasmin Khan-Singh

History of Training

It was in the 1950s that Michael Balint and his associates started training groups of doctors from family planning to use brief psychoanalytical skills in their everyday work. The proposal was not to import wholesale the psychotherapeutic techniques proper to another branch of medicine, but rather that each branch should aim to develop psychotherapeutic techniques appropriate to its own particular setting (1). Tom Main, being one of those associates, soon started his own groups in the 1960s, and over the next 40 years was closely involved in the training and development of these pioneering doctors. He had the innovative thinking to train leaders from within the membership, recognising that you did not need to be a psychoanalyst to lead such groups. The goal was not to breed mini-psychoanalysts, but doctors with the unique skill of being able to use brief, focussed, penetrative psychodynamic psychotherapy in tandem with their physical doctoring. In 1974, the Institute of Psychosexual Medicine (IPM) was founded and has continued to train interested health professionals to acquire the necessary skills to, first and foremost, benefit their patients.

Tom Main, in his paper 'Training for the acquisition of skills' (2) talked of the difficulties of such training, faced by not only those doing the training, but also those providing the training; how in the medical world there is no place for, and little value given to, the gathering of 'empathy' data (feelings and what effect that might have on the problem presented) from our patients. Now, 37 years on, there is a modest improvement in acknowledging these difficulties, e.g. training in communication skills or breaking bad news occurs in most branches of medicine now; however, there is still a way to go from learning scripted responses and behaviours to understanding, using and valuing the feelings from our patients.

Prue Tunnadine in 1997 (3) discussed 'How to become an accredited Seminar Leader'. She reminds us of the case material tempting one away from the discipline of group dynamics, and the rigid distinction between training (of the professional ego), and therapy (of dangerously fascinating personal material), only the former being the task of the Leaders' Workshop. At that time future seminar leaders were 'talent spotted' and invited by the director of training to lead a new group and present their work at the workshop. If the work they showed was adequate they would be accredited. There was a second way: a qualified member could independently set up a group and apply to the director of training to attend leaders' workshop to have their skills assessed for accreditation.

With the turn of the millennium came a time of self-enquiry by IPM members, considering the standards of training and assessments, the creation of the 'safe space' required for such training to take place for both trainees and seminar leaders, and how to make the training fit for purposes in the twenty-first century. A period of reflection, critical thinking and collective energy, with a consensus style of leadership led to development of guidance documents and robust reviewing and standardisation of methods of examinations. The dispelling of past myths, what 'should' or 'ought' to be done, has put the IPM in a position to consider specialist recognition, should that be a chosen route in the future.

Khan-Singh and Vaughan (4) discuss the changes over the period 2007–2012 in their article 'Growing up as a specialty'. A draft curriculum was completed, using Postgraduate Medical Education and Training Board (PMETB)/General Medical Council (GMC) principles with the doctor-patient relationship, use of the psychosomatic genital examination and experiential learning through seminar work, all taking centre stage. Expectations were set of our training structure, description of learning and what knowledge, skills, behaviour and engagement we would expect our future trainees and seminar leaders to achieve.

In the recent past, two significant events have taken place. The stepping down of Jasmin Khan-Singh, the Director of Training, in 2013 saw the advent of a three-member training committee as a replacement and in 2015 the decision was passed to allow nurses and allied health professionals to sit the Diploma examination. The training committee has introduced a 12-hour short course, held over a term or sometimes 2 days, which includes a combination of taught knowledge and seminar group work and is aptly named the Introductory Term. No doubt evaluation of these significant events and changes made will soon follow, as the next chapter of IPM training is written.

Training Programmes

The established training programmes offered by the IPM are summarised in Figure 27.1. At all levels of training it is skill-based training and there is no taught knowledge. It is also worth noting that healthcare practitioners train to diploma level.

Before discussing the details of these programmes, we ought to question the premise: is there a need for IPM training in 2018 and onwards?

Sexual dysfunction can have devastating and wide-reaching effects on individuals' well-being and ability to function in other areas of life, especially in forming relationships. A study of sexual attitudes and lifestyles in Britain in 2013 reported 42% of men and 51% of women aged 17–74 interviewed who had had sex in the previous year had experienced one or more sexual difficulties lasting a minimum of 3 months (5).

The commissioning document produced by the South West Expert Advisory Group (6) in 2016 states:

> People experiencing sexual dysfunction, if unable to access a Sexual Dysfunction Service, are very likely to access other services which will generally be unable to diagnose and/or treat the underlying problem, referring on to another service/specialist. It can also mean that people requiring sexual dysfunction interventions experience significant delays in accessing care and support as integrated patient pathways will generally not be in place.
>
> Differentiating between 'sexual health' and 'non-sexual health' aspects of sexual dysfunction is not useful or relevant in clinical practice, where both are clearly integrated in the same patient, professional and consultation. It is in essence 'body-mind' medicine and requires appropriately trained clinicians.
>
> It is the practitioner's training that will determine how they approach the patient and how many sessions they are likely to need and use for each patient, the latter having a cost impact.

It was the shift from being 'unconsciously incompetent' to 'consciously incompetent' that drove the early pioneers to seek training for the area they were not equipped to deal with; this uncomfortable awareness is still felt as keenly today by those working where sexual problems can be presented. Many a 'memorable case' by such doctors and their accounts of why they sought training can be read in the *Institute of Psychosexual Medicine Journal* (IPMJ) from the 50th journal onwards. There is no reason to suppose this drive for training has or will change significantly, until perhaps all clinicians that work in this field have been trained to a 'consciously competent' level, whereupon they can use the skills in their everyday work and refer appropriately. Furthermore, the IPM's existence of 44 years is a testimony to the need for training and its value to the practitioner and their patients.

Annual seminar evaluations from trainees of the IPM all support the need for the training, they talk of the utility of the skills gained being transferable to all their other areas of work, and comments on the effectiveness of this training are a common theme that runs through every year. (See Box 27.1.)

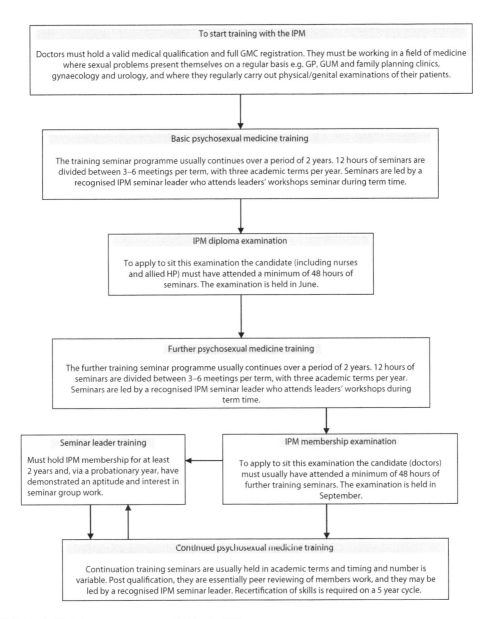

FIGURE 27.1 Training programmes provided by the IPM.

BOX 27.1: COMMENTS FROM ANNUAL SEMINAR EVALUATIONS

Many patients attend GUM clinics complaining of vaginal discharge and abdominal pain with negative findings. I began to realize that in some cases there was an underlying psychosexual element. I felt powerless to help such patients before IPM training. (Specialist Registrar GUM [SpR GUM])

I enjoyed IPM seminars because they stimulated parts of my brain that no other training has ever reached. (GP Principal)

IPM training made me more confident and hopefully to pick up problems I may have overlooked in the past. (Sexual and Reproductive HealthCare [SRH] Associate Specialist)

Training in psychosexual problems is part of the obstetrics and gynaecology, community sexual and reproductive health and genitourinary medicine curriculum, to varying degrees. GP training also requires some understanding and concentrates on communication skills between the doctor and patient. The IPM is needed to provide and support this training as experts in the field.

On a personal note, I can only share my experience: In all the many exams I have engaged with during my working life of 33 years, the learning experience that sticks out most for me is the training I received from the IPM. It was very hard and challenged me to look into myself while I tried to acquire the skills I needed. I had to acknowledge that I too have feelings and had to work out which was mine and which belonged to the patient. The first step necessary was an 'unlearning' of the medical model of being, so that paradoxically—a profound deep learning— the final result of training changed the very essence of the sort of doctor I became. I know that change and the new understanding instilled had enhanced effective patient care to the full benefit of all the patients I see. What a discovery – a truly holistic way of doctoring.

Who Should Consider Training?

The IPM Prospectus clarifies who will benefit from training (7):

> IPM training appeals to those who desire a deeper understanding than is offered in traditional education and recognise the need for an alternative approach when standard medical and surgical treatments have failed.
>
> Those who wish to train in psychosexual medicine must be practising in a field where sexual problems present themselves on a regular basis and where a physical examination of the genital area can be conducted. Such specialities are primary care, sexual and reproductive healthcare, genito-urinary medicine, gynaecology, urology, psychiatry and forensic medicine.
>
> Training is appropriate both for those who wish to improve their skills in managing patients with psychosexual problems in their everyday work setting, and for those who wish to gain a specialist qualification which accredits them to accept referrals.

For Which Type of Problem Is IPM Training Useful?

- Vaginismus, loss of libido, difficulties with orgasm
- Non-consummation and dyspareunia
- Erectile dysfunction, ejaculatory problems and other penile problems
- Chronic pelvic pain or genital pain, recurrent discharge with or without a physical cause
- Emotional and psychosexual sequelae of sexually transmitted infections
- Contraceptive-related problems (including the inability to use any method), repeated requests for abortions, effects of miscarriage
- Vasectomy and sterilisation requests with a hidden agenda of sexual problems
- Emotional and psychosexual effects of medical and surgical interventions, including miscarriage and termination of pregnancy.
- Psychosexual sequelae of sexual abuse
- Sexuality, cancer and terminal care
- Effects of ageing, disability or illness on sexuality
- Psychosexual problems related to infertility and ending of fertility
- Difficulties following childbirth

Institute of Psychosexual Medicine Seminar Training

Psychosexual medicine employs 'experiential learning' to foster an approach to the patient that simultaneously acknowledges the physical, psychological and social. HCPs are trained to 'listen' carefully, to use the imagination, to evaluate self-critically and to test the validity of professional intuition. They are learning to use brief interpretative therapy alongside their usual practice. They do this via the seminar training method – a meeting of interested HCPs, moderated and facilitated by a recognised IPM seminar leader.

The case-based discussion, centring on the doctor-patient relationship, acting as a learning tool for doctors to reflect on their practice has been long understood by Balint: he expected a 'Limited though considerable change in the personality of the doctor' as a result of successful training (8).

The Training (Basic) Seminar

This training of 2 years will enable doctors, nurses and allied health professionals to *recognise*, at a basic level, what is going on with the HCP-patient relationship, the defences of both practitioner and patient and to use the genital examination in a psychotherapeutic way. Seminar groups meet to discuss cases seen by group members, on a regular basis of 2- to 4-hour sessions.

The trainee learns about the feelings and atmosphere in the room and their use in the service of the clinical work. The trick is to recognise what is coming from the practitioner and what is a reflection of the patient. These skills can be used in the everyday work of the practitioner.

The Further Training (Advanced) Seminar

At the time of writing further training is only available for doctors. Some doctors may seek to make psychosexual medicine a field of special interest, and if they demonstrate enthusiasm and an aptitude, with supportive feedback discussion from their seminar leader, they can proceed to further training which may take up to 2 years or more.

In a further training seminar, doctors will continue to study the doctor-patient relationship, defences, etc. and will be more aware of the less conscious elements occurring in the consultation. The focus shifts from recognising to the *use of* unconscious material which should now be a part of each encounter. Further emphasis is placed on differential diagnosis and the selection of suitable cases for treatment by this method of brief psychosomatic therapy.

Doctors in further training may consider receiving referrals within their own local work setting but they will not have accreditation to do so until they have obtained the membership examination. See IPM Prospectus for further details (7).

Clinicians in training and beyond are encouraged to read the journal of the IPM, published twice annually and to attend the clinical and scientific meetings held in March and November, respectively. The meetings involve scientific presentations, including those from related specialties and schools, together with debates and case presentations, interspersed with seminar group time to allow case presentations and learning for all attenders.

Main (2) clarified the skills that need nurturing, during training, as *synaesthetic perceptiveness* to gather empathy data and *diacritic perceptiveness* to critically assess it. He tells us doctors are usually comfortable with the scientific approach, i.e. the diacritic (questioning and telling method), but the 'feeling' approach (tuning in to subjective truths felt by a whole living person) can be quite a challenge. But since no human being's distress is the same as that of any others, the practitioner faces each time a unique human being for whom general laws are not enough. The problem now is not general ignorance about mankind, but that the practitioner is utterly ignorant about this particular patient.

The average trainee must also face the fact that training in gaining a skill is slow, highly personal and time consuming, taking a good 15–18 months before any 'penny drops'. So perhaps it is of no surprise that some trainees seem to have a talent for the work and quickly pick up the skills. We all know this talent and recognise it when we meet it but no one word can describe it. The majority of trainees have to wait for a shift in understanding within themselves and a minority do not have or are unlikely to acquire the necessary perceptiveness. There are many reasons why the latter group exists; for some it is much too uncomfortable for them to make the inherent changes, for others they cannot let go of being the 'expert', for others still they cannot co-exist with the 'not knowing' and unfortunately they are unable to recognise their own shortfall; moreover as Main (2) has said 'one rarely finds this talent in high order in those whose main interest is in intellectual achievement'.

At this juncture it seems appropriate to issue a word of warning. This type of training should not be entered into lightly. It is a very challenging form of learning that reaches very deep, fundamentally changing the doctors in how they approach and view their patients, and their practise thereafter. For the trainees, the benefit gained by sharing their experiences in seminars far outweighs any pain (cognitive dissonance) they will feel as a result of the training. It is a process that produces *real learning*, as defined by Mulholland (9), via an observable change in the learner's ability to do, think or feel, or a combination of all three.

The training that Balint and Main were advocating can be given a name, according to the educational theory of today, and that is *transformative* learning (10). It is one of the highest forms of learning that can be achieved. Transformative learning involves helping adults to elaborate, create and transform their meaning schemes (beliefs, feelings, interpretations and decisions) through reflection on their content, the process by which they were learned and their premises (social context, history and consequences).

The method being used is group learning and the many benefits of group learning have become clear over the last few decades. The original study of groups was in the 1960s by Tuckmann (11), who extrapolated general concepts about group development, and summarised the four stages as forming, storming, norming and performing.

The aspects of *group learning* are comprehensively discussed and explored with reference to IPM seminar training by Khan-Singh (12). These include the promotion of deep learning through elaboration and reflection of knowledge, of higher-level skills such as reasoning and evaluation where problem solving is encouraged, interpersonal skills developed, exploration of attitudes, awareness and tolerance of other viewpoints occur and where members take responsibility for their own learning. Group size is of importance too and the IPM needs to be mindful when a group is too small or too large to function successfully. She concludes for the IPM that group learning is the very essence of their training and suggests in the world of studying and working with group dynamics, the IPM are credible experts in the field.

Seminar Leadership Training

The training of the seminar leader mirrors that of the IPM trainee, i.e. experiential learning.

The skills of leadership are achieved by attending seminars (leaders' workshops) with other seminar leaders. At the workshop the seminar leader presents the events and cases discussed during their seminar training groups. The focus is on understanding the group events/interactions and examining the skills of the leader in managing the group discussions and situations that arise out of the cases presented in the seminar. Seminar leaders are expected to be aware of the theoretical underpinning of group dynamics and leadership techniques and the emphasis in the workshop is the gaining of practical skills by experiential learning.

The seminar leader, like any group leader/tutor has many *roles*, depending on the task in hand. These roles are listed by the IPM in the seminar leader's job description, examples of which include providing a model of human behaviour, knowing the difference between training groups and therapeutic groups and recognising factors that prevent the group from working.

The list of *skills* required by the seminar leader is extensive (9), some of the more obvious ones are to do with leadership, being able to listen, question, observe, react, reinforce and summarise. The idea of the *superskill* is the crux of it and concerns learning when to use which skill. The seminar leader's lot is further complicated, and this is acknowledged by Skrine when she says:

> Life is not easy for the IPM Leader. She must be concerned not only with her understanding of the Doctor-Patient relationship but the group's understanding of this. (13)

Schon (14) in his book *Educating the Reflective Practitioner* describes the teachers of psychoanalytical practise that helps us to understand the seminar leader. He talks of

> Teachers unlike any they (the students) have known in the past, helping them to examine their own mental process and to detect the operation of unconscious tendencies.

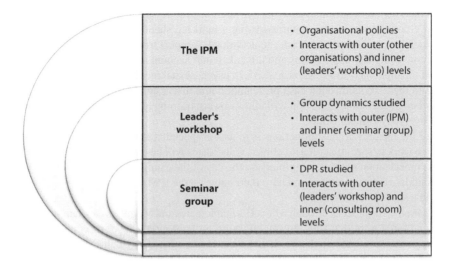

FIGURE 27.2   Parallel processes: travel up and down system levels.

This description resonates remarkably well with the IPM seminar leader and what they are learning to do.

The seminar leader job description also stipulates attending to the following:

- How does the patient conduct his/her life and deal with the reporting practitioner?
- How does the reporting practitioner deal with the patient?
- How does the group respond to practitioner and patient?
- How does the practitioner relate to the leader and the rest of the group?
- How does the group relate to the leader?

What is actually requiring attention is the concept of parallel processes or parallelism, at all the levels within the system, from the individual all the way up to the IPM as an organisation and possibly beyond. Each level will interact with and impact upon the inner and outer levels linked to it, in both directions, and provides the basis of the experiential learning for trainees and seminar leader alike. Figure 27.2 depicts three levels, but one can easily include the consulting room within the seminar group level and governing bodies engulfing the IPM organisational level.

Punter (15) reflects on leading the leaders' workshop and discusses these various working levels, their interaction with each other and the rich learning that can occur; as long as there is opening of the level's boundaries and that cultural identity does not get in the way. She describes the leaders' workshop functioning as a mirror reflecting the dynamics of the systems above and below it and as a group it straddles process and task; the task is to understand the IPM leaders' training groups using the process of the group in the service of the task. She hits the nail on the head when she thoughtfully states:

> I have seen the groups that I have led at the IPM trust that through exploring together in the group, wisdom will emerge and they have the wisdom that knowledge comes through not knowing in the moment of the group. (15; p. 13)

Examinations and Re-Certification

Comprehensive details on all examinations including objectives, eligibility criteria and format can be found on the IPM website (16). As discussed earlier, allied healthcare professionals can now sit the Diploma, if they so wish.

The examinations are a summative, criterion-referenced assessment based on the objectives of the examination. Standardisation is maintained using a marking sheet and a robust marking system, the details of which are available to candidates to download. A report from the candidate's seminar leader is requested on receiving any applications and it is taken into account as supportive evidence.

The aim of the diploma is to assess basic skills in psychosexual medicine. Candidates will be expected to demonstrate these skills through case presentation and discussion with the examiners on the day of the examination. Successful completion will allow onward training towards membership as well as using the skills in everyday clinical work.

The aim of the membership examinations is to assess specialist skills in psychosexual medicine and competence to work in specialist referral clinics. Candidates will be expected to demonstrate these skills through case presentation with the examiners on the day of the examination. Successful completion will allow the candidate to be accredited and have their name on the IPM Referrals List, which the public can access to find a specialist in their area.

Re-certification is the process through which IPM diplomates and Members can demonstrate to patients, colleagues and employers that they are maintaining an appropriate level of continuing professional development in psychosexual medicine. It is an electronic process, which occurs in line with GMC revalidation period of a 5-yearly cycle.

Future Concerns

There is a real concern that patients may come to harm, as currently any doctor can theoretically set themselves up as an 'expert' in sexual dysfunction by virtue of completing their Certificate of Completion of Specialist Training (CSST), without having undergone any specific training in the area. The IPM is the only training organisation with the ability to provide the unique 'body-mind' medicine training that is needed, as stated by the South West Expert Advisory Group. The IPM, to ensure protection of patients, must be ready to take this training role on when the GMC finalises how these specialist niche areas are to be recognised. This is most likely to take the form of 'credentialing', where standards of training, assessment and examinations will have to be determined and meet the requirements of the GMC. Thankfully, the ground work is already in place with the curriculum that was compiled back in 2007–2012, alongside the robust reviewing of IPM training and examinations. It will require future IPM members with the vision, willingness and drive to see it through so that patients will be find the appropriately trained practitioner.

Those of us working in the field have a duty to speak up for patients with sexual dysfunction as this group are very unlikely to complain (after all no patient wants to make public their 'intimate' distress) about the difficulties of being heard, the lack of services, and more worryingly inappropriate treatment or operations that they are put through.

Outcome research must be a priority, to compete with the over-importance attributed to evidence-based medicine. The trouble being that the evidence we hear of nowadays is really only provided for things that we can easily measure, can easily quantify, can do quickly, and can apply statistical analysis to it and so on. This is not the real world we live in and is at best only half the story. What the evidence basis totally forgets about is the artistic, humanities aspect of medicine and human beings; our individual patients and how they might feel about their problems and the impact of these feelings on the difficulties themselves. These are the very skills that IPM training endows and the IPM will have to fight to secure a value to the training.

Change is part of working in any field, but there is always a choice on the path(s) taken. The IPM, in its future forms, will do well to not forget the three essential characteristics of science: creativity, the habit of truth and the sense of human dignity, as described by Bronowski (17). I would add to this the need to always evaluate any changes that have been made, otherwise only chaos will ensue.

For further details on training, requesting the IPM prospectus or any queries, contact the IPM administrative secretary either via the IPM website (www.ipm.org.uk) or via email (admin@ipm.org.uk).

REFERENCES

1. Michael BE. *Psychotherapeutic Techniques in Medicine*. London: Tavistock Publications, 1961.
2. Main T. Training for the acquisition of knowledge or the development of skill? *Institute of Psychosex Med J* 2014;66:8–14.
3. Tunnadine P. Teaching psychosexual medicine becoming an accredited seminar leader. *IPMJ* 1997;14:10.
4. Khan-Singh J, Vaughan A. Growing up as a specialty: An update on education and training. *IPMJ* 2012;59:20 22.
5. Sexual Attitudes and Lifestyle Survey, 2013. Available from: www.natsal.ac.uk/media/823260/natsal_findings_final.pdf.
6. Commissioning Sexual Dysfunction Services, 2016. Available from: www.ipm.org.uk/91/sexual-dysfunction-service-commissioning-paper.
7. IPM Prospectus, 2014. Available from: www.ipm.org.uk/17/our-therapy.
8. Balint M. *The Doctor, His Patient and the Illness*. London: Pitman Medical Publications, 1956.
9. Mulholland H. Teaching small groups facilitating learning. *Hospital Update* 1994;20:382–384.
10. Kaufmann DM. Applying educational theory in practice. In P Cantillon, L Hutchinson, D Wood (Ed.), *ABC of Learning and Teaching in Medicine*. London: BMJ Publishing Group, 2003, 1–4.
11. Tuckman BW. Development sequence in small groups. *Psychol Bull* 1965;63:384–399.
12. Khan-Singh J. Aspects of training: Group learning. *IPMJ* 2008;49:20–24.
13. Skrine R. *Edited Transcripts of Leaders Workshops: Psychosexual Training and the Dr-Patient Relationship*. London: Montana Press, 1987.
14. Schon DA. *Educating the Reflective Practitioner. Chapter 9, Learning the Artistry of Psychoanalytic Practice*. Chichester: Wiley, 1987, 248.
15. Punter J. Reflections on leading the Leaders' workshop. *IPMJ* 2011;56:9–13.
16. IPM Examinations. Available from: www.ipm.org.uk/87/examinations.
17. Bronowski J. *Science and Human Values*. New York, NY: Harper Perennial, 1994.

Index